Marine Carotenoids in Inflammation and Cancer

Marine Carotenoids in Inflammation and Cancer

Editors

Elena Talero
Javier Ávila-Román

MDPI • Basel • Beijing • Wuhan • Barcelona • Belgrade • Manchester • Tokyo • Cluj • Tianjin

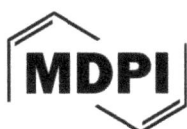

Editors
Elena Talero
Universidad de Sevilla
Spain

Javier Ávila-Román
Universidad de Sevilla
Spain

Editorial Office
MDPI
St. Alban-Anlage 66
4052 Basel, Switzerland

This is a reprint of articles from the Special Issue published online in the open access journal *Marine Drugs* (ISSN 1660-3397) (available at: https://www.mdpi.com/journal/marinedrugs/special_issues/Carotenoids_Inflammation_Cancer).

For citation purposes, cite each article independently as indicated on the article page online and as indicated below:

LastName, A.A.; LastName, B.B.; LastName, C.C. Article Title. *Journal Name* **Year**, *Volume Number*, Page Range.

ISBN 978-3-0365-2516-7 (Hbk)
ISBN 978-3-0365-2517-4 (PDF)

© 2021 by the authors. Articles in this book are Open Access and distributed under the Creative Commons Attribution (CC BY) license, which allows users to download, copy and build upon published articles, as long as the author and publisher are properly credited, which ensures maximum dissemination and a wider impact of our publications.

The book as a whole is distributed by MDPI under the terms and conditions of the Creative Commons license CC BY-NC-ND.

Contents

About the Editors vii

Preface to "Marine Carotenoids in Inflammation and Cancer" ix

Helena M. Amaro, Rita Barros, Tânia Tavares, Raquel Almeida, Isabel Sousa Pinto, Francisco Xavier Malcata and Ana Catarina Guedes
Gloeothece sp.—Exploiting a New Source of Antioxidant, Anti-Inflammatory, and Antitumor Agents
Reprinted from: 2021, *19*, 623, doi:10.3390/md19110623 1

Shohei Tsuji, Shinsuke Nakamura, Takashi Maoka, Tetsuya Yamada, Takahiko Imai, Takuya Ohba, Tomohiro Yako, Masahiro Hayashi, Ken Endo, Masanao Saio, Hideaki Hara and Masamitsu Shimazawa
Antitumour Effects of Astaxanthin and Adonixanthin on Glioblastoma
Reprinted from: *Mar. Drugs* 2020, *18*, 474, doi:10.3390/md18090474 19

Suhn Hyung Kim and Hyeyoung Kim
Transcriptome Analysis of the Inhibitory Effect of Astaxanthin on *Helicobacter pylori*-Induced Gastric Carcinoma Cell Motility
Reprinted from: *Mar. Drugs* 2020, *18*, 365, doi:10.3390/md18070365 35

Micaela Giani, Yoel Genaro Montoyo-Pujol, Gloria Peiró and Rosa María Martínez-Espinosa
Halophilic Carotenoids and Breast Cancer: From Salt Marshes to Biomedicine
Reprinted from: *Mar. Drugs* 2021, *19*, 594, doi:10.3390/md19110594 49

Javier Ávila-Román, Sara García-Gil, Azahara Rodríguez-Luna, Virginia Motilva and Elena Talero
Anti-Inflammatory and Anticancer Effects of Microalgal Carotenoids
Reprinted from: *Mar. Drugs* 2021, *19*, 531, doi:10.3390/md19100531 71

Eshak I. Bahbah, Sherief Ghozy, Mohamed S. Attia, Ahmed Negida, Talha Bin Emran, Saikat Mitra, Ghadeer M. Albadrani, Mohamed M. Abdel-Daim, Md. Sahab Uddin and Jesus Simal-Gandara
Molecular Mechanisms of Astaxanthin as a Potential Neurotherapeutic Agent
Reprinted from: *Mar. Drugs* 2021, *19*, 201, doi:10.3390/md19040201 121

Antia G. Pereira, Paz Otero, Javier Echave, Anxo Carreira-Casais, Franklin Chamorro, Nicolas Collazo, Amira Jaboui, Catarina Lourenço-Lopes, Jesus Simal-Gandara and Miguel A. Prieto
Xanthophylls from the Sea: Algae as Source of Bioactive Carotenoids
Reprinted from: *Mar. Drugs* 2021, *19*, 188, doi:10.3390/md19040188 137

Elena Catanzaro, Anupam Bishayee and Carmela Fimognari
On a Beam of Light: Photoprotective Activities of the Marine Carotenoids Astaxanthin and Fucoxanthin in Suppression of Inflammation and Cancer
Reprinted from: *Mar. Drugs* 2020, *18*, 544, doi:10.3390/md18110544 169

Yasin Genç, Hilal Bardakci, Çiğdem Yücel, Gökçe Şeker Karatoprak, Esra Küpeli Akkol, Timur Hakan Barak and Eduardo Sobarzo-Sánchez
Oxidative Stress and Marine Carotenoids: Application by Using Nanoformulations
Reprinted from: *Mar. Drugs* 2020, *18*, 423, doi:10.3390/md18080423 191

About the Editors

Elena Talero, full professor in pharmacology, received her PhD degree with European Mention from the University of Seville (Spain) in 2009 under the supervision of Prof. V. Motilva and Dr. S. Sánchez-Fidalgo. During her predoctoral period, Elena joined the laboratory of Prof. Alfredo Martinez (Cellular, Molecular and Developmental Neurobiology Department, Instituto Cajal, Madrid) for 5 months as well as the Division of Preclinical Oncology (School of Medical and Surgical Sciences, University of Nottingham, UK) for 3 months under the supervision of Prof. S. Watson. In 2011, she worked as a postdoc on several projects with Prof. Chris Paraskeva at Bristol University (UK) for 6 months.

Her current research interests focus on understanding inflammation as an essential component in the multifactorial origin of different diseases, with a special emphasis on intestinal bowel disease, skin inflammation, and associated tumor processes. Her research focuses on finding new bioactive compounds of marine or terrestrial origins for the treatment and/or prevention of these pathologies.

Javier Ávila-Román, assistant professor, received his PhD degree in pharmacy in 2014 from the University of Seville (Spain). He worked as assistant professor in the Faculty of Biology and as a researcher in the Faculty of Pharmacy from 2010 to 2017. During this period, he studied the role of natural products isolated from microalgae, mainly oxylipins (OXL), in inflammatory bowel diseases (IBD) and associated colon cancer. He moved in 2017 to Rovira i Virgili University in Tarragona (Spain) and worked as a postdoctoral researcher in the Nutrigenomic Group at the Department of Biochemistry and Biotechnology in the Faculty of Chemistry for 3 years. Currently, he is an assistant professor in the Faculty of Pharmacy at the Universidad de Sevilla.

His current research interests focus on natural and nutritional products, more specifically, on the anti-inflammatory activity of these bioactive products in IBD and inflammatory skin diseases, as well as on deciphering their role in the organism and their molecular mechanisms.

Preface to "Marine Carotenoids in Inflammation and Cancer"

Acute inflammation is a highly regulated biological response that can arise in organisms in response to pathogens, toxic agents, or tissue damage. This inflammation is accompanied by oxidative conditions triggered at the site of the injury to combat infection or damage, with the aim of removing harmful stimuli and restoring tissue homeostasis. However, uncontrolled acute inflammation and oxidative stress can lead to a chronic inflammatory state, which is believed to play an important role in the pathogenesis of many diseases, including cancer. Currently, the need to find new anti-inflammatory and anticancer compounds has given rise to a vast number of studies in the marine environment, which represents an excellent source to isolate bioactive molecules, such as carotenoids, due to their antioxidant and anti-inflammatory activities.

In this Special Issue, the reported products are the main carotenoids (β-carotene, lutein, astaxanthin, canthaxanthin, zeaxanthin, and fucoxanthin) found in marine organisms such as microalgae, macroalgae, cyanobacteria, and archaea, and other minor carotenoids found in some of these groups of microorganisms (bacterioruberin, cryptoxanthin, adonixanthin, siphonaxanthin, sioxanthin, and myxol). This Special Issue covers both the in vitro and in vivo evaluation of marine carotenoids with anti-inflammatory and anticancer activities as well as clinical trials conducted in humans. Among the properties of carotenoids discussed in this book, it is worth highlighting the potential of astaxanthin and its precursor metabolite, adonixanthin, since oral administration of these carotenoids has shown beneficial effects on glioblastoma for the first time by suppressing cell proliferation and migration. In addition, astaxanthin has been shown to inhibit *Helicobacter pylori*-induced gastric carcinoma cell motility and, consequently, cancer progression through the inhibition of cytoskeleton reorganization. In addition, a carotenoid-containing lipid extract of *Gloeothece* sp. has demonstrated antioxidant, anti-inflammatory, and anticancer properties in vitro.

Additionally, this book compiles some complete reviews, with one of them covering current knowledge of marine carotenoids as anti-inflammatory and anticancer agents. Another review on haloarchaea has shown that a rare carotenoid, bacterioruberin, has an antioxidant role in a breast cancer environment and is being considered a promising drug in this type of cancer. Furthermore, fucoxanthin and astaxanthin have shown photoprotective activities in skin diseases and skin cancer. Moreover, astaxanthin has been shown to be a good therapeutic agent in neurological and neuroinflammatory diseases. Another review reported the beneficial effects of oral administration of xanthophylls (fucoxanthin, astaxanthin, lutein, and zeaxanthin) in many oxidative and inflammatory pathologies, as well as their bioavailability in the human body. Finally, given the low bioavailability of carotenoids when consumed, this Special Issue compiles the current studies on advanced nanoformulations that act as carotenoid carriers leading them to target sites.

Elena Talero, Javier Ávila-Román
Editors

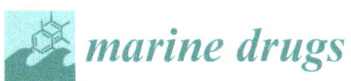

Article

Gloeothece sp.—Exploiting a New Source of Antioxidant, Anti-Inflammatory, and Antitumor Agents

Helena M. Amaro [1], Rita Barros [2,3,4], Tânia Tavares [5,6], Raquel Almeida [2,3,4,7], Isabel Sousa Pinto [1,7], Francisco Xavier Malcata [6,8] and Ana Catarina Guedes [1,*]

[1] CIIMAR—Interdisciplinary Centre of Marine and Environmental Research, University of Porto, Terminal de Cruzeiros de Leixões, Av. General Norton de Matos, s/n, 4450-208 Matosinhos, Portugal; lena.amaro@gmail.com (H.M.A.); isabel.sousa.pinto@gmail.com (I.S.P.)
[2] i3S—Institute for Innovation and Health Research, University of Porto, Rua Alfredo Allen, 208, 4200-135 Porto, Portugal; rita.barros@gmail.com (R.B.); ralmeida@ipatimup.pt (R.A.)
[3] IPATIMUP—Institute of Pathology and Molecular Immunology, University of Porto, Rua Júlio Amaral de Carvalho, 45, 4200-135 Porto, Portugal
[4] FMUP—Faculty of Medicine, University of Porto, Alameda Prof. Hernâni Monteiro, 4200-319 Porto, Portugal
[5] LAQV-REQUIMTE, Department of Chemical Sciences, Faculty of Pharmacy, University of Porto, Rua Jorge Viterbo Ferreira, 228, 4050-313 Porto, Portugal; tsgtavares@gmail.com
[6] LEPABE—Laboratory of Engineering of Environmental, Biotechnology and Energy Process, Rua Dr. Roberto Frias, s/n, 4200-465 Porto, Portugal; fmalcata@fe.up.pt
[7] FCUP—Faculty of Science, University of Porto, Rua do Campo Alegre, s/n, 4169-007 Porto, Portugal
[8] Department of Chemical Engineering, University of Porto, Rua Dr. Roberto Frias, s/n, 4200-465 Porto, Portugal
* Correspondence: acatarinaguedes@gmail.com; Tel.: +351-22-340-18-00

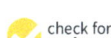

Citation: Amaro, H.M.; Barros, R.; Tavares, T.; Almeida, R.; Pinto, I.S.; Malcata, F.X.; Guedes, A.C. *Gloeothece* sp.—Exploiting a New Source of Antioxidant, Anti-Inflammatory, and Antitumor Agents. *Mar. Drugs* **2021**, *19*, 623. https://doi.org/10.3390/md19110623

Academic Editors: Elena Talero and Javier Ávila-Román

Received: 30 September 2021
Accepted: 26 October 2021
Published: 4 November 2021

Publisher's Note: MDPI stays neutral with regard to jurisdictional claims in published maps and institutional affiliations.

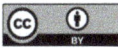

Copyright: © 2021 by the authors. Licensee MDPI, Basel, Switzerland. This article is an open access article distributed under the terms and conditions of the Creative Commons Attribution (CC BY) license (https://creativecommons.org/licenses/by/4.0/).

Abstract: Bioactive lipidic compounds of microalgae, such as polyunsaturated fatty acids (PUFA) and carotenoids, can avoid or treat oxidation-associated conditions and diseases like inflammation or cancer. This study aimed to assess the bioactive potential of lipidic extracts obtained from *Gloeothece* sp.–using Generally Recognized as Safe (GRAS) solvents like ethanol, acetone, hexane:isopropanol (3:2) (HI) and ethyl lactate. The bioactive potential of extracts was assessed in terms of antioxidant (ABTS$^{\bullet+}$, DPPH$^{\bullet}$, $^{\bullet}$NO and O$_2^{\bullet}$ assays), anti-inflammatory (HRBC membrane stabilization and Cox-2 screening assay), and antitumor capacity (death by TUNEL, and anti-proliferative by BrdU incorporation assay in AGS cancer cells); while its composition was characterized in terms of carotenoids and fatty acids, by HPLC-DAD and GC-FID methods, respectively. Results revealed a chemopreventive potential of the HI extract owing to its ability to: (I) scavenge $^{-}$NO$^{\bullet}$ radical (IC$_{50}$, 1258 ± 0.353 µg·mL^{-1}); (II) inhibit 50% of COX-2 expression at 130.2 ± 7.4 µg·mL^{-1}; (III) protect 61.6 ± 9.2% of lysosomes from heat damage, and (IV) induce AGS cell death by 4.2-fold and avoid its proliferation up to 40% in a concentration of 23.2 ± 1.9 µg·mL^{-1}. Hence, *Gloeothece* sp. extracts, namely HI, were revealed to have the potential to be used for nutraceutical purposes.

Keywords: lutein; β-carotene; linolenic acid; linoleic acid; lipidic compounds; carotenoids; PUFAs

1. Introduction

The first reports on cyanobacteria date back to the time of Aztecs who used *Spirulina* (*Arthrospira platensis, A. maxima*) as food [1]. Nowadays the potential application of cyanobacteria in our daily lives has been well documented. Such microscopic organisms are indeed a universal source of a vast array of chemical products with applications in the feed, food, nutritional, cosmetic, and pharmaceutical industries [1–3]. The last decades have witnessed the massive development in the production of cyanobacteria through the improvement of processing methods, with particular emphasis on the extraction of high-value compounds to be used as nutraceuticals and pharmaceuticals [1,4].

Nevertheless, the exploitation of prokaryotic and eukaryotic microalgae is restricted to a few strains and most species remain largely unexplored. So far, till 2019, 260 families of bioactive compounds were identified in cyanobacteria with a wide range of applications, e.g., agriculture, pharmacology, cosmetology, or in the food industry; belonging to 10 different classes: alkaloids, depsipeptides, lipopeptides, macrolides/lactones, peptides, terpenes, polysaccharides, lipids, polyketides, and others [5]. Additionally, 14 major activities have been listed from the literature, among them are cytotoxicity, anti-inflammatory, and antioxidant, activities, at which bioactivities are particularly attributed to carotenoids, chlorophylls, mycosporine-like amino acids, and phycocyanins [5].

Extensive research efforts during the last decades revealed that continued oxidative stress may activate mechanisms that lead to chronic inflammation—which, in turn, could mediate chronic diseases like cancer. Oxidative stress occurs due to an imbalance between the production of free radicals, such as reactive oxygen species (ROS), and their elimination by natural protective mechanisms, such as antioxidants molecules. This imbalance may lead to injury of vital biomolecules, cells, and eventually the whole organism [6]. Therefore, the search for antioxidants or radical scavengers able to neutralize the harmful effects of oxidative stress has been in order, as they would prevent or treat inflammation or cancer [7,8].

Cancer is nowadays the 6th leading single cause of death worldwide [9]. This disease occurs due to an imbalance between the rate of cell proliferation and apoptosis; thus, an ideal therapy would be based on the ability to restore this balance, by either reducing cancer cell growth and/or promoting cancer cell death [10]. Gastric cancer ranks as the 5th most common type of cancer, and is the 3rd in cancer-related death [11]; its development has been frequently associated with severe inflammation caused by bacterium *Helicobacter pylori* [12].

It should be emphasized that it was found long ago that oxidative stress, chronic inflammation, and cancer development are closely related, particularly in what concerns their activation pathways—which entail the production of several inflammatory signaling molecules, like prostaglandins (PGs) as well as oxygen- and nitrogen-derived free radicals, as schematized in Figure 1 [7], a key characteristic of tumor promoters is their ability to recruit inflammatory cells and to stimulate them to generate ROS [7,13]. On the other hand, ROS are usually generated during mitochondrial metabolism and play an important role in cell signaling and homeostasis. ROS such as NO$^\bullet$, are produced during the inflammatory process [14] in response to inflammatory stimuli (e.g., cytokines or pathogens)—and some cases of deregulated inflammatory responses; thus may accordingly promote a state of chronic oxidative stress and inflammation [15].

The triggering of the inflammatory pathway by lipopolysaccharides (LPS) causes rapid activation of NOX2 and NADPH oxidase, and release of internal $O_2^{\bullet-}$. This radical triggers, in turn, NF-κB phosphorylation, by activating several enzymes—namely cyclooxygenase 2 (COX-2), and iNOS which induce the release of PGE2, free radicals like $O_2^{\bullet-}$ and NO, and the chemokine MCP-1. Other activation products of NF-κB include anti-apoptotic factors, cell cycle regulators, and adhesion molecules—which may be related to cancer cells' survival, proliferation, adhesion, invasion and metastasis, and angiogenesis [16]. Of note, the release of such mediators, like cytokines, may be regulated by secretory lysosomes. Indeed, secretory lysosomes can secrete or degrade inflammatory cytokines in the regulation of cytokine release, thus positively and negatively regulating the inflammation, having a feedback mechanism to adjust the balance of the inflammatory response in cells and organelles. Furthermore, involvement of a lysosomal membrane protein in the activation of NF-κB and other pathways suggests that the lysosomal compartments may play a central role in the inflammatory signaling network—and accordingly, provide a theoretical basis for the development of anti-inflammatory drug combinations consisting of a lysosomal inhibitor [17], see Figure 1.

Another common strategy followed in the formulation of anti-inflammatory agents is based on suppressing of production of inflammatory mediators, such as COX-2 inhibitors, that interfere with the initiation and progression of inflammation-associated diseases [18]. PGs were found in several kinds of tumors, like gastric cancer [19] or colon adenocarcinoma [20]; causing tumorigenic effects, such as stimulation of cell growth and angiogenesis, inhibition of apoptosis, and suppression of the immune system. Several studies also indicate that COX-2 inhibitors can reduce the risk of development of colon, lung, or skin cancer [21–23], and namely improve therapeutic effects on human cancers in combination with chemotherapeutic [24].

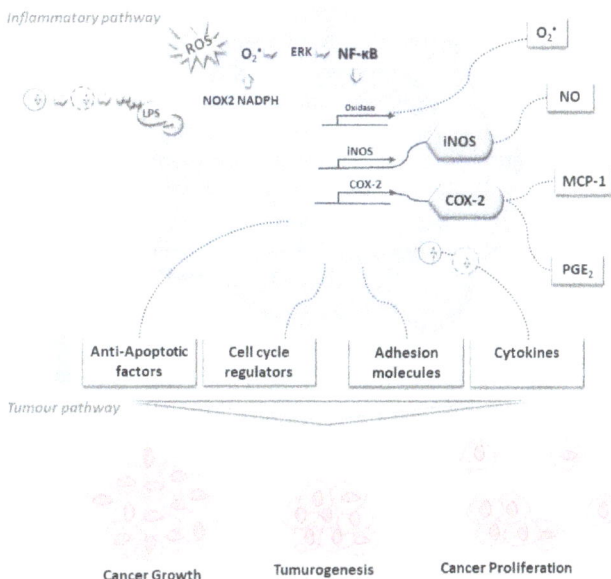

Figure 1. Brief schematic representation of how oxidative stress, inflammation, and cancer development may be correlated. After the lipopolysaccharide (LPS) inflammatory activation pathway in a macrophage cell, secretory lysosomes ( ) secrete or degrade inflammatory cytokines in regulating cytokines released by immune cells through a feedback mechanism. Phosphorylation of NF-κB activates several enzymes, e.g., cyclooxygenase(COX-2), oxidase, and iNOS, thus inducing the release of prostaglandins (PGE2), $O_2^{\bullet-}$ and other molecules like anti-apoptotic factors, cell cycle regulators, adhesion molecules that are likely to be related to tumorogenesis, cancer cell growth and proliferation. The unbalanced increase of the former may lead to tumorogenesis and (among other events) cancer growth and proliferation.

In practice, the synthetic drugs used to treat these disorders may bring about severe side effects; hence is important to find compounds from biological sources, such as cyanobacteria, lacking adverse effects [25]. Carotenoids and PUFA from microalgal sources have indeed been claimed to have anti-cancer and anti-inflammatory properties, having sometimes an antioxidant-based mechanism of action [26–28]. Some of them have even been proposed for the treatment and prevention of such chronic diseases [29,30]. Epidemiological studies suggest that carotenoids can prevent free radical-dependent oxidation of LDL, cholesterol, proteins or DNA, by capturing free radicals and thus reducing stress induced by ROS [31]. Furthermore, PUFA, namely n-3 PUFA, was described to hold antioxidant and anti-inflammatory effects [32–34].

In the particular case of cancer, some strategies of chemoprevention can be accomplished by incorporating antioxidant compounds in the diet, which would block or delay cancer development, either in the initial phase of carcinogenesis or at the stage of progression of neoplastic cells to cancer [35]. A clear example is β-carotene, which protective effect against cancer was intimately associated with its antioxidant role [2] and COX-2 suppression abilities [36]. Moreover, the potential of microalgal lipidic components as chemopreventive agents was observed in colon, skin, and stomach cancer [2]. Also, other carotenoids such as violaxanthin, zeaxanthin, lutein, and fucoxanthin, or ethanol-based carotenoids-extracts, isolated from microalgae, exhibited antiproliferative activity against different cancer cells [27,35,37–40].

For this study, a scarcely studied prokaryotic colonial microalga was selected, *Gloeothece* sp., with promising bioactive lipidic composition [41]. This study aimed to exploit the bioactive potential of its lipid extracts, as a new source of antioxidant, anti-inflammatory, and antitumor compounds—thus forecasting a possible application in the food and nutraceutical industry. Hence, GRAS (Generally Recognized as Safe) solvents—ethanol, acetone, ethyl lactate, and a mixture (3:2) of hexane/isopropanol, were selected to extract lipidic bioactive compounds from *Gloeothece* sp. [42,43].

2. Results

2.1. Biochemical Composition of Extracts

Gloeothece sp. extracts may have the potential of application in the nutraceutical industry, due to their content in bioactive compounds as carotenoids, polyunsaturated fatty acids (PUFA), or phenolic compounds. First, a crude characterization of extracts composition in terms of each family of compounds (m_C/m_E, %) was done, as depicted in Figure 2.

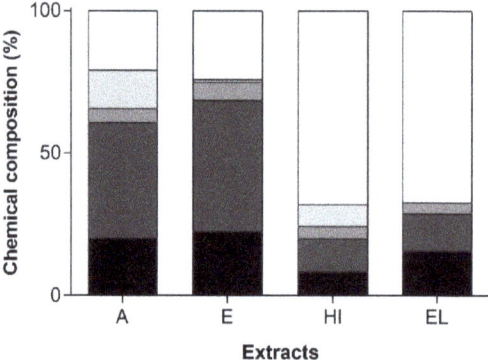

Figure 2. *Gloeothece* sp. extract's composition (m_C/m_E, %) in terms of ■ MUFA, ■ PUFA, ■ carotenoids, □ phenolic compounds, and other unidentified compounds, obtained with acetone (A), ethanol (E), hexane:isopropanol (1:1, v/v) (HI) and ethyl lactate (EL).

It can be observed that A and E extracts are mainly composed of fatty acids, ca. 60 and 66%, respectively, most of them PUFA (more than 40%). Extract A also exhibited the highest percent composition in phenolic compounds (13%, m_C/m_E), followed by HI extract (ca. 8%, m_C/m_E). The contents of carotenoids were ca. 4% in all extracts, except for E, which reaches 6.5%.

A detailed fatty acids composition, available in Table 1, reveals different profiles in monounsaturated (MUFA) and polyunsaturated (PUFA) fatty acids, either in terms of concentration ($\mu g_{Fatty\ Acid} \cdot mg_{Extract}^{-1}$) and content (%, $m_{Fatty\ Acid}/m_{Total\ Fatty\ Acid}$).

Concerning the MUFA C18:1 n9 c+t (oleic acid, OA), this is the one present in higher content and the 3rd in terms of all fatty acids. Its content in all extracts ranges between 14.4 (E) and 17.4% (EL), having a higher concentration in extract A, $53.796 \pm 2.918\ \mu g_{Fatty\ Acid} \cdot mg_{Extract}^{-1}$—i.e., approximately half of concentration in E, and one quarter in HI and EL.

In terms of PUFA, E and A exhibited a higher content, 40.7 and 46.0% (m_{FA}/m_{TFA}), respectively. In another way, HI and EL accounted for 80 and 71.3 (%, m_{FA}/m_{TFA}), respectively, in saturated fatty acids (data not shown).

Table 1. Fatty acid concentration ($\mu g_{Fatty\ Acid} \cdot mg_{Extract}^{-1}$) ± standard deviation and content ($m_{Fatty\ Acid}/m_{Total\ Fatty\ Acid}$, %) in each *Gloeothece* sp. extracts, E—ethanol extract, A—acetone extract; HI (3:2)—Hexane:Isopropanol (3:2, v/v) extract, and EL—ethyl lactate, in terms of monounsaturated fatty acids (MUFA) and polyunsaturated fatty acids (PUFA).

Fatty Acids	Fatty Acids Concentration and Content ($\mu g_{FA} \cdot mg_E^{-1}$, %($m_{FA}/m_{TFA}$))			
	E	A	HI (3:2)	EL
C14:1	0.520 ± 0.002 0.3	1.495 ± 0.013 1.3	0.937 ± 0.001 2.3	0.607 ± 0.020 3.3
C16:1	1.046 ± 0.053 0.7	2.426 ± 0.158 1.7	0.994 ± 0.023 2.7	0.869 ± 0.092 3.7
C17:1	6.849 ± 0.012 4.3	19.154 ± 2.152 5.3	2.517 ± 0.099 6.3	1.017 ± 0.187 7.3
C18:1 n9 c+t	22.812 ± 1.118 14.4	53.796 ± 2.918 15.4	12.910 ± 2.598 [a] 16.4	12.767 ± 1.980 [a] 17.4
C22:1 n9	0.184 ± 0.010 [a] 0.3	0.849 ± 0.043 0.2	0.202 ± 0.057 [a] 2.3	0.317 ± 0.016 3.3
Σ MUFA	31.412 20.0	76.870 22.4	17.559 8.5	15.577 15.6
C18:2 n6 t	24.242 ± 0.597 15.3	59.711 ± 3.278 16.3	11.683 ± 1.432 17.3	6.240 ± 1.510 26.4
C18:2 n6 c	0.406 ± 0.025 0.3	0.984 ± 0.012 1.3	0.308 ± 0.083 [a] 2.3	0.337 ± 0.008 [a] 3.3
C18:3n6	1.934 ± 0.030 1.2	1.467 ± 0.039 [a] 2.2	1.250 ± 0.152 [b] 3.2	1.267 ± 0.196 [a,b] 4.2
C18:3 n3	37.233 ± 0.685 23.4	96.765 ± 5.713 24.4	13.216 ± 0.225 25.4	4.575 ± 1.437 18.3
C20:2	0.498 ± 0.009 0.25	0.724 ± 0.205 [a] 1.3	0.943 ± 0.701 [a] 2.3	0.289 ± 0.014 3.3
C20:5 n3	0.344 ± 0.023 [a] 0.2	- -	0.283 ± 0.105 [a] 2.2	0.462 ± 0.071 3.2
Σ PUFA	64.160 40.7	159.651 46.0	27.682 11.5	13.170 13.2

[a,b] Same lowercase letters for the same fatty acid mean no significant difference between extracts ($p < 0.05$).

Among PUFA, C18:3 n3 (α-linolenic acid, ALA) attained the highest content in all extracts, between 23.4 (E) and 26.4 (EL) % (m_{FA}/m_{TFA}); but with a higher concentration in A (96.765 ± 5.713 $\mu g_{FA} \cdot mg_E^{-1}$); followed by E (37.233 ± 0.685 $\mu g_{FA} \cdot mg_E^{-1}$), HI (13.216 ± 0.225 $\mu g_{FA} \cdot mg_E^{-1}$), and EL (4.575 ± 1.437 $\mu g_{FA} \cdot mg_E^{-1}$). In other way, the PUFA C18:2 n6 t (linoleic acid, LA) attained the highest concentration, 6.240 ± 1.510 $\mu g_{FA} \cdot mg_E^{-1}$, in the EL extracts. Note that conjugated linoleic acid (CLA, C18:2 n6 t + C18:2 n6 c), also in high content (%, m_{FA}/m_{TFA}) and concentration ($\mu g_{FA} \cdot mg_E^{-1}$) in E, (15.5%, 60.695 $\mu g_{FA} \cdot mg_E^{-1}$), followed by EL (6.6%, 6.577 $\mu g_{FA} \cdot mg_E^{-1}$), HI (5%, 11.991 $\mu g_{FA} \cdot mg_E^{-1}$), and A (1.5%, 24.648 $\mu g_{FA} \cdot mg_E^{-1}$). Furthermore, C20:5 n3, (eicosapentaenoic acid, EPA) was detected in EL and HI extracts, in concentration of 0.462 ± 0.071 and 0.283 ± 0.105 $\mu g_{FA} \cdot mg_E^{-1}$, respectively.

Observing the carotenoid profile and concentration (see Figure 3), extract A—besides having the highest concentration in total carotenoids, contains a quite different profile from the others, while E and HI profiles appeared to be similar. In another way, EL contains the fewest carotenoids and lowest content. Lutein is the most abundant carotenoid in all extracts, being ca. 35% more concentrated in A (10.73 ± 0.59 $\mu g_{carot} \cdot mg_E^{-1}$) than in E and HI, and 69% more than in EL, 3.19 ± 0.22 $\mu g_{carot} \cdot mg_E^{-1}$. Neoxanthin is the second most abundant xanthophyll, with 3.21 ± 0.23 $\mu g_{carot} \cdot mg_E^{-1}$ in A, i.e., 1.5-fold that of E, 2.1-fold of HI, and 4.1-fold of EL. Moreover, A is the only extract than contains zeaxanthin 1.07 ± 0.12 $\mu g_{carot} \cdot mg_E^{-1}$, and the highest concentration of α-carotene, i.e., 0.53 ± 0.04 $\mu g_{carot} \cdot mg_E^{-1}$, and β-carotene, i.e., 1.60 ± 0.03 $\mu g_{carot} \cdot mg_E^{-1}$.

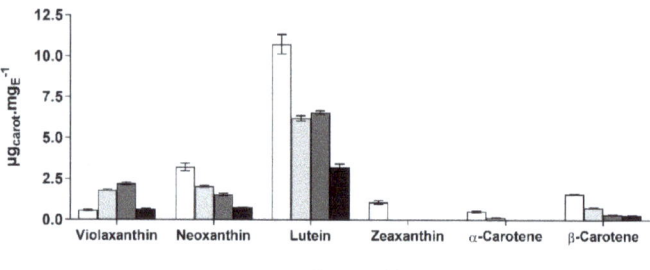

Figure 3. Carotenoid profile and content ($\mu g_{carotenoids} \cdot mg_{Extract}^{-1}$) in each *Gloeothece* sp. extract, ☐ Acetone (A), ▨ Ethanol (E), ▪ Hexane:Isopropanol (3:2) (HI) and ■ Ethyl Lactate (EL) extracts.

2.2. Antioxidant Capacity of Lipidic Extracts

The extracts were tested for their total antioxidant capacity (via ABTS$^{\bullet+}$ and DPPH$^{\bullet}$ methods), and specific radical antioxidant capacity for radicals $O_2^{\bullet-}$ and $^{\bullet}NO$.

As observed in Table 2, all extracts exhibited total antioxidant capacity—although in some assays the IC$_{50}$ values could not be estimated within the range of concentrations tested, such as $O_2^{\bullet-}$ assay.

Table 2. Comparison of antioxidant capacity of *Gloeothece* sp. extracts (average ± standard deviation), against the radicals ABTS$^{+\bullet}$, DPPH$^{\bullet}$, $^{\bullet}NO^-$ and $O_2^{\bullet-}$, expressed in terms of IC$_{50}$ ($mg_{Extract} \cdot mL^{-1}$), and values of IC50 values (average ± standard deviation) of extracts on cell viability, according to sulforhodamine B (SRB) assay for gastric cancer cell lines, AGS.

Solvents	Antioxidant Capacity IC$_{50}$ ($mg_E \cdot mL^{-1}$)				SRB IC$_{50}$ ($\mu g_E \cdot mL^{-1}$)
	ABTS$^{\bullet+}$	DPPH$^{\bullet}$	$O_2^{\bullet-}$	$^{\bullet}NO^-$	
Ethanol	0.259 ± 0.074 a,b	1.538 ± 0.012	nd	0.637 ± 0.024	241.0 ± 22.5 a
Acetone	0.217 ± 0.009 a	0.978 ± 0.032	nd	0.284 ± 0.090	114.4 ± 6.4
HI 3:2 (v/v)	0.283 ± 0.034 b	nd	nd	1.258 ± 0.353	23.2 ± 1.9
Ethyl lactate	5.809 ± 0.203	4.016 ± 1.256	nd	nd	209.3 ± 11.0 a

a,b Means within the same column, without a common superscript, are significantly different ($p < 0.05$). HI—Hexane: isopropanol (3:2) v/v; nd—not determined.

No significant differences were found between E and A extracts ($p < 0.05$) in ABTS$^{\bullet+}$ assay, and A extract exhibited the lowest IC$_{50}$ in DPPH$^{\bullet}$ and $^{\bullet}NO^-$ assays. Although the IC$_{50}$ for EL extract at $^{\bullet}NO^-$ assay could not be calculated in the range of concentrations tested, it was revealed to have antioxidant capacity.

2.3. Antitumoral Features of Lipidic Extracts

Among the available cancer adenocarcinoma cell lines, AGS highlights as being the gastric line most used in vitro study models [44]. Hence, antitumor capacities of all extracts were evaluated through different assays, using AGS cell line as a model. First, the cancer cell viability was evaluated by Sulforhodamine B assay, and IC$_{50}$ was determined for each extract. The IC$_{50}$ values of each extract were then used to determine whether the extracts were able to promote cell death via TUNEL assay; and whether the extracts were able to inhibit cancer cell proliferation, via cell proliferation BrdU assay.

2.3.1. Evaluation of Cancer Cell Viability by Sulforhodamine B Assay

Sulforhodamine B assay (SRB) uses the protein-binding dye SRB to indirectly assess cell growth [45,46].

Despite DMSO being widely described to be cytotoxic depending on its concentration—yet, it was used to suspend extracts at low and non-cytotoxic concentrations. DMSO was thus titrated in these cell lines and, it was found that a concentration of 0.25% (v/v) was innocuous to AGS cells (data not shown).

For each extract, a dose-response curve was established, allowing determination of the extract's concentration causing a cell growth inhibition of 50%, as shown in Table 2.

From the results calculated in Table 2, HI extract outstands for its lowest IC_{50} values, reaching values 5- to 10-fold lower when compared to the other extracts. IC50 values determined for each extract were then used to perform the cancer cell death and proliferation assays.

2.3.2. Evaluation of Cancer Cell Death via TUNEL Assay

TUNEL is a common method for detecting DNA fragmentation that may result from cell death, either by apoptosis or necrosis [47]. Induction of DNA fragmentation in AGS cells, treated with the different extracts, at their IC_{50} by 48 h of treatment, was examined using TUNEL. The results produced (Figure 4) show that treatment with all four extracts results in a significantly increased cell death ($p < 0.05$), yet a stronger effect was observed for HI extract—which increased AGS cells death by c.a. of 4-fold.

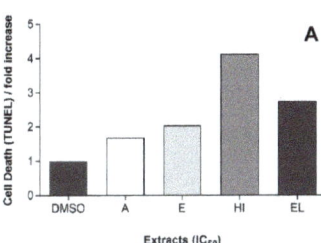 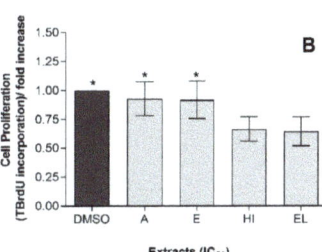

Figure 4. Antitumoral features of *Gloeothece* sp. lipidic extracts (**A**) AGS cell death, quantified by fold increase ☐ Acetone (A), ☐ Ethanol (E), ▨ hexane:isopropanol (3:2) (HI) and ■ Ethylic lactate (EL) extracts; and, (**B**) AGS cell proliferation, quantified by fold increase by Acetone (A), Ethanol (E), hexane:isopropanol (3:2) (HI) and Ethylic lactate (EL) extracts, using DMSO as a negative control. Bars with a common character are significantly not different ($p < 0.05$) from the DMSO control.

2.3.3. Evaluation of Cancer Cell Proliferation

Assessment of cell proliferation by BrdU assay is based on the incorporation of BrdU into their replicating DNA, which can further be detected by immunofluorescence. For a quantitative approach, samples were analyzed by flow cytometry. Results revealed an anti-proliferative effect of the HI and EL extracts upon AGS, via 40% of inhibition of proliferation in ca., while cells treated with the E or A extracts behaved no differently from the negative control with DMSO (Figure 4), i.e., exhibited no antiproliferative effect.

2.4. Anti-Inflammatory Potential of Lipidic Extracts

The mechanism of inflammation can be partially triggered via the release of ROS, from activated neutrophils and macrophages, thus leading to damage in macromolecules causing, namely, lipid peroxidation of membranes. ROS spread inflammation by stimulating the release of cytokines, regulated by lysosomes, which in turn stimulate the recruitment of additional neutrophils and macrophages. Lysosome structure conveys a physical and functional interface among cell organelles, as it plays a role in negative or positive modulation of the production of inflammatory cytokines [17,48]. Furthermore, free radicals are mediators that induce or sustain inflammatory processes; hence their neutralization by antioxidants and radical scavengers are fundamental to reducing inflammation [49]. In this context, extracts from *Gloeothece* sp. were screened for their potential anti-inflammatory features, by resorting to two different assays, one reflecting the stabilization of extracts on Human red blood cell (HRBC) membrane induced by heat, and another that ascertains the capacity of such extracts to inhibit the human enzyme COX-2.

2.4.1. Human Red Blood Cell (HRBC) Membrane Stabilization Assay

This assay allows the characterization of the capacity of *Gloeothece* sp. extracts to protect erythrocytes from hemolysis when heat is supplied. Since the erythrocyte membrane is quite similar to the lysosomal one, indirectly is possible to conclude if any *Gloeothece* sp. extract holds any capacity in the stabilization of lysosomal membranes [50], and so, if they have the potential to be used as a non-steroidal drug—the common anti-inflammatory drug that inhibits lysosomal enzymes or stabilizes their membrane.

Results show that the HI 3:2 (v/v) extract is the most promising as it exhibits a protection capacity of 61.6 ± 9.6%; nonetheless, EL extract also appears to hold some potential in protecting HRBC membranes. Conversely, the E and A extracts did not show significant protective capacity (see Table 3).

Table 3. Anti-inflammatory potential of *Gloeothece* sp. lipidic extracts, upon the protection of HRBC membranes (average ± standard deviation) from heat, expressed in percentage of stabilization and IC50 (average ± standard deviation) values of extracts obtained at of COX-2 enzymatic activity inhibition.

Solvents	HRBC Stabilization (%)	COX-2 Enzymatic Activity Inhibition IC$_{50}$ ($\mu g_E \cdot mL^{-1}$)
Acetone	-	116.8 ± 7.7
Ethanol	-	198.3 ± 15.2
HI 3:2 (v/v)	61.6 ± 9.2	130.2 ± 7.4
Ethyl lactate	14.8 ± 4.3	-

2.4.2. Cox Human Inhibitory Assay

Cyclooxygenases (COXs) catalyze reactions that lead to the formation of pro-inflammatory prostaglandins (PG), thromboxanes, and prostacyclins. Hence, the ability of extracts to inhibit the conversion of AA to Prostaglandin H2 (PGH2) via inhibition of COX-2 was determined. All concentrations tested exhibit anti-inflammatory activity in vitro, by inhibiting PG production in a dose-dependent manner. However, the extracts exhibited different behaviors within the range of concentrations tested, data not shown.

While A and EL at lower extract concentration induces a higher inhibition, a linear percent of inhibition is of E concentration was observed, whereas a non-significantly percentage of inhibition variation was detected with HI concentration. In terms of total inhibition capacity of COX-2 enzymatic activity, one notices that A, E, and HI performed equally well beyond 50% with no significant differences between them ($p < 0.05$); however, the corresponding IC50 values (see Table 3) revealed that A and HI extracts attained the lowest values, without significant differences ($p < 0.05$).

2.5. Cytotoxicity

For a putative application of *Gloeothece* sp. extracts as a nutraceutical ingredient, it is mandatory that extracts do not exhibit any cytotoxicity to non-cancer cells. Therefore, cytotoxicity effects upon HCMEC cells were assessed after 24 h (see Figure 5A) and 48 h (see Figure 5B), using DMSO 1% as a negative control. Results show that A extract is cytotoxic, although its cytotoxicity decreases after 48 h. However, promising results were observed concerning the E extract, since there was no evidence of cytotoxicity at all concentrations tested. On the other hand, both HI and EL extracts were not lethal up to 100 $\mu g \cdot mL^{-1}$; the highest concentrations tested were toxic, although toxicity decreases with time.

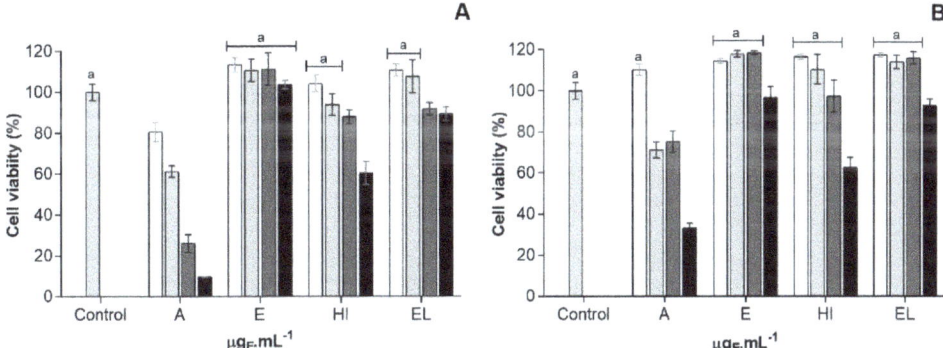

Figure 5. Cytotoxicity evaluation of Acetone (A), Ethanol (E), Hexane:Isopropanol (3:2) (HI) and Ethyl Lactate (EL) *Gloeothece* sp. extracts, against HCMEC cell line, tested at ☐ 50, ☐ 100, ▓ 200 and ■ 300 µg·mL^{-1}, by 24 h (**A**) and 48 h (**B**). Bars marked with the same letter in the same superscript have no significant difference relative to the control ($p < 0.05$).

3. Discussion

Drugs commonly used to treat inflammation and cancer raise severe side effects, such as toxicity and decreased life quality [51,52]. In this regard, this work aimed at making a preliminary test of *Gloeothece* sp. extracts to be eventually used as a natural source in nutraceuticals, and/or as a potential chemopreventive agent—based on the composition in carotenoids and PUFA, coupled with antioxidant, antitumoral, and anti-inflammatory features. Pearson correlations were calculated (data not shown) between composition (carotenoids and PUFA) and bioactive features, however possible synergetic effects among the molecules, that were not possible to measure, may contribute to its bioactive potential. Hence, these features will be discussed separately, and then in an integrated manner.

3.1. Antioxidant Capacity of Lipidic Crude Extracts

The antioxidant capacity of cyanobacterial carotenoids is well established—particularly concerning lutein and β-carotene [27,29,30,53], and long-chain fatty acids such ω3 PUFA [30,32]. Analyzing the extract contents in PUFA (see Table 1), carotenoids (see Figure 2) and, it results of total antioxidant capacity, it is possible to correlate extract concentration of carotenoids and PUFA with antioxidant bioactivity—at which A extract, stands out due to its lowest IC$_{50}$ values at all antioxidant assays. As observed previously, lutein probably contributes the most to said bioactivity, owing to its higher concentration [54]. However, other carotenoids (e.g., β-carotene and neoxanthin) should not be overlooked owing to their concentrations, as well as such PUFA as 18:1 n9, 18:2 n6, and 18:3 n3 based on the IC$_{50}$ values of *Gloeothece* sp. extracts (A > E > HI > EL). Particularly, a correlation was found with C18:2 n6 ($r = 1$, $p < 0.083$).

Concerning the specific radical's scavenger capacity, results reveal the same trend, particularly in NO$^{\bullet}$ assay, in which the lowest IC$_{50}$ was again observed in the A extract. The high concentration of total carotenoids and PUFA, namely lutein and C18:2 n6, may account for their important antioxidant role ($r = 1$, $p < 0.083$), as reported before [55–57].

Although the IC$_{50}$ values for the O$_2^{\bullet-}$ assay could not be found at the tested concentrations, some scavenging effects were detected at E and EL extracts—data not shown.

Hence, owing to the antioxidant scavenging capacity of A and E extracts against NO$^{\bullet}$ and O$_2^{\bullet-}$ radicals in vitro, a similar capacity is expected in vivo—with a preventive role of chronic inflammatory diseases, cancer, or neurodegenerative disorders [58,59].

3.2. Antitumoral Features of Cyanobacterial Extracts

Unlike observed with antioxidant capacity, the most promising extracts, in terms of inducing AGS cell death and cell proliferation, are HI and EL extracts; where it cannot be established a clear correlation of antitumor capacity and high content in carotenoids and fatty acids.

Despite a possible interaction of all extracts' compounds, some evidence relate such bioactivities with some compounds identified in *Gloeothece* sp. extracts, such as phenolic compounds. Although these compounds have not been characterized, the content in aromatic compounds is described to exert effects in bioactivities, particularly in antitumor and anti-inflammatory agents [60].

From a nutraceutical point of view, dietary supplementation of β-carotene in animal models of colon carcinogenesis has revealed anticancer capacities for that compound [61], as well as growth-inhibitory and pro-apoptotic effects in human colon cancer cell lines [36]. It has also been demonstrated that such chemopreventive activity is dose-dependent, a high dose proving to be harmful and likely to have a proliferative effect upon some cancer cells lines [1]; this may explain why the HI and EL extracts, characterized by the lowest levels of β-carotene and lowest IC50 values, exhibited the best results upon cancer cell death and proliferation. Additionally, such xanthophylls, violaxanthin have been found to possess antiproliferative activity against different cancer cells [35], and in fact, HI extract exhibited the highest level of violaxanthin.

Some PUFA, particularly ω-3, have been reported to possess in vitro and in vivo anticancer effects, via modulation of tumor growth or increase of cell death rate [62,63], this is the particular case of EPA, able to inhibit some cancer cell lines proliferation in a dose-dependent and time-dependent manner [62]. However, particular attention should go to LA. Studies reveal that treatment of AGS and MKN cells with linoleic acid (C18:2n6), in which EL extract has the higher content, led to an increase in a proapoptotic protein expression and a decrease of an anti-apoptotic protein expression, as well as inhibits the production of PGE2 and activity of telomerase by suppressing COX-2 and hTERT expression, in a dose-dependent manner [64,65], which may be in line with our results in AGS cell death. Indeed, in our study, a correlation was found between cell death and C18:2n6 content ($r = 1$, $p < 0.083$).

It should be noted that the antitumoral IC_{50} value for the HI extract (23.2 ± 1.9 µg·mL^{-1}) is lower than other hexanoic extracts reported before for human colon carcinoma cell line (HCT116), for example for *Chlorella ellipsoidea* and *C. vulgaris* which IC_{50} value was ca. 41µg·mL^{-1} and equivalent to the one obtained with pure lutein (21.02 ± 0.85 µg·mL^{-1}) [39]. Also, correlation was found for AGS cell proliferation and content of C18:1 n9, C18:2 n6, C18:3 n3 and β-carotene contents ($r = 1$, $p < 0.083$).

3.3. Anti-Inflammatory Potential of Lipidic Crude Extracts

The anti-inflammatory potential of *Gloeothece* sp. extracts was assessed by two assays. In the HRBC assay, HI extracts stood out in terms of inhibition capacity of 61%; hence, this HI extract may potentially stabilize cell membrane and thus prevent stress-induced decay, as well as stabilize the lysosomal membrane. This feature is crucial in the prevention of an anti-inflammatory response induced by the release of lysosomal constituents, which cause further tissue inflammation and damage upon extracellular release [50].

As seen before, the ability to inactivate COX-2 is indicative of the potential of an extract to be used as an anti-inflammatory drug. All extracts of *Gloeothece* sp. exhibited that ability, some of them having a dose-dependent response, like E extracts. However, extract A exhibited the best performance at a concentration of 75 µg·mL^{-1}, inhibiting in ca. 57% of COX-2 enzymatic activity; however, the possible application of A extracts use must be discarded due to its cytotoxicity to HCMEC cells. Nonetheless, HI extract follows as most promising due to ca. 48% of inactivation capacity and with no cytotoxicity associated.

A number of anti-inflammatory molecules obtained from microalgae have been shown to display high antioxidant capacity, that is in the composition of A and HI, such as β-carotene, lutein, zeaxanthin, and ω3 PUFA [66]. Some of the anti-inflammatory ability could be attributed to violaxanthin. This xanthophyll isolated from *C. ellipsoidea* showed anti-inflammatory activity when it was tested on LPS-stimulated RAW 264.7

mouse macrophages, by inhibiting NF-κB activation and NO and prostaglandin E2 (PGE2) production [67].

3.4. Potential of Application of Gloeothece sp. Extracts

Chemoprevention consists of the use of pharmaceutical drugs, or nutritional supplements to reduce the risk of developing or having a recurrence of cancer. Several in vitro and animal studies showed the chemopreventive properties of a few metabolites from microalgae (e.g., carotenoids, fatty acids, polysaccharides, and proteins), namely against colon and skin cancer [2].

Performance recorded for *Gloeothece* sp. extracts, particularly the A and HI shows that they are a promising source in the eventual formulation of some nutraceutical products bearing antioxidant, anticancer, and anti-inflammatory capacities. But despite the notable antioxidant features of the A extract, particularly its ability to inhibit the radical NO•, its potential application as a nutraceutical is limited due to its cytotoxicity.

Experimental and epidemiological evidence reported before suggests that anti-inflammatory drugs may also decrease the incidence of some types of cancer, as well as tumor burden and volume [68,69]. An attempt to provide a global overview of the potential of action of HI and A extracts is conveyed by Figure 6.

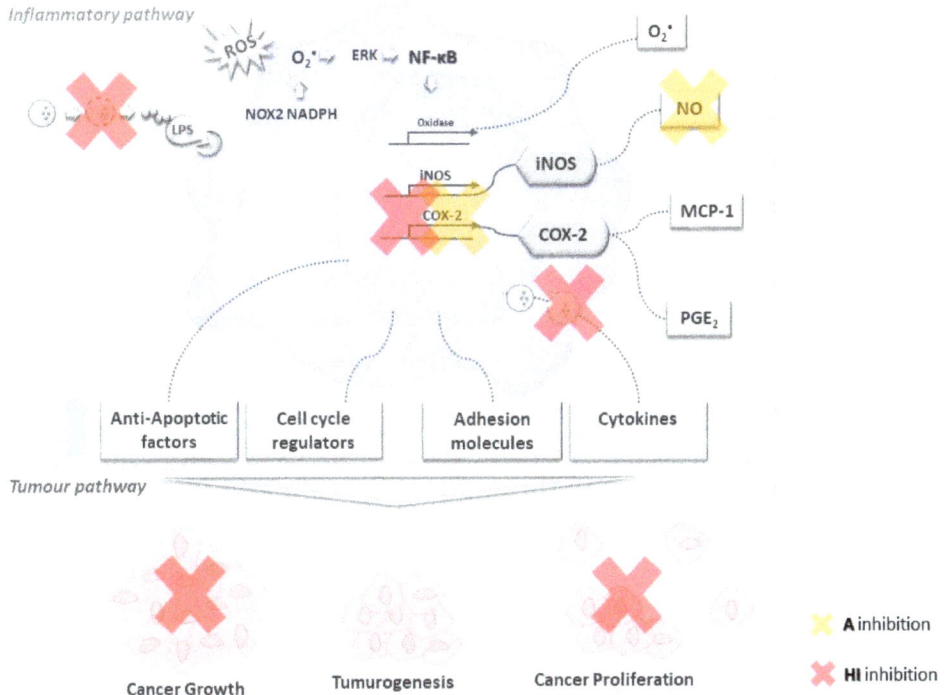

Figure 6. Schematic representation of how the HI (red cross) and A (yellow cross) extracts may modulate oxidative stress, inflammation, and cancer development. The HI extract protects membranes of secretory lysosomes, thus avoiding the release of inflammatory cytokines and consequent feedback mechanism. The phosphorylation of NF-κB is activated. A is able to reduce the produced NO radicals. HI and A are able to suppress cyclooxygenase (COX-2), and subsequent release of prostaglandins (PGE2), as well as anti-apoptotic factors, cell cycle regulators, adhesion molecules related to tumorogenesis, cancer cell growth, and proliferation. HI extract is able to inhibit cancer-related events such as cancer growth and proliferation.

Hence, the HI extracts of *Gloethece* sp. appeared to be the most promising as a chemopreventive agent in the nutraceutical industry because of their features as (1) antioxidant namely high total antioxidant capacity and scavenging capacity against ⁻NO• radical; (2) antitumor induction of cell death upon AGS cells, along with anti-proliferative effects; and (3) anti-inflammatory, namely inability to inhibit COX-2 expression while protecting lysosomes.

4. Materials and Methods

4.1. Microorganism Source and Biomass Production

Gloeothece sp. (ATCC 27152) was purchased from ATCC—American Type Culture Collection (USA), and kept at 25 °C, using Blue Green (BG11) as culture medium [70]. For biomass production, in 4 L batch culture, first, a pre-inoculum, with an initial optical density of 0.1 at 680 nm, was cultivated for 10 days in 800 mL of BG11 medium, buffered at pH 8 with Tri-(hydroxymethyl)-aminomethane hydrochloride (Tris-HCl)—ensuring that the microorganism was at the exponential growth phase at the time of inoculation for biomass production. Hence, biomass production was started with an initial optical density of 0.1 in BG11 medium buffered at pH 8 and was produced for 14 days under a continuous illumination with fluorescent BIOLUX lamps, with an intensity of 150 $\mu mol_{photon} \cdot m^{-2} \cdot s^{-1}$, and air bubbling at a flow rate of 0.5 $L \cdot min^{-1}$. Biomass was then collected by centrifugation at $18 \times g$ for 10 min, the supernatant was rejected and pellet freeze-dried, and stored under gaseous nitrogen until analyses were performed.

4.2. Extract Preparation

Extracts from *Gloeothece* sp. were obtained from 200 mg of lyophilized biomass, using four alternative food-grade solvents (Fisher Chemical, New Hampshire, EUA): ethanol (E), acetone (A), a mixture (3:2) of hexane/isopropanol (HI), and ethyl lactate (EL), as previously tested [41].

4.3. Chemical Characterization of Extracts

Fatty acids and carotenoids are among the most widely known bioactive compounds found in microalgae, which possess a high interest in the nutraceutical and pharmaceutical markets; hence, solvent extracts were evaporated and residue composition was determined for each *Gloeothece* sp. extract, as detailed below.

4.3.1. Profile and Content of Polyunsaturated Fatty Acids

The weighted residue was submitted to direct transesterification to produce fatty acid methyl esters according to the acidic method described by Lepage and Roy [71], after modifications introduced by Cohen et al. [72] using acetyl chloride (Sigma-Aldrich, St. Louis, MO, USA) as catalyst. The internal standard used was heptadecanoic (C17:0, Sigma-Aldrich, St. Louis, MO, USA) acid and esters were analyzed in a Varian Chrompack CP-3800 gas chromatograph (GC), using a flame ionization detector, and quantified with the software Varian Star Chromatography Workstation (USA, Version 5.50). Helium was employed as the carrier gas in splitless mode and the silica CP-WAX 52 CB (Agilent) column was used. The injector and detector were maintained at 260 and 280 °C, respectively, and the oven heating program was the same as described before [42]. To identify PUFA, chromatographic grade standards of fatty acids were used in methyl ester form CRM47885 (Supelco, St. Louis, MO, USA). Concentrations of each polyunsaturated fatty acid (PUFAs) were determined and mean values were used as a datum point.

4.3.2. Profile and Content of Carotenoids

To determine the content in carotenoids of the extracts, high-performance liquid chromatography (HPLC) was applied as an analytical technique as detailed before [54]. The residue was weighed and resuspended in acetone: acetonitrile (9:1); 8-β-apo-carotenol (Sigma-Aldrich, St. Louis, MO, EUA) was used as internal standard. Standards were purchased from CarotNature, Lutein (No. 0133, Xanthophyll, (3R,3'R,6'R)-β,ε-Carotene-3,3'-diol with 5% Zeaxanthin with 96% purity), β-carotene (No. 0003, β, β-carotene) with 96% purity) and β-apo-carotenol (No. 0482, 8'-Apo-β-caroten-8'-al) with 97% purity). The elution times of the chromatographic standards were: 14.4 min for lutein and 34.4 min for β-carotene. Identification was by comparison of retention times and UV–visible photo-diode array spectra, following the procedure by Guedes [54].

4.4. Antioxidant Effects of Lipidic Extracts

The antioxidant capacity of each extract was evaluated via four spectrophotometric assays: two assessed total antioxidant capacity (ABTS$^{+\bullet}$, DPPH$^\bullet$); while the other two were more specific for two biological radicals, superoxide ($O_2^{\bullet-}$) and nitric oxide ($^\bullet NO^-$)—with the later be known to be correlated with inflammation processes.

A positive control, Trolox, was used to validate the antioxidant capacity of extracts and putatively establish a calibration curve but comparing the antioxidant capacity of the extracts, their IC_{50} values were established. A dilution series was accordingly prepared for each extract, with concentrations ranging from 0.440 to 7 mg·mL^{-1}—for ethanol, acetone, and HI extracts, and from 1.5 to 24 mg·mL^{-1} for ethyl lactate extract, in Phosphate Buffered Saline (PBS) containing 5% of DMSO. Each antioxidant assay was performed in triplicate, as described in the following sub-sections.

4.4.1. ABTS$^{+\bullet}$ Scavenging Capacity

The total antioxidant capacity was determined as the capacity to decrease the absorbance of blue/green chromophore 2,2'-Azino-bis (3-ethylbenzothiazoline-6-sulfonic acid) (ABTS$^{\bullet+}$) (Alfa Aesar, Massachusetts, US). Absorbance was accordingly determined at 734 nm, upon the reaction of the extract with ABTS$^{\bullet+}$ for 6 min—as previously optimized by Guedes et al. [54].

4.4.2. DPPH$^\bullet$ Scavenging Capacity

The antioxidant capacity was determined, in triplicate, by reacting each extract with 2,2-diphenyl-1-picrylhydrazyl (DPPH$^\bullet$) (Sigma-Aldrich (St. Louis, MO, USA), after an incubation period of 30 min at room temperature in dark. The scavenging reaction was monitored at 515 nm, as implemented before by Amaro et al. [41].

4.4.3. Superoxide Radical ($O_2^{\bullet-}$) Scavenging Capacity

Superoxide radicals are generated by the NADH/PMS system. The extract antioxidant capacity was determined by monitoring the absorbance of the reaction mixture, at 560 nm and room temperature, for 2 min, as previously performed by Amaro et al. [41].

4.4.4. Nitric Oxide Radical ($^\bullet NO^-$) Scavenging Capacity

Each extract was incubated with sodium nitroprusside, for 60 min at room temperature, in the light. Griess reagent was added afterward, and the chromophore reaction was carried out in the dark for 10 min; absorbance was read at 562 nm [41].

4.5. Anticancer Effects of Gloeothece sp. Extract

4.5.1. Cancer Cell Culture

Human gastric carcinoma cell line AGS CRL-1739 (obtained from ATCC, USA) derived from fragments of a tumor resected from a patient who had received no prior therapy, were maintained in RPMI1640 (Invitrogen, Thermo Fisher Scientific, Waltham, MA, USA) supplemented with 10% FBS (Lonza, Basel, Switzerland) and kept at 37 °C, in a humidified 5% CO_2 incubator.

4.5.2. Cancer Cell Viability Sulforhodamine B Assay

Solvents of each extract were evaporated by rotavapor and extracts resuspended with the minimum amount of dimethyl sulfoxide (DMSO) (AppliChem, Darmstadt, Germany), thus producing in concentrations of 130, 150, 120, and 450 mg·mL^{-1}, for acetone, ethanol, HI and ethyl lactate extracts, respectively.

AGS cells in a concentration of 1×10^4 were seeded in 96-wells plates and treated for 48 h with different concentrations of microalgal extracts (0 to 550 µg·mL^{-1} whenever possible) or DMSO (AppliChem, Darmstadt, Germany) as negative treatment control (0.05% v/v). As a positive control, DMSO 100%, was used to validate the antitumoral capacity of extracts. Then cells were fixed by the addition of 50 µL of cold 50% trichloroacetic acid (Merck Millipore, Kenilworth, NJ, USA) to each well, and incubating the plates at 4 °C for 1 h. Next the fixation step, the plates were washed three times with deionized water and dried at room temperature. The cells were then stained with 50 µL of 4% sulforhodamine B (SRB) (Sigma-Aldrich, St. Louis, MO, USA) in 1% acetic acid (Mallinckrodt Baker, Deventer, The Netherlands) for 30 min and then washed three times with deionized water. After the plates were dry, the cells were solubilized with 100 µL of 10 mM unbuffered Tris Base (Sigma-Aldrich, St. Louis, MO, USA), and the optical density at 510 nm was measured using the fluorimeter SynergyTM 4 Multi-Mode Microplate Reader (Biotek, Winooski, VT, USA). Results were plotted as dose-response curves, and the IC$_{50}$ for each extract was found and expressed as µg$_E$·mL^{-1}.

4.5.3. Cancer Cell Death TUNEL Assay

AGS cells were cultured in 6-well plates in a concentration of 7.5×10^5, and treated for 48 h with the microalgal extracts at the IC$_{50}$ found at the SRB assay, for 48 h. DMSO (AppliChem, Darmstadt, Germany) was used as a positive control treatment. Cells were washed and trypsinized and the pellet obtained was fixed in 3 mL of ice-cold methanol for 15 min. Then, cells were washed and resuspended in 500 µL of PBS. Incubation with TUNEL reaction mix (1:9:10 concerning the Dilution Buffer reagent, according to manufacture instructions—In Situ Cell Death Detection Kit Fluorescein, Roche, Mannheim, Germany) was done for 1 h, at 37 °C, in the dark. Then, data were acquired using a BD Accuri C6 flow cytometer (BD Biosciences, San Jose, CA, USA).

4.5.4. Cancer Proliferative Assay

AGS cells were cultured in 6-well plates containing a concentration of 7.5×10^5 and treated with the extracts at the IC$_{50}$ found at the SRB assay, for 48 h, using DMSO (AppliChem, Darmstadt, Germany) as positive control treatment. 5-Bromo-2′-deoxyuridine (BrdU) (BrdU labeling and detection kit 1, Roche, Mannheim, Germany) was incorporated in the cell culture medium at the ratio of 1:1000, and underwent incubation for 1 h, at 37 °C. Straightaway the following incubation, the cells were harvested, washed with PBS, fixed in 1 mL of ice-cold methanol for 30 min, washed again, and resuspended in 500 µL of PBS. This was followed by the incubation with 1 mL of HCl 4 M (Mallinckrodt Baker, Deventer, The Netherlands), for 20 min, two washing steps with PBS, a blocking step (PBS containing 0.5% Tween 20 and 0.05% BSA), and finally 1 h incubation at room temperature with the primary antibody against BrdU (1:20, Bu20a, Dako, Glostrup, Denmark). Next, the cells were further washed with PBS and incubated with the secondary antibody labeled with FITC (1:200, polyclonal rabbit anti-mouse, Dako, Glostrup, Denmark), for 30 min at room temperature washed two times and resuspended in 500 µL of PBS. Data acquisition was performed with a BD Accuri C6 flow cytometer (BD Biosciences, San Jose, CA, USA).

4.6. Anti-Inflammatory Effects of Extracts

To assess the anti-inflammatory potential of the lipidic extracts, two assays were performed. The Human red blood cell (HRBC) membrane stabilization assay, induced by heat, was used first; it allowed to observe if any extract holds the potential to stabilize lysosomal membranes. The second assay is specific to a prostaglandin-endoperoxide synthase, human COX-2 enzymatic activity inhibition—and helps conclusion on whether any extract has the potential to be used as a non-steroidal anti-inflammatory agent. The study was conducted according to the guidelines of the Declaration of Helsinki, and approved by the Institutional Ethics Committee of CIIMAR (protocol code 001/2020 and date of approval 8 June 2020).

4.6.1. Human Red Blood Cell (HRBC) Membrane Stabilization Assay

Human fresh blood was collected intravenously to heparinized tubes, from a healthy volunteer that was not taking any non-steroidal anti-inflammatory drugs (NSAIDs) for 2 weeks before the experiment. Blood was centrifuged at $700\times g$ for 10 min and supernatant (plasma) was removed. Hence human red blood cells (HRBC) were washed three times with an equal volume of isotonic PBS (10 mM sodium phosphate buffer(Alfa Aesar, Massachusetts, US) pH 7.4) and then reconstituted at 40% (v/v) suspension. Salicylic acid at 500 µg mL^{-1} was used for positive control and PBS with 20% of DMSO (AppliChem, Darmstadt, Germany) for negative control.

Each extract, prepared as explained in Section 2.2, at concentrations of 130, 150, 120, and 450 mg·mL^{-1}, for A, E, HI, and EL, respectively, were resuspended in PBS containing 20% of DMSO, and then mixed in 1:1 (v/v) with a solution of HRBC in 2% in PBS. Samples were incubated at 56 °C for 20 min, cooled in tap water, and centrifuged at $700\times g$ for 5 min, and the supernatant was collected. The absorbance of the supernatant was measured spectrophotometrically at 560 nm using a microplate reader (Thermofisher GO, New Hampshire, EUA) [73]. The percentage of inhibition was calculated for each extract as:

$$\% \text{ inhibition} = [(Abs_E - Abs_{EB}) - Abs_C]/Abs_C \times 100 \qquad (1)$$

where Abs_E denotes supernatant absorbance after reaction with extract; Abs_{EB} denotes extract absorbance at 560 nm; and Abs_C denotes the control absorbance of PBS with 20% of DMSO.

4.6.2. Cox Human Inhibitory Screening Assay

The anti-inflammatory potential of the extracts was assessed via an enzyme inhibitory assay—inhibition of COX-2 enzymatic activity, using the COX-2 Enzyme Activity Assay Kit (Cayman Chemical, Michigan, MI, US), according to the manufacturer's instructions. Dried lipidic extracts were diluted in DMSO, and assayed at different concentrations—75, 125, and 250 µg·mL^{-1}.

In this assay, arachidonic acid (AA) served as a substrate for the human recombinant COX-2 enzyme, thus leading to the production of prostaglandin. The assay measures PGF2α produced by SnCl2 reduction of COX-derived PGH2. The PGF2α levels produced in the presence versus absence of test products were quantified through an enzyme immunoassay—using an antibody that binds to all major prostaglandin compounds, results are expressed in percent of inhibition, calculated according to kit instructions.

4.7. Cytotoxicity Evaluation

Cytotoxicity of the extracts was evaluated by measuring the viability of Human Cardiac Microvascular Endothelial Cells (HCMEC) obtained from the American Type Culture Collection (ATCC). Cells were seeded in a 96-well plate with a final concentration of 10×10^4 cells mL^{-1} with Dulbecco's Modified Eagle Medium (DMEM) (Sigma-Aldrich (St. Louis, MO, USA) for 24 h.

The cellular viability was assessed by the mitochondrial-dependent reduction of 3-(4,5-dimethylthiazole-2-yl)-2,5-diphenyltetrazolium bromide (MTT) (Sigma-Aldrich (St. Louis, MO, USA) to formazan, quantified by optical density measurement at 510 nm, as described by Lopes et al. [74]. Several concentrations of the extracts were tested: 50, 100, 200, and 300 µg·mL^{-1}—using DMSO 1% as negative control and DMSO 20% as the positive control. The assay was independently repeated four times, with duplicate extracts. Cytotoxicity was expressed as a percentage of cell viability, considering the values of the negative control as 100% viability.

Author Contributions: Conceptualization: H.M.A., A.C.G.; Methodology: H.M.A., A.C.G., R.B. and T.T.; Formal analysis and investigation: H.M.A., R.B. and T.T.; Writing—original draft preparation: H.M.A.; Writing—review and editing: A.C.G., R.B., I.S.P., F.X.M.; Funding acquisition: I.S.P., F.X.M. and R.A.; Supervision: A.C.G., F.X.M. and I.S.P. All authors have read and agreed to the published version of the manuscript.

Funding: This research was supported by national funds through FCT—Foundation for Science and Technology within the scope of UIDB/04423/2020, granted to CIIMAR and UIDB/00511/2020 granted to LEPABE funded by national funds through FCT/MCTES (PIDDAC).

Institutional Review Board Statement: The study was conducted according to the guidelines of the Declaration of Helsinki, and approved by the Institutional Ethics Committee of CIIMAR (protocol code 001/2020 and date of approval 8 June 2020).

Informed Consent Statement: Informed consent was obtained from all subjects involved in the study.

Conflicts of Interest: The authors declare no conflict of interest.

References

1. García, J.L.; de Vicente, M.; Galán, B. Microalgae, old sustainable food and fashion nutraceuticals. *Microb. Biotechnol.* **2017**, *10*, 1017–1024. [CrossRef] [PubMed]
2. Talero, E.; Garcia-Maurino, S.; Avila-Roman, J.; Rodriguez-Luna, A.; Alcaide, A.; Motilva, V. Bioactive Compounds Isolated from Microalgae in Chronic Inflammation and Cancer. *Mar. Drugs* **2015**, *13*, 6152–6209. [CrossRef] [PubMed]
3. Panjiar, N.; Mishra, S.; Yadav, A.N.; Verma, D.P. Functional Foods from Cyanobacteria: An Emerging Source for Functional Food Products of Pharmaceutical Importance. In *Microbial Functional Foods and Nutraceuticals*, 1st ed.; Gupta, V.K., Ed.; Wiley-Blackwell: Hoboken, NJ, USA, 2017.
4. Olaizola, M. Commercial development of microalgal biotechnology: From the test tube to the marketplace. *Biomol. Eng.* **2003**, *20*, 459–466. [CrossRef]
5. Demay, J.; Bernard, C.; Reinhardt, A.; Marie, B. Natural Products from Cyanobacteria: Focus on Beneficial Activities. *Mar. Drugs* **2019**, *17*, 320. [CrossRef]
6. Ghosh, N.; Das, A.; Chaffee, S.; Roy, S.; Sen, C.K. Reactive Oxygen Species, Oxidative Damage and Cell Death. In *Immunity and Inflammation in Health and Disease*; Chatterjee, S., Jungraithmayr, W., Bagchi, D., Eds.; Academic Press: Cambridge, MA, USA, 2018; pp. 45–55.
7. Reuter, S.; Gupta, S.C.; Chaturvedi, M.M.; Aggarwal, B.B. Oxidative stress, inflammation, and cancer: How are they linked? *Free Radic. Biol. Med.* **2010**, *49*, 1603–1616. [CrossRef]
8. Arulselvan, P.; Fard, M.T.; Tan, W.S.; Gothai, S.; Fakurazi, S.; Norhaizan, M.E.; Kumar, S.S. Role of Antioxidants and Natural Products in Inflammation. *Oxid. Med. Cell Longev.* **2016**, *2016*, 5276130. [CrossRef]
9. WHO. The Top 10 Causes of Death. Available online: https://www.who.int/news-room/fact-sheets/detail/the-top-10-causes-of-death (accessed on 26 January 2021).
10. Labi, V.; Erlacher, M. How cell death shapes cancer. *Cell Death Dis.* **2015**, *6*, e1675. [CrossRef]
11. Rawla, P.; Barsouk, A. Epidemiology of gastric cancer: Global trends, risk factors and prevention. *Prz. Gastroenterol.* **2019**, *14*, 26–38. [CrossRef]
12. Díaz, P.; Valenzuela Valderrama, M.; Bravo, J.; Quest, A.F.G. Helicobacter pylori and Gastric Cancer: Adaptive Cellular Mechanisms Involved in Disease Progression. *Front. Microbiol.* **2018**, *9*, 5 [CrossRef]
13. Frenkel, K. Carcinogen-mediated oxidant formation and oxidative DNA damage. *Pharmacol. Ther.* **1992**, *53*, 127–166. [CrossRef]
14. Lopez-Lazaro, M. Role of Oxygen in Cancer: Looking Beyond Hypoxia. *Anti-Cancer Agents Med. Chem.* **2009**, *9*, 517–525. [CrossRef]
15. Pashkow, F.J.; Watumull, D.G.; Campbell, C.L. Astaxanthin: A novel potential treatment for oxidative stress and inflammation in cardiovascular disease. *Am. J. Cardiol.* **2008**, *101*, 58d–68d. [CrossRef]
16. Liu, T.; Zhang, L.; Joo, D.; Sun, S.-C. NF-κB signaling in inflammation. *Signal Transduct. Target. Ther.* **2017**, *2*, 17023. [CrossRef]
17. Ge, W.; Li, D.; Gao, Y.; Cao, X. The Roles of Lysosomes in Inflammation and Autoimmune Diseases. *Int. Rev. Immunol.* **2014**, *34*, 415–431. [CrossRef]
18. Hadad, N.; Levy, R. The synergistic anti-inflammatory effects of lycopene, lutein, β-carotene, and carnosic acid combinations via redox-based inhibition of NF-κB signaling. *Free Radic. Biol. Med.* **2012**, *53*, 1381–1391. [CrossRef] [PubMed]
19. Echizen, K.; Hirose, O.; Maeda, Y.; Oshima, M. Inflammation in gastric cancer: Interplay of the COX-2/prostaglandin E2 and Toll-like receptor/MyD88 pathways. *Cancer Sci.* **2016**, *107*, 391–397. [CrossRef] [PubMed]
20. Gustafsson, A.; Andersson, M.; Lagerstedt, K.; Lonnroth, C.; Nordgren, S.; Lundholm, K. Receptor and enzyme expression for prostanoid metabolism in colorectal cancer related to tumor tissue PGE2. *Int. J. Oncol.* **2010**, *36*, 469–478.
21. Shukla, Y.; George, J. Combinatorial strategies employing nutraceuticals for cancer development. *Ann. N. Y. Acad. Sci.* **2011**, *1229*, 162–175. [CrossRef] [PubMed]

22. Ming, M.E. The Search for a chemoprevention agent effective against melanoma: Considerations and challenges. *J. Investig. Dermatol.* **2011**, *131*, 1401–1403. [CrossRef] [PubMed]
23. Baron, J.A. Statins and the colorectum: Hope for chemoprevention? *Cancer Prev. Res.* **2010**, *3*, 573–575. [CrossRef]
24. Li, S.; Jiang, M.; Wang, L.; Yu, S. Combined chemotherapy with cyclooxygenase-2 (COX-2) inhibitors in treating human cancers: Recent advancement. *Biomed. Pharmacother.* **2020**, *129*, 110389. [CrossRef] [PubMed]
25. El-Shemy, H.A.; Aboul-Enein, A.M.; Aboul-Enein, K.M.; Fujita, K. Willow Leaves' Extracts Contain Anti-Tumor Agents Effective against Three Cell Types. *PLoS ONE* **2007**, *2*, e178. [CrossRef]
26. Tanaka, T.; Shnimizu, M.; Moriwaki, H. Cancer Chemoprevention by Carotenoids. *Molecules* **2012**, *17*, 3202. [CrossRef]
27. Guedes, A.C.; Amaro, H.M.; Malcata, F.X. Microalgae as sources of high added-value compounds—a brief review of recent work. *Biotechnol. Prog.* **2011**, *27*, 597–613. [CrossRef] [PubMed]
28. Niranjana, R.; Gayathri, R.; Nimish Mol, S.; Sugawara, T.; Hirata, T.; Miyashita, K.; Ganesan, P. Carotenoids modulate the hallmarks of cancer cells. *J. Funct. Foods* **2015**, *18*, 968–985. [CrossRef]
29. Zuluaga, M.; Gueguen, V.; Pavon-Djavid, G.; Letourneur, D. Carotenoids from microalgae to block oxidative stress. *BioImpacts BI* **2017**, *7*, 1–3. [CrossRef] [PubMed]
30. Richard, D.; Kefi, K.; Barbe, U.; Bausero, P.; Visioli, F. Polyunsaturated fatty acids as antioxidants. *Pharmacol. Res.* **2008**, *57*, 451–455. [CrossRef]
31. Gong, M.; Bassi, A. Carotenoids from microalgae: A review of recent developments. *Biotechnol. Adv.* **2016**, *34*, 1396–1412. [CrossRef]
32. Guermouche, B.; Soulimane-Mokhtari, N.A.; Bouanane, S.; Merzouk, H.; Merzouk, S.; Narce, M. Effect of Dietary Polyunsaturated Fatty Acids on Oxidant/Antioxidant Status in Macrosomic Offspring of Diabetic Rats. *BioMed Res. Int.* **2014**, *2014*, 9. [CrossRef]
33. Tatsumi, Y.; Kato, A.; Sango, K.; Himeno, T.; Kondo, M.; Kato, Y.; Kamiya, H.; Nakamura, J.; Kato, K. Omega-3 polyunsaturated fatty acids exert anti-oxidant effects through the nuclear factor (erythroid-derived 2)-related factor 2 pathway in immortalized mouse Schwann cells. *J. Diabetes Investig.* **2019**, *10*, 602–612. [CrossRef]
34. Tortosa-Caparrós, E.; Navas-Carrillo, D.; Marín, F.; Orenes-Piñero, E. Anti-inflammatory effects of omega 3 and omega 6 polyunsaturated fatty acids in cardiovascular disease and metabolic syndrome. *Crit. Rev. Food Sci. Nutr.* **2017**, *57*, 3421–3429. [CrossRef] [PubMed]
35. Castro-Puyana, M.; Pérez-Sánchez, A.; Valdés, A.; Ibrahim, O.H.M.; Suarez-Álvarez, S.; Ferragut, J.A.; Micol, V.; Cifuentes, A.; Ibáñez, E.; García-Cañas, V. Pressurized liquid extraction of Neochloris oleoabundans for the recovery of bioactive carotenoids with anti-proliferative activity against human colon cancer cells. *Food Res. Int.* **2017**, *99*, 1048–1055. [CrossRef] [PubMed]
36. Palozza, P.; Serini, S.; Maggiano, N.; Tringali, G.; Navarra, P.; Ranelletti, F.O.; Calviello, G. beta-Carotene downregulates the steady-state and heregulin-alpha-induced COX-2 pathways in colon cancer cells. *J. Nutr.* **2005**, *135*, 129–136. [CrossRef] [PubMed]
37. Cha, K.H.; Koo, S.Y.; Lee, D.-U. Antiproliferative Effects of Carotenoids Extracted from Chlorella ellipsoidea and Chlorella vulgaris on Human Colon Cancer Cells. *J. Agric. Food Chem.* **2008**, *56*, 10521–10526. [CrossRef]
38. Sheu, M.J.; Huang, G.J.; Wu, C.H.; Chen, J.S.; Chang, H.Y.; Chang, S.J.; Chung, J.G. Ethanol extract of Dunaliella salina induces cell cycle arrest and apoptosis in A549 human non-small cell lung cancer cells. *In Vivo* **2008**, *22*, 369–378.
39. Pasquet, V.; Morisset, P.; Ihammouine, S.; Chepied, A.; Aumailley, L.; Berard, J.B.; Serive, B.; Kaas, R.; Lanneluc, I.; Thiery, V.; et al. Antiproliferative activity of violaxanthin isolated from bioguided fractionation of Dunaliella tertiolecta extracts. *Mar. Drugs* **2011**, *9*, 819–831. [CrossRef]
40. Neumann, U.; Derwenskus, F.; Flaiz Flister, V.; Schmid-Staiger, U.; Hirth, T.; Bischoff, S.C. Fucoxanthin, A Carotenoid Derived from *Phaeodactylum tricornutum* Exerts Antiproliferative and Antioxidant Activities In Vitro. *Antioxidants* **2019**, *8*, 183. [CrossRef]
41. Amaro, H.M.; Fernandes, F.; Valentão, P.; Andrade, P.B.; Sousa-Pinto, I.; Malcata, F.X.; Guedes, A.C. Effect of Solvent System on Extractability of Lipidic Components of *Scenedesmus obliquus* (M2-1) and *Gloeothece* sp. on Antioxidant Scavenging Capacity Thereof. *Mar. Drugs* **2015**, *13*, 6453–6471. [CrossRef]
42. Amaro, H.M.; Guedes, A.C.; Preto, M.A.C.; Sousa-Pinto, I.; Malcata, F.X. *Gloeothece* sp. as a Nutraceutical Source-An Improved Method of Extraction of Carotenoids and Fatty Acids. *Mar. Drugs* **2018**, *16*, 327. [CrossRef]
43. European Union. Directive 2009/32/EC of the European Parliament and of the Council of 23 April 2009 on the approximation of the laws of the Member States on extraction solvents used in the production of foodstuffs and food ingredients. *Off. J. Eur. Union* **2009**, *L 141*, 3–11.
44. Bargiela-Iparraguirre, J.; Prado-Marchal, L.; Fernandez-Fuente, M.; Gutierrez-Gonzalez, A.; Moreno-Rubio, J.; Munoz-Fernandez, M.; Sereno, M.; Sanchez-Prieto, R.; Perona, R.; Sanchez-Perez, I. MCHK1 expression in Gastric Cancer is modulated by p53 and RB1/E2F1: Implications in chemo/radiotherapy response. *Sci. Rep.* **2016**, *6*, 21519. [CrossRef] [PubMed]
45. Vichai, V.; Kirtikara, K. Sulforhodamine B colorimetric assay for cytotoxicity screening. *Nat. Protoc.* **2006**, *1*, 1112–1116. [CrossRef]
46. Azevedo, C.M.; Afonso, C.M.; Soares, J.X.; Reis, S.; Sousa, D.; Lima, R.T.; Vasconcelos, M.H.; Pedro, M.; Barbosa, J.; Gales, L.; et al. Pyranoxanthones: Synthesis, growth inhibitory activity on human tumor cell lines and determination of their lipophilicity in two membrane models. *Eur. J. Med. Chem.* **2013**, *69*, 798–816. [CrossRef] [PubMed]
47. Elmore, S. Apoptosis: A Review of Programmed Cell Death. *Toxicol. Pathol.* **2007**, *35*, 495–516. [CrossRef] [PubMed]
48. Lawrence, R.E.; Zoncu, R. The lysosome as a cellular centre for signalling, metabolism and quality control. *Nat. Cell Biol.* **2019**, *21*, 133–142. [CrossRef] [PubMed]

49. Lavanya, R.; Maheshwari, S.U.; Harish, G.; Raj, J.B.; Kamali, S.; Hemamalani, D.; Varma, J.B.; Reddy, C.U. Investigation of in-vitro anti-inflammatory, anti-platelet and anti-arthritic activities in the leaves of Anisomeles malabarica Linn. *Res. J. Pharm. Biol. Chem. Sci.* **2010**, *1*, 745–752.
50. Murugesh, N.; Vembar, S.; Damodaran, C. Studies on erythrocyte membrane IV: In vitro haemolytic activity of oleander extract. *Toxicol. Lett.* **1981**, *8*, 33–38. [CrossRef]
51. Lee, J.L.; Mukhtar, H.; Bickers, D.R.; Kopelovich, L.; Athar, M. Cyclooxygenases in the skin: Pharmacological and toxicological implications. *Toxicol. Appl. Pharmacol.* **2003**, *192*, 294–306. [CrossRef]
52. Palesh, O.; Scheiber, C.; Kesler, S.; Mustian, K.; Koopman, C.; Schapira, L. Management of side effects during and post-treatment in breast cancer survivors. *Breast J.* **2018**, *24*, 167–175. [CrossRef]
53. Dutot, M.; Fagon, R.; Rousseau, D.; Rat, P. Antioxidant and Anti-Inflammatory Effects of PUFA-Rich Marine Oils: Application to the Ocular Surface. *Investig. Ophthalmol. Vis. Sci.* **2009**, *50*, 919.
54. Guedes, A.C.; Amaro, H.M.; Pereira, R.D.; Malcata, F.X. Effects of temperature and pH on growth and antioxidant content of the microalga Scenedesmus obliquus. *Biotechnol. Prog.* **2011**, *27*, 1218–1224. [CrossRef]
55. He, R.-R.; Tsoi, B.; Lan, F.; Yao, N.; Yao, X.-S.; Kurihara, H. Antioxidant properties of lutein contribute to the protection against lipopolysaccharide-induced uveitis in mice. *Chin. Med.* **2011**, *6*, 38. [CrossRef] [PubMed]
56. Stringham, J.M.; Stringham, N.T. Nitric Oxide and Lutein: Function, Performance, and Protection of Neural Tissue. *Foods* **2015**, *4*, 678–689. [CrossRef]
57. Moraes, M.L.; Ribeiro, A.M.L.; Santin, E.; Klasing, K.C. Effects of conjugated linoleic acid and lutein on the growth performance and immune response of broiler chickens. *Poult. Sci.* **2016**, *95*, 237–246. [CrossRef]
58. Pacher, P.; Beckman, J.S.; Liaudet, L. Nitric oxide and peroxynitrite in health and disease. *Physiol. Rev.* **2007**, *87*, 315–424. [CrossRef] [PubMed]
59. Hu, Y.; Xiang, J.; Su, L.; Tang, X. The regulation of nitric oxide in tumor progression and therapy. *J. Int. Med. Res.* **2020**, *48*, 0300060520905985. [CrossRef]
60. Christodoulou, M.I.; Kontos, C.K.; Halabalaki, M.; Skaltsounis, A.L.; Scorilas, A. Nature promises new anticancer agents: Interplay with the apoptosis-related BCL2 gene family. *Anticancer Agents Med. Chem.* **2014**, *14*, 375–399. [CrossRef]
61. Choi, S.Y.; Park, J.H.; Kim, J.S.; Kim, M.K.; Aruoma, O.I.; Sung, M.K. Effects of quercetin and beta-carotene supplementation on azoxymethane-induced colon carcinogenesis and inflammatory responses in rats fed with high-fat diet rich in omega-6 fatty acids. *Biofactors* **2006**, *27*, 137–146. [CrossRef]
62. Bie, N.; Han, L.; Meng, M.; Zhang, Y.; Guo, M.; Wang, C. Anti-tumor mechanism of eicosapentaenoic acid (EPA) on ovarian tumor model by improving the immunomodulatory activity in F344 rats. *J. Funct. Foods* **2020**, *65*, 103739. [CrossRef]
63. Biondo, P.D.; Brindley, D.N.; Sawyer, M.B.; Field, C.J. The potential for treatment with dietary long-chain polyunsaturated n-3 fatty acids during chemotherapy. *J. Nutr. Biochem.* **2008**, *19*, 787–796. [CrossRef]
64. Kwon, J.I.; Kim, G.Y.; Park, K.Y.; Ryu, C.H.; Choi, Y.H. Induction of apoptosis by linoleic acid is associated with the modulation of Bcl-2 family and Fas/FasL system and activation of caspases in AGS human gastric adenocarcinoma cells. *J. Med. Food* **2008**, *11*, 1–8. [CrossRef] [PubMed]
65. Choi, Y.H. Linoleic Acid-Induced Growth Inhibition of Human Gastric Epithelial Adenocarcinoma AGS Cells is Associated with Down-Regulation of Prostaglandin E2 Synthesis and Telomerase Activity. *J. Cancer Prev.* **2014**, *19*, 31–38. [CrossRef]
66. Montero-Lobato, Z.; Vázquez, M.; Navarro, F.; Fuentes, J.L.; Bermejo, E.; Garbayo, I.; Vílchez, C.; Cuaresma, M. Chemically-Induced Production of Anti-Inflammatory Molecules in Microalgae. *Mar. Drugs* **2018**, *16*, 478. [CrossRef]
67. Soontornchaiboon, W.; Joo, S.S.; Kim, S.M. Anti-inflammatory Effects of Violaxanthin Isolated from Microalga *Chlorella ellipsoidea* in RAW 264.7 Macrophages. *Biol. Pharm. Bull.* **2012**, *35*, 1137–1144. [CrossRef]
68. Mazhar, D.; Ang, R.; Waxman, J. COX inhibitors and breast cancer. *Br. J. Cancer* **2006**, *94*, 346–350. [CrossRef]
69. Zappavigna, S.; Cossu, A.M.; Grimaldi, A.; Bocchetti, M.; Ferraro, G.A.; Nicoletti, G.F.; Filosa, R.; Caraglia, M. Anti-Inflammatory Drugs as Anticancer Agents. *Int. J. Mol. Sci.* **2020**, *21*, 2605. [CrossRef]
70. Stanier, R.Y.; Kunisawa, R.; Mandel, M.; Cohen-Bazire, G. Purification and properties of unicellular blue-green algae (order Chroococcales). *Bacteriol. Rev.* **1971**, *35*, 171–205. [CrossRef] [PubMed]
71. Lepage, G.; Roy, C.C. Direct transesterification of all classes of lipids in a one-step reaction. *J. Lipid Res.* **1986**, *27*, 114–120. [CrossRef]
72. Cohen, Z.; Vonshak, A.; Richmond, A. Effect on environmental conditions on fatty acids composition of the red alga *Phorphyridium cruentum*: Correlation to growth rate. *J. Phycol.* **1988**, *24*, 328–332. [CrossRef]
73. Moualek, I.; Iratni Aiche, G.; Mestar Guechaoui, N.; Lahcene, S.; Houali, K. Antioxidant and anti-inflammatory activities of *Arbutus unedo* aqueous extract. *Asian Pac. J. Trop. Biomed.* **2016**, *6*, 937–944. [CrossRef]
74. Lopes, G.; Sousa, C.; Silva, L.R.; Pinto, E.; Andrade, P.B.; Bernardo, J.; Mouga, T.; Valentao, P. Can phlorotannins purified extracts constitute a novel pharmacological alternative for microbial infections with associated inflammatory conditions? *PLoS ONE* **2012**, *7*, e31145. [CrossRef] [PubMed]

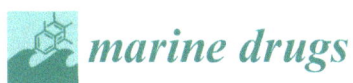

Article

Antitumour Effects of Astaxanthin and Adonixanthin on Glioblastoma

Shohei Tsuji [1], Shinsuke Nakamura [1,*], Takashi Maoka [2], Tetsuya Yamada [1,3], Takahiko Imai [1], Takuya Ohba [1], Tomohiro Yako [1], Masahiro Hayashi [4], Ken Endo [5], Masanao Saio [6], Hideaki Hara [1] and Masamitsu Shimazawa [1]

1. Department of Biofunctional Evaluation, Molecular Pharmacology, Gifu Pharmaceutical University, Gifu 501-1196, Japan; tsuji.yakkou@gmail.com (S.T.); yamada.yakkou@gmail.com (T.Y.); imai.yakkou@gmail.com (T.I.); ohba.yakkou@gmail.com (T.O.); yako.yakkou@gmail.com (T.Y.); hidehara@gifu-pu.ac.jp (H.H.); shimazawa@gifu-pu.ac.jp (M.S.)
2. Research Institute for Production Developent Division of Food Function and Chemistry, Kyoto 606-0805, Japan; maoka@mbox.kyoto-inet.or.jp
3. Department of Neurosurgery, Gifu University School of Medicine, Gifu 501-1194, Japan
4. Department of HPM Research & Development, Biotechnology R&D Group, High Performance Materials Company, ENEOS Corporation, Yokohama 231-0815, Japan; hayashi.masahiro@eneos.com
5. Department of HPM Business Promotion Group V, Business promotion Group, High Performance Materials Company, ENEOS Corporation, Tokyo 108-8005, Japan; endo.ken@eneos.com
6. Graduate School of Health Sciences, Gunma University, Gunma 371-8514, Japan; saio@gunma-u.ac.jp
* Correspondence: nakamuras@gifu-pu.ac.jp; Tel./Fax: +81-58-230-8100/8105

Received: 22 July 2020; Accepted: 16 September 2020; Published: 18 September 2020

Abstract: Several antitumour drugs have been isolated from natural products and many clinical trials are underway to evaluate their potential. There have been numerous reports about the antitumour effects of astaxanthin against several tumours but no studies into its effects against glioblastoma. Astaxanthin is a red pigment found in crustaceans and fish and is also synthesized in *Haematococcus pluvialis*; adonixanthin is an intermediate product of astaxanthin. It is known that both astaxanthin and adonixanthin possess radical scavenging activity and can confer a protective effect on several damages. In this study, we clarified the antitumour effects of astaxanthin and adonixanthin using glioblastoma models. Specifically, astaxanthin and adonixanthin showed an ability to suppress cell proliferation and migration in three types of glioblastoma cells. Furthermore, these compounds were confirmed to transfer to the brain in a murine model. In the murine orthotopic glioblastoma model, glioblastoma progression was suppressed by the oral administration of astaxanthin and adonixanthin at 10 and 30 mg/kg, respectively, for 10 days. These results suggest that both astaxanthin and adonixanthin have potential as treatments for glioblastoma.

Keywords: brain; cancer; oral administration; *paracoccsu carotinifaciens*; xanthophyll carotenoid

1. Introduction

Glioblastoma is one of the most lethal types of brain tumour; it arises from glial cells [1,2]. The standard treatment for glioblastoma is a combination of chemotherapy and radiotherapy following the surgical removal of tumour tissue [3]. However, glioblastomas generally show a poor prognosis and short survival time, rarely longer than 14 months [4]. The poor prognosis is attributed to chemoresistance to temozolomide, the first-line drug for the treatment of glioblastoma [5]. Therefore, it is essential that novel drugs are developed that possess an antitumour effect based on different mechanisms to those of temozolomide. However, the development of novel drugs for glioblastoma has been limited by the blood–brain barrier (BBB) issue [6]. Recent studies have shown that certain compounds derived from natural products, such as curcumin and resveratrol, can cross the BBB and have an antitumour effect against glioblastoma [7,8]. Both powerful antitumour effects and transferability to brain tissues are essential requirements for any new treatments for glioblastoma.

In this study, we focused on a xanthophyll carotenoid, astaxanthin, and its intermediate product, adonixanthin (Figure 1) [9]. Astaxanthin, a red pigment that occurs naturally in shrimp, crab, and salmon [10], is a powerful antioxidant and has shown some protective effects in various oxidative stress and disease models [11–15]. Adonixanthin has similarly powerful antioxidative effects [9,16]. Crucially, it has been reported that, in mouse models, both astaxanthin and adonixanthin have the ability to cross the BBB to reach the brain tissue and can protect vessels in the brain from cerebral ischaemia and haemorrhage [17,18]. However, there have been no reports that either astaxanthin or adonixanthin have antitumour effects against glioblastoma. It is known that astaxanthin has antitumour effects against oral cancer, bladder carcinogenesis, colon carcinogenesis, leukaemia, and hepatocellular carcinoma [19–23]; however, the mechanisms for this antitumour activity of astaxanthin are yet to be fully clarified. It has been reported that the antitumour effect of astaxanthin and adonixanthin are mediated by multiple mechanisms, including JAK-2/STAT-3, NF-κB, ERK, AKT (PKB), PPARγ, and Nrf2 [24].

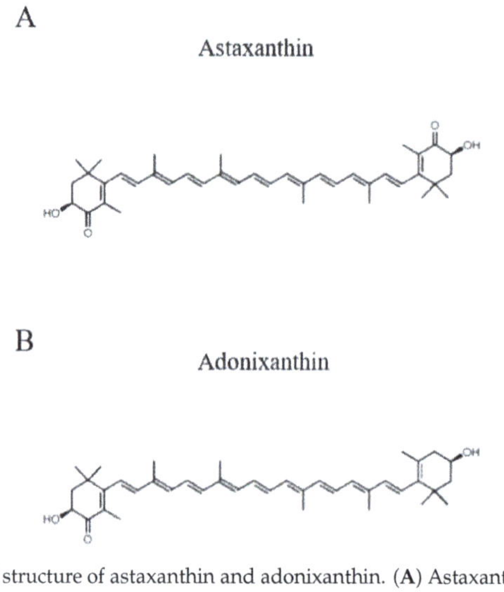

Figure 1. The chemical structure of astaxanthin and adonixanthin. (**A**) Astaxanthin (**B**) Adonixanthin.

The purpose of this study was to clarify whether astaxanthin and adonixanthin have antitumour effects against glioblastoma following their oral administration. Furthermore, we aimed to verify whether orally administered astaxanthin or adonixanthin can be absorbed by the brain tissue. We investigated the antitumour mechanisms of astaxanthin and adonixanthin using glioblastoma cells.

2. Results

2.1. Astaxanthin and Adonixanthin Suppressed the Growth of Glioblastoma Cells

Robust cell viability is an important characteristic of tumour cells. We performed a cell viability assay using the murine glioblastoma cell line GL261 and the human glioblastoma cell line U251MG. Both astaxanthin and adonixanthin showed antitumour effects against GL261 and U251MG cells, in a concentration-dependent manner (Figure 2A,B). In GL261 cells, astaxanthin and adonixanthin suppressed cell viability at concentrations of more than 5 and 0.1 μM (Figure 2A). In U251MG cells, astaxanthin and adonixanthin suppressed cell viability at concentrations of more than 1 and 0.1 μM (Figure 2B). Moreover, we performed the BrdU cell proliferation assay to determine whether the results of cell viability by astaxanthin and adonixanthin (Figure 2A,B) are based on proliferation.

Astaxanthin and adonixanthin at the 10 µM treatment for 72 h reduced the number of BrdU-positive cells (Figure 2C,D). The BrdU-positive cell rates were 60.56 ± 1.40% (control group), 19.17 ± 1.77% (temozolomide group), 49.13 ± 2.66% (astaxanthin group), and 41.31 ± 1.51% (adonixanthin group).

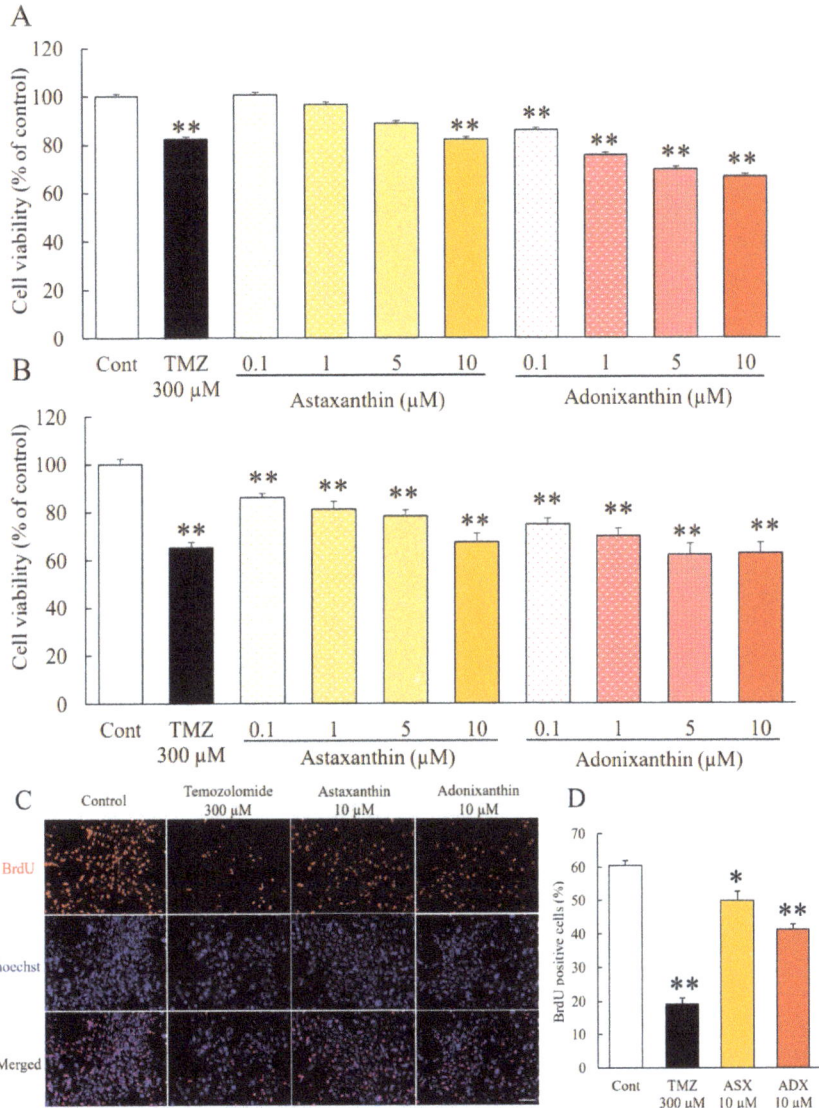

Figure 2. Cell viability of the mouse and human glioblastoma cell line with astaxanthin and adonixanthin. (**A**, **B**) These graphs show the cell viability of GL261 (mouse glioblastoma cell line) and U251MG (human glioblastoma cell line) treated for 96 h with temozolomide, astaxanthin, or adonixanthin. Data are shown as mean ± SEM (n = 6). ** p < 0.01 vs. control group (Tukey's test). (**C**) These images show the representative photographs of the BrdU assay 96 h after treatment of temozolomide, astaxanthin, or adonixanthin in GL261. (**D**) This graph shows the BrdU-positive cells (%). Data are shown as mean ± SEM (n = 6). * p < 0.05, ** p < 0.01 vs. control group (Student's t-test). TMZ; temozolomide.

2.2. Astaxanthin and Adonixanthin Suppressed the Migration of Glioblastoma Cells

In addition to cell viability, cell migration is also important for tumour enlargement. We performed a wound healing assay using the murine glioblastoma cell line GL261 and the human glioblastoma cell line U251MG. Astaxanthin and adonixanthin suppressed cell migration by 8.84 ± 2.09% and 13.74 ± 4.01% in GL261, respectively (Figure 3A,B). Astaxanthin and adonixanthin suppressed cell migration by 21.15 ± 1.84% and 26.32 ± 5.14% in U251MG, respectively, at a concentration of 10 μM (Figure 3C,D).

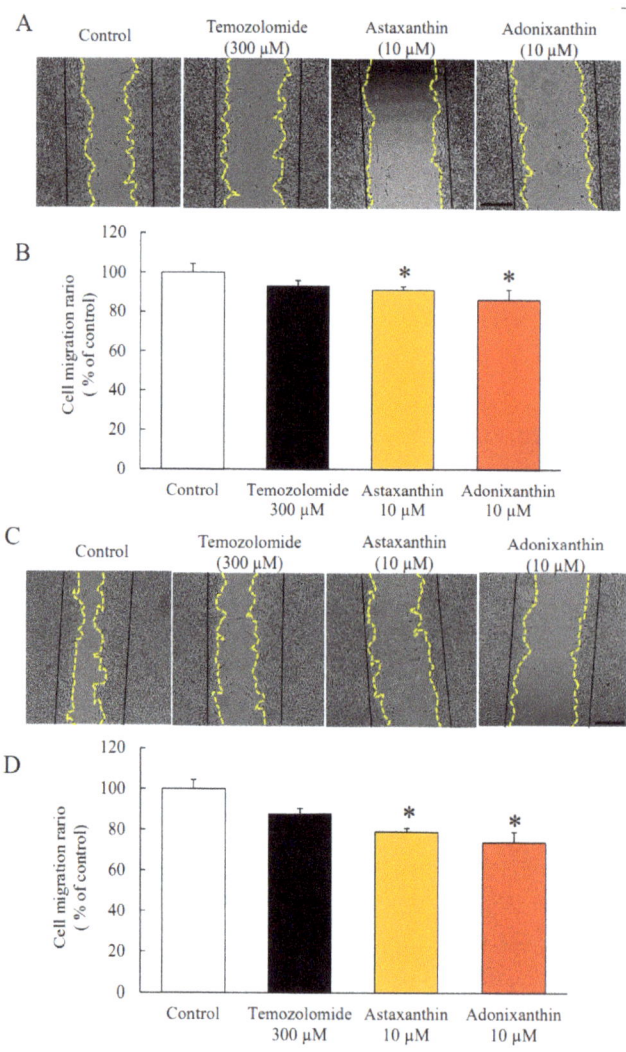

Figure 3. Wound healing assay with astaxanthin and adonixanthin in human glioblastoma cell U251MG and mouse glioblastoma cell line GL261. (**A**,**C**) These images show representative photographs of the wound healing assay 48 h after treatment of temozolomide, astaxanthin, or adonixanthin in GL261 (**A**) and U251MG (**B**). (**B**,**D**) These bar graphs show the cell migration abilities of GL261 (**B**) and U251MG (**D**). Data are shown as mean ± SEM (n = 3). * p < 0.05 vs. control group (Student's t-test). Migration area ratio = (0 h scratch area—48 h non migration area)/0 h scratch area. (Original magnification × 20). The scale bars are 500 μm.

2.3. Astaxanthin and Adonixanthin Decreased the Expression of Some Proteins to Promote Cell Growth and Migration

We performed immunoblotting to reveal the mechanisms of the antitumour effects of astaxanthin and adonixanthin. In general, the phosphorylation of ERK1/2 and Akt are accelerated during tumour progression in many types of tumour [25,26]. The phosphorylation of ERK1/2 and Akt were decreased 6 h post-treatment with astaxanthin and adonixanthin (Figure 4A,B). Both astaxanthin and adonixanthin treatment for 48 h increased the phosphorylation of p38 mitogen-activated protein kinase: MAPK (Figure 4C). To elucidate the antitumour effect of astaxanthin and adonixanthin, we confirmed the expression of cyclin D1 (cell cycle-related protein) and p27 (cyclin-dependent kinase inhibitor). As a result, both astaxanthin and adonixanthin treatment for 48 h decreased the expression of cyclinD1 (Figure 4D) and increased the expression of p27 (Figure 4E). Next, we focused on some proteins that are related to cell migration (Matrix metalloproteinase-2, -9: MMP-2, -9, and fibronectin). Treatment with astaxanthin and adonixanthin for 48 h decreased MMP-2 expression (Figure 4F) but not MMP-9 expression (Figure 4G). Interestingly, adonixanthin also decreased the expression of fibronectin (Figure 4H).

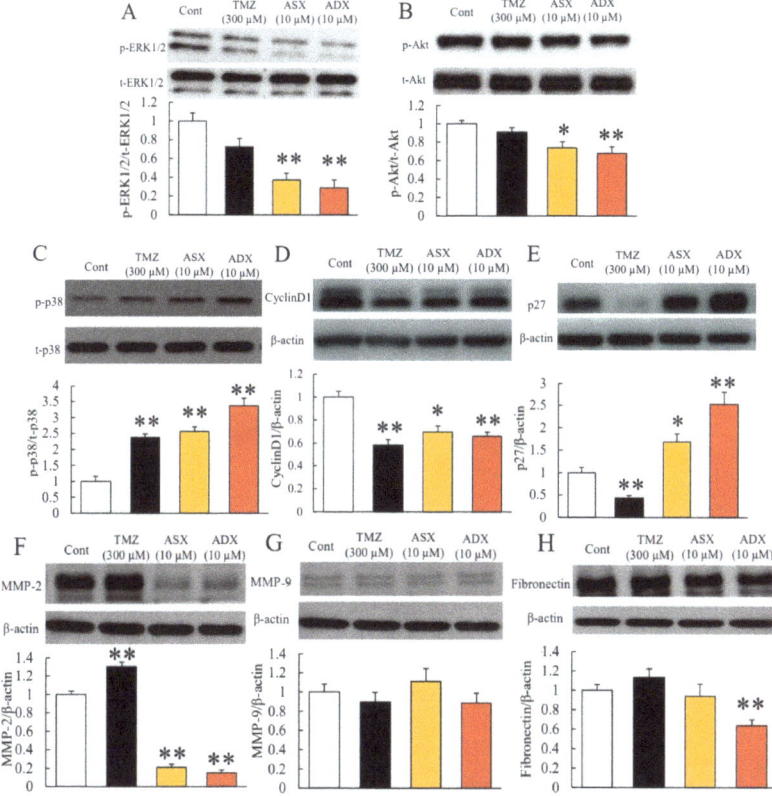

Figure 4. Expression of some proteins related to tumour progression after treatment of astaxanthin and adonixanthin in the mouse glioblastoma cell line. (**A,B**) The quantitative data of the expression levels of p-ERK1/2 and p-Akt in the mouse glioblastoma cell line GL261 at 6 h after treatment of 300 μM temozolomide, 10 μM astaxanthin, or 10 μM adonixanthin. Both astaxanthin and adonixanthin reduced the expression of p-ERK1/2 and p-Akt. Data are shown as mean ± SEM (n = 5 or 6). * $p < 0.05$, ** $p < 0.01$ vs. control group (Student's t-test). (**C~H**) The quantitative data of expression levels of p-p38, p38,

cyclin D1, p27, MMP-2, -9, and fibronectin, in the mouse glioblastoma cell line GL261 at 48 h after treatment of 300 μM temozolomide, 10 μM astaxanthin, or 10 μM adonixanthin. Data are shown as mean ± SEM ($n = 6$). * $p < 0.05$, ** $p < 0.01$ vs. control group (Student's t-test). ASX; astaxanthin, ADX; adonixanthin, TMZ; temozolomide.

2.4. Astaxanthin and Adonixanthin Decreased the Production of Reactive Oxygen Species (ROS)

In previous reports, the presence of ROS was shown to promote tumour progression via the phosphorylation of ERK1/2 and Akt [27,28]. Therefore, we performed an ROS assay to investigate the effects of astaxanthin and adonixanthin on the level of intracellular ROS. Both astaxanthin and adonixanthin decreased the amount of intracellular ROS, with the effect of adonixanthin stronger than that of astaxanthin (Figure 5A). We also verified the expression of NADPH oxidase 4 (Nox4), which is a representative factor to produce ROS. Adonixanthin significantly decreased the expression of Nox4, whereas astaxanthin produced no change in Nox4 expression (Figure 5B).

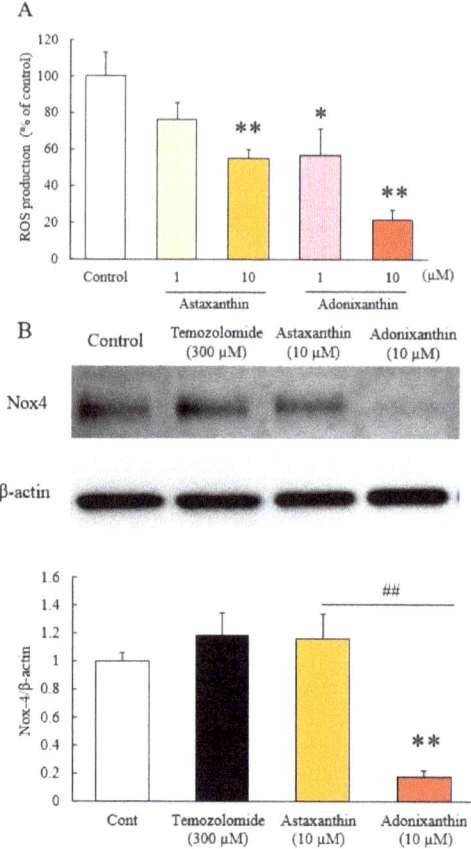

Figure 5. The amount of ROS and expression of Nox-4 after treatment of astaxanthin and adonixanthin in the mouse glioblastoma cell line. (**A**) ROS production was measured by an ROS detecting probe (5-(and-6)-chloromethyl—2′,7′-dichlorodihydrofluorescein diacetate, acetyl ester: CM-H$_2$DCFDA). Treatment of astaxanthin and adonixanthin at 1 and 10 μM reduced the amount of ROS in GL261. Data are shown as mean ± SEM ($n = 6$). * $p < 0.05$, ** $p < 0.01$ vs. control group (Tukey's test). (**B**) Immunoblot analysis and quantification of Nox4 at 6h after treatment of temozolomide. Data are shown as mean ± SEM ($n = 6$). ** $p < 0.01$ vs. control group (Student's t-test) and ## $p < 0.01$ vs. astaxanthin 10 μM group (Student's t-test).

2.5. Concentrations of Astaxanthin and Adonixanthin in Murine Serum and Tissues

Following the oral administration of astaxanthin, the concentration of *trans*- or *cis*-astaxanthin in the serum was 6.04 ± 1.16 and 13.35 ± 3.78 ng/mL, respectively. Astaxanthin was not detected in the serum in pretreatment samples (Table 1). Adonixanthin was also only detected in the treated group. The levels of *trans*- and *cis*- adonixanthin were 34.72 ± 3.00 and 35.02 ± 5.01 ng/mL, respectively (Table 1). In the adonixanthin-treated group, the *trans*-isomer was detected significantly more frequently compared with its detection in the astaxanthin-treated group.

Table 1. The concentrations of astaxanthin and adonixanthin in the murine serum.

	Astaxanthin		Adonixanthin	
Compounds	Pre-treatment	4 h After the Final Oral Administration	Pre-treatment	4 h after the Final Oral Administration
trans-Astaxanthin	N.D.	6.04 ± 1.16		
cis-Astaxanthin	N.D.	13.4 ± 3.78		
trans-Adonixanthin			N.D.	34.7 ± 3.00
cis-Adonixanthin			N.D.	35.02 ± 5.01

Data are shown as mean ± SEM (n = 4). ng/mL. N.D.; not detected.

As shown in Table 2, following oral administration of astaxanthin or adonixanthin, these compounds were absorbed in each region of the brain in mice. *Trans*-astaxanthin was detected at 5.22 ± 0.87, 5.06 ± 1.85, 11.37 ± 3.14, and 12.28 ± 1.07 ng/g in the cerebral cortex, the cerebellum, the striatum, and the hippocampus of astaxanthin-treated mice, respectively. *Cis*-astaxanthin was detected at 3.62 ± 1.56, 2.43 ± 1.58, 3.76 ± 2.06, and 2.61 ± 2.67 ng/g in the cerebral cortex, the cerebellum, the striatum, and the hippocampus of astaxanthin-treated mice, respectively. *Trans*-adonixanthin was detected at 3.24 ± 0.44, 2.85 ± 1.05, 2.90 ± 1.87, and 3.63 ± 2.10 ng/g in the cerebral cortex, the cerebellum, the striatum, and the hippocampus of adonixanthin-treated mice, respectively. There was no *cis*-astaxanthin in any of the brain tissues. Furthermore, neither astaxanthin nor adonixanthin were detected in the brains of the vehicle-treated group.

Table 2. The concentrations of astaxanthin and adonixanthin in the murine tissues.

Brain Tissues	Astaxanthin		Adonixanthin	
	trans	cis	trans	cis
Cerebral cortex	5.22 ± 0.87	3.62 ± 1.56	3.24 ± 0.44 *	N.D.
Cerebellum	5.06 ± 1.85	2.43 ± 1.58	2.85 ± 1.05	N.D.
Striatum	11.37 ± 3.14	3.76 ± 2.06	2.90 ± 1.87	N.D.
Hippocampus	12.28 ± 1.07 *	2.61 ± 1.33	3.63 ± 2.10	N.D.

Data are shown as mean ± SEM (n = 4). ng/g. * $p < 0.05$ vs. *cis*-forms group (Mann–Whitney U-test). N.D.; not detected.

2.6. The Effects of Astaxanthin and Adonixanthin on Body Weight

To investigate systemic influences following the administration of astaxanthin and adonixanthin, we explored changes in the body weight of mice. The weight of vehicle-, astaxanthin-, and adonixanthin-treated mice at pretreatment was 34.33 ± 2.04, 34.28 ± 1.93, and 34.22 ± 2.67 g, respectively. After 10 days of administration, the weight of vehicle-, astaxanthin-, and adonixanthin-treated mice was 34.72 ± 2.05, 35.50 ± 1.95, and 36.15 ± 2.05 g, respectively (Supplementary Material Figure S5). No significant changes in body weight were observed in mice treated with either astaxanthin or adonixanthin.

2.7. Astaxanthin and Adonixanthin Showed Antitumour Effects in a Murine Orthotopic Glioblastoma Model

We investigated whether astaxanthin and adonixanthin exhibited antitumour effects in a murine orthotopic glioblastoma model. Treatment with astaxanthin and adonixanthin at 10 and 30 mg/kg for 10 days, respectively, significantly suppressed tumour enlargement (Figure 6A,B).

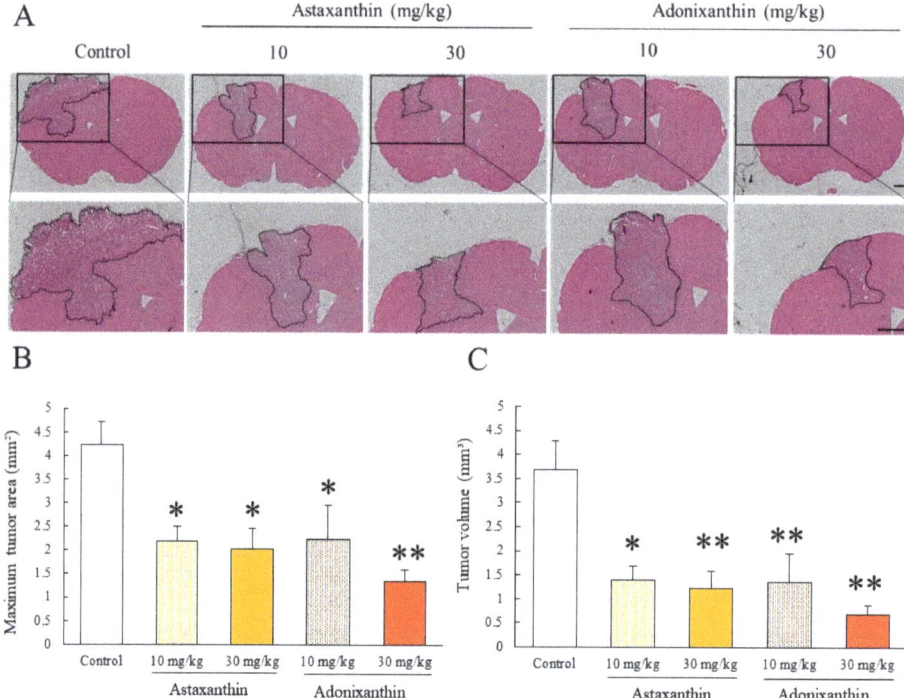

Figure 6. The antitumour effect of astaxanthin and adonixanthin in the murine orthotopical glioblastoma model. (**A**) These images were representative photographs of haematoxylin and eosin staining of the coronal section. Control, $n = 11$; astaxanthin 10, 30 mg/kg treated: $n = 9, 8$; adonixanthin 10, 30 mg/kg treated: $n = 8, 10$. The scale bars are 1 mm. (**B,C**) These bar graphs show the tumour area and volume at 2 weeks after GL261 cell injection. The oral administration of astaxanthin and adonixanthin suppressed the glioblastoma progression in an in vivo glioblastoma model. Data are shown as mean ± SEM ($n = 8$–11). * $p < 0.05$, ** $p < 0.01$ vs. control group (Tukey's test).

3. Discussion

Astaxanthin and adonixanthin, synthesized in marine organisms [10], have antitumour properties [9] and a therapeutic effect on the central nervous system [18,29]. However, there are no reports about their effects for glioma. In the present study, we demonstrated the antitumour effects of these compounds in both in vitro and in vivo glioblastoma models.

Astaxanthin and adonixanthin inhibited both cell proliferation and migration in human and mouse glioblastoma cells (Figures 2 and 3). Next, in order to elucidate the antitumour mechanism of astaxanthin and adonixanthin, the expression of proteins related to tumour progression and the degree of ROS production were examined using the mouse glioblastoma cell line GL261. Astaxanthin and adonixanthin were found to reduce the expression of phosphorylated ERK1/2 and phosphorylated Akt (Figure 3A,B). It was shown that astaxanthin exhibited an antitumour effect in an oral cancer model via the suppression of phosphorylation of ERK1/2 and Akt [19]. Similarly, it is presumed that astaxanthin and adonixanthin also have an antitumour effect against glioblastoma through the inhibition of the phosphorylation of ERK1/2 and Akt. Furthermore, astaxanthin and adonixanthin increased the expression of phosphorylated p38 (Figure 4C). The phosphorylation of p38 can lead to cell damage and cell cycle arrest [30]. Therefore, the antitumour effects of both astaxanthin and adonixanthin were involved in increasing the expression of phosphorylated p38. To elucidate the antitumour effect of these compounds, we confirmed the expression of cell cycle-related protein cyclin D1, and apoptosis-related protein Bcl-2. These compounds decreased the expression of cyclin D1 (Figure 4D) but not Bcl2 (Supplementary Material Figure S4b). In fact, these compounds did not induce cell death in GL261 (Supplementary Material Figure S4a) and decreased the cell proliferation in GL261 (Figure 2C,D). Moreover, these compounds increased the expression of p27, a cyclin-dependent kinase inhibitor (Figure 4E). In a previous report, the phosphorylation of ERK1/2 and Akt increased the expression of cyclinD1 and decreased the expression of p27 [31–33]. These results indicate that the antitumour effect of both astaxanthin and adonixanthin may be mediated by not cell death but cell cycle arrest. Temozolomide significantly reduced the expression of p27 (Figure 4E). This may be due to a feedback to the potent cell cycle arrest effect of temozolomide, as previously reported [34]. Additionally, adonixanthin reduced the expression of MMP-2 and fibronectin, downstream of ERK1/2 and Akt signalling (Figure 4E,G). In addition, both astaxanthin and adonixanthin decreased the mRNA level of fibronectin (Supplementary Material Figure 3). These results indicate that adonixanthin could affect ERK1/2 and Akt signalling upstream. In MMP9, the reason why there were no changes in the expression (Figure 3F) may be that it is an inflammation-related enzyme, the expression of which is low in the normal condition.

To elucidate the active site of both compounds, we examined their effect on ROS, which is important for the regulation of both ERK1/2 and Akt phosphorylation [35]. In the past, it has been reported that ROS promote tumour progression via the phosphorylation of ERK1/2 and Akt [27,30]. Therefore, we evaluated the level of ROS in glioblastoma cells following treatment with both compounds for 6 h. Both compounds greatly reduced the levels of intracellular ROS (Figure 5A). Astaxanthin and adonixanthin have been reported to possess radical scavenging properties [9], and the reduction of reactive oxygen species in glioblastoma cells shown in this study may also include the direct antioxidant activity of these compounds. Nox4 is a key factor involved in the regulation of ROS production and is upregulated in glioblastoma compared with other nicotinamide adenine dinucleotide phosphate: NADPH oxidase isoforms [36]. Only adonixanthin significantly suppressed the expression of Nox4 (Figure 5B). As the effect of adonixanthin on intracellur ROS in glioblastoma cells, it is considered that adonixanthin may inhibit the expression of ROS production-related factors, such as Nox4.

We examined whether astaxanthin and adonixanthin can be delivered to the brain following oral administration, using healthy mice. We confirmed that both compounds were delivered to the brain, that astaxanthin was detected at a higher concentration than adonixanthin in the brain tissue, and that the *cis*-form of adonixanthin was not detected at all in any brain tissues (Table 2). Conversely, adonixanthin was detected at high levels in mouse tissues other than the brain (Supplementary Material Table S1). It is suggested that orally administered adonixanthin mainly affects the peripheral tissues due to the difference in the distribution of adonixanthin. In this study, we used structurally stable *trans*-isomers of both astaxanthin and adonixanthin. The *trans*-form of astaxanthin and adonixanthin is converted to the *cis*-form in the blood following oral administration [37]. The differences in the structure between the *cis*- and *trans*-forms may affect their antitumour activity, and although the *cis*-form of astaxanthin has been reported to show greater antioxidant activity than the *trans*-form [38], the detailed mechanism underlying this remains unknown. In addition, the concentrations of astaxanthin and adonixanthin detected in the brain were approximately 30 and 10 nM, respectively. These concentrations correspond to one-third and one-tenth of the minimum concentration (0.1 µM) used in the cell proliferation test, as shown in Figure 2A,B. In glioblastoma pathology, invasive glioblastoma cells degrade the basement membrane around blood vessels and cause disruption of the blood–brain barrier. As a result, the transferability to the brain of immune cells and chemotherapeutic drugs is increased [39,40]. In a study using a glioma rat model, it was reported that translocation of a magnetic resonance imaging

(MRI) contrast agent increased about five times in tumour tissues compared with its translocation in healthy tissues [41]. Therefore, it is inferred that astaxanthin and adonixanthin administered orally accumulate in glioblastoma tissues at higher concentrations compared with their accumulation in healthy tissues.

Next, using an in vivo glioblastoma mouse model, we examined whether the oral administration of astaxanthin and adonixanthin exhibited an antitumour effect on glioblastoma. Both astaxanthin and adonixanthin significantly suppressed tumour growth in this in vivo glioblastoma model (Figure 6). These results showed that astaxanthin and adonixanthin transferred to the brain by oral administration exert an antitumour effect on glioblastoma. Although adonixanthin tended to have a greater effect than astaxanthin in this in vitro study (Figures 2–5), astaxanthin and adonixanthin showed a comparable antitumour effect in the in vivo glioblastoma model. These results may reflect differences both in transferability to the brain and the ratio of isoforms of astaxanthin or adonixanthin.

In conclusion, these findings suggest that the oral administration of astaxanthin and adonixanthin, respectively, could be potentially useful treatments for glioblastoma.

4. Materials and Methods

4.1. Reagents

Both astaxanthin and adonixanthin obtained from *Paracoccsu carotinifaciens* were provided by ENEOS Corporation (Tokyo, Japan). Adonixanthin is an intermediate compound between zeaxanthin and astaxanthin [42,43]. These compounds were dissolved by dimethyl sulfoxide, DMSO (FUJIFILM Wako Pure Chemical Corporation, Osaka, Japan), on in vitro and diffused by olive oil (FUJIFILM Wako Pure Chemical Corporation, Osaka, Japan) on in vivo. In the in vitro study, the final concentration of DMSO in all the groups was 0.1%.

4.2. Cell Line and Culture Condition

The human glioblastoma cell line U251MG was purchased from European Collection of Authenticated Cell Cultures (ECACC; London, the United Kingdom). The murine glioblastoma cell line GL261 was kindly provided by Dr. Saio, Graduate School of Health Sciences, Gunma University. The human glioblastoma cell line U87MG was obtained from American Type Culture Collection (ATCC). These cells were cultured in Dulbecco's Modified Eagle Medium (DMEM) with low glucose (Nacalai Tesque, Tokyo, Japan) supplemented with 10% foetal bovine serum (FBS; Valeant, Costa Mesa, CA, USA), 100 units/mL penicillin, and 100 mg/mL streptomycin at 37 °C in 5% CO_2. Cells were passaged by trypsinization and used within 10 passages.

4.3. Cell Viability

U251MG, GL261, or U87MG cells were seeded onto 96-well plates at a density of 2×10^3 cells/well with DMEM supplemented with 10% FBS and then incubated for 24 h, after which the culture medium was changed to DMEM containing 10% FBS. Then, astaxanthin, adonixanthin or temozolomide (Tokyo Chemical Industry Co., Ltd., Tokyo, Japan) were added to the culture. Cell proliferation was determined using the CCK-8 assay according to the manufacturer's instructions (Dojindo, Kumamoto, Japan). After each incubation, 10 μL of CCK-8 solution were added to each well. Plates were incubated for 3 h for 37 °C, and the absorbance was read at 450 nm with a reference wavelength of 630 nm using a Varioscan Flash 2.4 microplate reader (Thermo Fisher Scientific, Waltham, MA, USA).

4.4. BrdU (Bromodeoxyuridine) Cell Proliferation Assay

GL261 cells were seeded onto 96-well plates at a density of 2×10^3 cells/well with DMEM supplemented with 10% FBS and then incubated for 24 h, after which the culture medium was changed to DMEM containing 10% FBS. Then, astaxanthin, adonixanthin, or temozolomide (Tokyo Chemical Industry Co., Ltd., Tokyo, Japan) were added to the culture. After 72 h of culture, the culture medium was changed to DMEM containing 10% FBS and treated with BrdU at 10 µM for 3 h. After that, immunocytochemistry was performed according to the protocol of anti-BrdU antibody (abcam, ab6326).

4.5. Cell Migration Assay

The cell migration assay was conducted as previously described [44].

GL261 cells and U251 cells (2.0×10^4 cells per well) were plated in a 12-well plate (BD Biosciences, Tokyo, Japan) with culture medium supplemented with 10% FBS. After 24 h of incubation, the medium was changed to DMEM containing 1% FBS. After 6 h, wounds were scratched by a P1000 pipette tip and washed with phosphate-buffered saline (PBS) to eliminate cell debris. Then, fresh medium was added with 10 µM astaxanthin or adonixanthin. Pictures were taken at 48 h and these scratched areas were measured using an All-in-One Fluorescence Microscope (BZ-X710; Keyence, Osaka, Japan). The cell migration rate was measured the area of the wound before migration (S0) and after migration (S1) and calculated S1/(S0−S1) × 100. The control group was then standardized to be 100%. Wound widths at 0 h were created within 1 to 1.5 mm and data were excluded if they were not suitable for that width.

4.6. Immunoblotting

GL261 cell was seeded at 2.5×10^4 cells per well in 24-well plates with culture medium supplemented with 10% FBS. After 24 h of incubation, the medium was changed to DMEM containing 10% FBS and 0.1%DMSO PBS, 300 µM temozolomide, 10 µM astaxanthin, or 10 µM adonixanthin was added for 6 and 48 h. Cells were lysed in a special buffer (RIPA buffer R0278; Sigma-Aldrich, St. Louis, MO, USA) with a protease inhibitor cocktail (Sigma-Aldrich), phosphatase inhibitor cocktails 2 and 3 (Sigma-Aldrich), and sample buffer (Wako, Osaka, Japan). The protein concentration was determined by comparison with a known concentration of bovine serum albumin using the BCA Protein Assay Kit (Thermo Fisher Scientific). The amount of total protein was 2 µg. Equal amounts of protein in sample buffer containing 10% 2-mercaptoethanol were subjected to sodium dodecyl sulphate polyacrylamide gel electrophoresis (SDS-PAGE) in 5–20% gradient gels (SuperSep Ace; Wako), and the separated proteins were transferred to polyvinylidene difluoride membrane (Immobilon-P; Merck Millipore Corporation, Bedford, MA, USA). After blocking for 30 min with Blocking One-P (Nacalai Tesque), we incubated the membranes with primary antibodies overnight at 4 °C. The primary antibodies were a rabbit anti-phospho-p44/42 MAPK; ERK1/2 (T202/Y204) 197G2 (4377S, Cell signalling, diluted 1:1000), a rabbit anti-p44/42 MAPK; ERK1/2 (9102S, Cell signalling, diluted 1:1000), a rabbit anti-phospho-Akt (S473) 193H12 (4058S, Cell signalling, diluted 1:1000), a rabbit anti-Akt (9272S, Cell signalling, diluted 1:1000), a rabbit anti-phospho-p38 MAPK (T180/Y182) (9211S, Cell signalling, diluted 1:1000), a rabbit anti-p38 MAPK (9212S, Cell signalling, diluted 1:1000), a rabbit anti-mmp-2 (AB19167, Chemicon®, diluted 1:1000), a rabbit anti-mmp-9 (AB19016, Chemicon®, diluted 1:1000), a rabbit anti-fibronectin (ab2413, abcam, diluted 1:1000), a rabbit anti-cyclin D1 (2978, Cell signalling, diluted 1:1000), a mouse anti-p27 (sc-1641, Santa Cluz, diluted 1:500), a rabbit anti-Nox4 (NB110-5849SS, Novus, diluted 1:500), a mouse anti-Bcl-2 (sc-7382, Santa Cluz, diluted 1:500), and a mouse anti-β-actin antibody (#A2228, Sigma-Aldrich, diluted 1:1000).

After that, the membrane was incubated with the following secondary antibodies: a goat anti-rabbit IgG, or a goat anti-mouse IgG antibody (Thermo Fisher Scientific, diluted 1:1000). The band intensity was measured using an Immuno Star LD (Wako). Band intensity was measured using an LAS-4000 UV mini Luminescent Image Analyzer (Fujifilm, Tokyo Japan) and Multi Gauge Version 3.0 (Fujifilm). The phosphorylation of ERK1/2, Akt, and p38 MAPK was measured by normalizing against total ERK1/2, total Akt, and total p38 MAPK. Equal loading was confirmed using β-actin as controls for phosphoprotein signals.

4.7. Quantitative Real-Time Reverse Transcription Polymerase Chain Reaction Analysis (qRT-PCR)

To evaluate the effect of astaxanthin and adonixanthin on the expression of *Fibronectin* mRNA expression, we performed quantitative real-time reverse transcription polymerase chain reaction (qRT-PCR) analysis. GL261 cell was seeded at 2.5×10^4 cells well in 24-well plates with culture medium supplemented with 10% FBS. After 24 h of incubation, the medium was changed to DMEM containing 10% FBS and 0.1% DMSO PBS, 300 µM temozolomide, 10 µM astaxanthin, or 10 µM adonixanthin was added for 48 h. After 48 h of treatment, RNA was isolated from GL261 cells using Nucleo Spin RNA II (Takara, Shiga, Japan). RNA concentrations were determined using NanoVue Plus (GE Healthcare Japan, Tokyo, Japan). Single-strand cDNAs were synthesized from the isolated RNAs via reverse transcription with a PrimeScript RT Reagent Kit (Perfect Real Time; Takara). Quantitative real-time RT-PCR was performed using TB Green Premix Ex Taq II (Tli RNaseH Plus; Takara) and a TP800 Thermal Cycler Dice Real Time System (Takara). All procedures were carried out in accordance with the manufacturer's instructions. The PCR primer sequences for *Fibronectin* were as follows: 5'-CGA GGT GAC AGA GAC CAC AA-3' (forward) and 5'-CTG GAG TCA AGC CAG ACA CA -3' (reverse). β-actin (internal control) was as follows: 5'-CAT CCG TAA AGA CCT CTA TGC CAA C-3' (forward) and 5'-ATG GAG CCA CCG ATC CAC A-3' (reverse). The cycling conditions were in accordance with the manufacturer's protocol. The results are expressed as relative gene expression levels normalized to that of β-actin.

4.8. Cell Death Assay

GL261 cells were seeded onto 96-well plates at a density of 2×10^3 cells/well with DMEM supplemented with 10% FBS and then incubated for 24 h, after which the culture medium was changed to DMEM containing 10% FBS. Then, astaxanthin, adonixanthin, or temozolomide (Tokyo Chemical Industry Co., Ltd., Tokyo, Japan) were added to the culture. Cell death was measured by Hoechst 33,342 (Invitrogen, Carlsbad, CA, USA) and propidium iodide (Invitrogen). At 96 h after treatment, the Hoechst 33,342 and propidium iodide were added to the medium to final concentrations of 8.1 and 1.5 µM, respectively, for 15 min. Images of stained cells were captured with a Lionheart™ FX Automated Microscope (BioTek, Tokyo, Japan). The percentage of propidium iodide-positive cells was determined by distinguishing Hoechst 33,342 and propidium iodide fluorescence.

4.9. Reactive Oxygen Species Assay

Intracellular radical activation within GL261 cells was measured with 5-(and-6)-chloromethyl—2',7'-dichlorodihydrofluorescein diacetate, acetyl ester (CM-H_2DCFDA; Thermo Fisher Scientific, MA, USA). Six hours after treatment of temozolomide, astaxanthin, or adonixanthin, CM-H_2DCFDA was added to the culture medium and incubated at 37 °C for 1 h under shading in GL261. Fluorescence was measured using a Varioscan Flash 2.4 microplate reader (Thermo Fisher Scientific, MA, USA) at 485 (excitation)-535 nm (emission). Measurements were performed 0, 30, and 60 min after the addition of CM-H_2DCFDA.

4.10. Animals

All experimental design and procedures were approved by the murine experiment committees of Gifu Pharmacological University and were in compliance with ARRIVE (Animal Research: Reporting in Vivo Experiments) guidelines. These experiments were approved by the animal experiment committees of Gifu Pharmaceutical University, Japan (Ethic nos. 2018-099, 2019-065). For all experiments, male C57BL/6J mice (8 weeks old; body weight 22~27 g) and male ICR mice (6 weeks old; body weight 25~28 g) purchased from Japan SLC, Inc. (Hamamatsu, Shizuoka, Japan) were used. Animals were housed at 24 ± 2 °C under a 12-h light-dark cycle. Food and water were available to all animals ad libitum. All experimental procedures and outcome assessments were performed in a blinded manner.

4.11. Murine orthotopic Glioblastoma Model

Murine glioblastoma cell (GL261) transplantation was performed as previously described [39]. Briefly, mice received an intracranial injection of 1×10^5 cells in 2 µL of PBS using a Hamilton microliter syringe at the following coordinates: 1 mm anterior, 2 mm lateral (left of middle) to bregma, at a depth of 3 mm from the dural surface. This protocol was completed using a stereotactic frame.

4.12. In Vivo Drug Treatment

In the experiment of the murine orthotopic glioblastoma model, oral administration of each astaxanthin (10 and 30 mg/kg) and adonixanthin (10 and 30 mg/kg) was initiated 3 days after intracranial injection of GL261 cells and was continued for 10 days. In the experiment of the brain tissue absorption with oral astaxanthin or adonixanthin, after one week of adaptation, ICR mice were randomly divided into the following three groups: control group, astaxanthin group (50 mg/kg), and adonixanthin group (50 mg/kg). Mice were orally administered each reagent suspended in olive oil (5 mL/kg) by the daily single dose for 10 days. The control group was treated by olive oil alone (5 mL/kg).

Since 50 mg/kg is known to be a dose of astaxanthin that does not show adverse effects even with long-term administration, this dose of astaxanthin and adonixanthin was used in the distribution experiment of this study. Moreover, it was reported that the oral administration of astaxanthin at 25 mg/kg inhibited hippocampal inflammation in diabetic mice [45]. Thus, we set up a dose similar to that in the present study.

4.13. Mouse Brain Analysis on In Vivo Glioblastoma Model

Mice were euthanized and transcranial perfused with cold saline for 2 min at room temperature. After that, the perfusate was changed to 0.1 M phosphate buffer (PB; pH 7.4) containing 4% paraformaldehyde (PFA, Wako Pure Chemicals, Osaka, Japan) for 3 min. Brains were fixed in 4% paraformaldehyde, embedded in paraffin (Leica Biosystems, Wetzlar, Germany), cut into 5-μm sections, and processed for haematoxylin-eosin (HE) staining. Pictures were taken using an All-in-One Fluorescence Microscope (BZ-X710; Keyence, Osaka, Japan). We assessed the maximum cross-sectional area of the tumour and tumour volume as described previously [46].

4.14. Collecting Blood and Tissues

In mice, blood samples were collected under anaesthesia by using sodium pentobarbital (50 mg/kg, 10 mL/kg, *i.p*). To separate serum and from blood, we centrifuged at 1700 g for 10 min. After mice were euthanized by exsanguination under deep anaesthesia, tissues, such as brain, were picked. Furthermore, the cerebral cortex, cerebellum, striatum, and hippocampus were separated from the whole brain.

All samples, including serum and tissues, were stored at −80 °C until the analysis of astaxanthin and adonixanthin was performed.

4.15. Analysis of Astaxanthin and Adonixanthin

Carotenoid fraction was collected from blood and some tissues by silica gel HPLC using a Cosmosil 5SL-II column with acetone:hexane (2:8, *v/v*) for the mobile phase at a flow rate of 1.0 mL/min as described above. This fraction was evaporated to dryness, dissolved in isopropanol: hexane (4:96, *v/v*), and subjected to chiral HPLC. Identification of each carotenoid was performed by authentic carotenoids obtained from Paracoccus (ENEOS Corporation, Tokyo, Japan) by our routine methods [47] and the content of each carotenoid was calculated from peak areas by comparison with the authentic samples.

4.16. Statistical Analysis

All data are presented as mean ± standard error of the mean (SEM). We performed the experiments assuming normality and selected an appropriate statistical analysis method depending on the presence or absence of equal variance. Specifically, student's t-test or Welch's test was used in the case of equal or non-equal variance under Bonferroni correction in Figure 2D, Figure 3, Figure 4, Figure 5B, and Figures S3–S5. We used a one-way analyses of variance (ANOVA) followed by Tukey's test or Games-Howell's test for multiple comparisons in Figure 2A, Figure 2B, Figure 5A, Figure 6, Figures S1 and S2; and the Mann–Whitney U-test for two-group comparisons in Table 2 and Supplementary Material Table S1. These statistics were performed by SPSS Statistics (IBM, Armonk, NY, USA) software. $p < 0.05$ was considered statistical significance.

Supplementary Materials: The following are available online at http://www.mdpi.com/1660-3397/18/9/474/s1, Figure S1, Supplemental Figure 1. Cell viability of mouse and human glioblastoma cell line with astaxanthin and adonixanthin., Figure S2, Cell viability of human glioblastoma cell line U87MG with astaxanthin and adonixanthin, Figure S3, Expression of Fibronectin mRNA after 48 h treatment of astaxanthin and adonixanthin in mouse glioblastoma cell line. Figure S4, The effect of astaxanthin and adonixanthin for cell death. Figure S5, The effects of astaxanthin and adonixanthin on body weight. Table S1: Astaxanthin or adonixanthin levels in the mouse tissues without brain.

Author Contributions: Conceptualization, S.T., S.N., H.H. and M.S. (Masamitsu Shimazawa); Data curation, S.T., S.N. and M.S. (Masamitsu Shimazawa); Formal analysis, S.T.; Funding acquisition, H.H.; Investigation, S.T., T.M., T.Y. (Tetsuya Yamada), T.I., T.O. and T.Y. (Tomohiro Yako); Methodology, S.T., S.N., H.H. and M.S. (Masamitsu Shimazawa); Project administration, S.N. and H.H.; Resources, M.H., K.E. and M.S. (Masanao Saio); Software, S.T.; Supervision, S.N. and H.H.; Validation, S.N. and M.S. (Masamitsu Shimazawa); Visualization, S.T., S.N., H.H. and M.S. (Masamitsu Shimazawa); Writing—original draft, S.T.; Writing—review & editing, S.N., M.S., H.H. and M.S. (Masamitsu Shimazawa). All authors have read and agreed to the published version of the manuscript.

Funding: Dr. Hara had grants from ENEOS Corporation (Tokyo, Japan). The other authors declare no competing financial interest.

Conflicts of Interest: This study was funded by ENEOS Corporation (Tokyo, Japan). M.K. and K.E are employees of ENEOS Corporation.

References

1. Friedman, H.S.; Kerby, T.; Calvert, H. Temozolomide and treatment of malignant glioma. *Clin. Cancer Res.* **2000**, *6*, 2585–2597.
2. Stupp, R.; Taillibert, S.; Kanner, A.A.; Kesari, S.; Steinberg, D.M.; Toms, S.A.; Taylor, L.P.; Lieberman, F.; Silvani, A.; Fink, K.L.; et al. Maintenance Therapy With Tumor-Treating Fields Plus Temozolomide vs Temozolomide Alone for Glioblastoma: A Randomized Clinical Trial. *JAMA* **2015**, *314*, 2535–2543. [CrossRef] [PubMed]
3. Stupp, R.; Mason, W.P.; Van Den Bent, M.J.; Weller, M.; Fisher, B.; Taphoorn, M.J.B.; Belanger, K.; Brandes, A.A.; Marosi, C.; Bogdahn, U.; et al. Radiotherapy plus concomitant and adjuvant temozolomide for glioblastoma. *N. Engl. J. Med.* **2005**, *352*, 987–996. [CrossRef] [PubMed]
4. Ostrom, Q.T.; Gittleman, H.; Liao, P.; Rouse, C.; Chen, Y.; Dowling, J.; Wolinsky, Y.; Kruchko, C.; Barnholtz-Sloan, J. CBTRUS statistical report: Primary brain and central nervous system tumors diagnosed in the United States in 2007–2011. *Neuro. Oncol.* **2014**, *16*, iv1–iv63. [CrossRef] [PubMed]
5. Lacroix, M.; Abi-Said, D.; Fourney, D.R.; Gokaslan, Z.L.; Shi, W.; DeMonte, F.; Lang, F.F.; McCutcheon, I.E.; Hassenbusch, S.J.; Holland, E.; et al. A multivariate analysis of 416 patients with glioblastoma multiforme: Prognosis, extent of resection, and survival. *J. Neurosurg.* **2001**, *95*, 190–198. [CrossRef] [PubMed]
6. Warren, K.E. Beyond the blood: Brain barrier: The importance of central nervous system (CNS) pharmacokinetics for the treatment of CNS tumors, including diffuse intrinsic pontine glioma. *Front. Oncol.* **2018**, *8*, 239. [CrossRef]
7. Zhao, M.; Zhao, M.; Fu, C.; Yu, Y.; Fu, A. Targeted therapy of intracranial glioma model mice with curcumin nanoliposomes. *Int. J. Nanomed.* **2018**, *13*, 1601–1610. [CrossRef]
8. Clark, P.A.; Bhattacharya, S.; Elmayan, A.; Darjatmoko, S.R.; Thuro, B.A.; Yan, M.B.; Van Ginkel, P.R.; Polans, A.S.; Kuo, J.S. Resveratrol targeting of AKT and p53 in glioblastoma and glioblastoma stem-like cells to suppress growth and infiltration. *J. Neurosurg.* **2017**, *126*, 1448–1460. [CrossRef]
9. Maoka, T.; Yasui, H.; Ohmori, A.; Tokuda, H.; Suzuki, N.; Osawa, A.; Shindo, K.; Ishibashi, T. Anti-oxidative, anti-tumor-promoting, and anti-carcinogenic activities of adonirubin and adonixanthin. *J. Oleo Sci.* **2013**, *62*, 181–186. [CrossRef]
10. Miki, W.; Yamaguchi, K.; Konosu, S. Comparison of carotenoids in the ovaries of marine fish and shellfish. *Comp. Biochem. Physiol. Part B Biochem.* **1982**, *71*, 7–11. [CrossRef]

11. Nakajima, Y.; Inokuchi, Y.; Shimazawa, M.; Otsubo, K.; Ishibashi, T.; Hara, H. Astaxanthin, a dietary carotenoid, protects retinal cells against oxidative stress in-vitro and in mice in-vivo. *J. Pharm. Pharmacol.* **2008**, *60*, 1365–1374. [CrossRef] [PubMed]
12. Nishioka, Y.; Oyagi, A.; Tsuruma, K.; Shimazawa, M.; Ishibashi, T.; Hara, H. The antianxiety-like effect of astaxanthin extracted from Paracoccus carotinifaciens. *BioFactors* **2011**, *37*, 25–30. [CrossRef] [PubMed]
13. Murata, K.; Oyagi, A.; Takahira, D.; Tsuruma, K.; Shimazawa, M.; Ishibashi, T.; Hara, H. Protective Effects of Astaxanthin from Paracoccus carotinifaciens on Murine Gastric Ulcer Models. *Phyther. Res.* **2012**, *26*, 1126–1132. [CrossRef] [PubMed]
14. Otsuka, T.; Shimazawa, M.; Nakanishi, T.; Ohno, Y.; Inoue, Y.; Tsuruma, K.; Ishibashi, T.; Hara, H. The protective effects of a dietary carotenoid, astaxanthin, against light-induced retinal damage. *J. Pharmacol. Sci.* **2013**, *123*, 209–218. [CrossRef]
15. Otsuka, T.; Shimazawa, M.; Inoue, Y.; Nakano, Y.; Ojino, K.; Izawa, H.; Tsuruma, K.; Ishibashi, T.; Hara, H. Astaxanthin Protects Against Retinal Damage: Evidence from In Vivo and In Vitro Retinal Ischemia and Reperfusion Models. *Curr. Eye Res.* **2016**, *41*, 1465–1472. [CrossRef]
16. Inoue, Y.; Shimazawa, M.; Nagano, R.; Kuse, Y.; Takahashi, K.; Tsuruma, K.; Hayashi, M.; Ishibashi, T.; Maoka, T.; Hara, H. Astaxanthin analogs, adonixanthin and lycopene, activate Nrf2 to prevent light-induced photoreceptor degeneration. *J. Pharmacol. Sci.* **2017**, *134*, 147–157. [CrossRef]
17. Pan, L.; Zhou, Y.; Li, X.F.; Wan, Q.J.; Yu, L.H. Preventive treatment of astaxanthin provides neuroprotection through suppression of reactive oxygen species and activation of antioxidant defense pathway after stroke in rats. *Brain Res. Bull.* **2017**, *130*, 211–220. [CrossRef]
18. Iwata, S.; Imai, T.; Shimazawa, M.; Ishibashi, T.; Hayashi, M. Protective e ff ects of the astaxanthin derivative, adonixanthin, on brain hemorrhagic injury. *Brain Res.* **2018**, *1698*, 130–138. [CrossRef]
19. Kavitha, K.; Kowshik, J.; Kishore, T.K.K.; Baba, A.B.; Nagini, S. Astaxanthin inhibits NF-κB and Wnt/β-catenin signaling pathways via inactivation of Erk/MAPK and PI3K/Akt to induce intrinsic apoptosis in a hamster model of oral cancer. *Biochim. Biophys. Acta Gen. Subj.* **2013**, *1830*, 4433–4444. [CrossRef]
20. Tanaka, T.; Morishita, Y.; Suzui, M.; Kojima, T.; Okumura, A.; Mori, H. Chemoprevention of mouse urinary bladder carcinogenesis by the naturally occurring carotenoid astaxanthin. *Carcinogenesis* **1994**, *15*, 15–19. [CrossRef]
21. Nagendraprabhu, P.; Sudhandiran, G. Astaxanthin inhibits tumor invasion by decreasing extracellular matrix production and induces apoptosis in experimental rat colon carcinogenesis by modulating the expressions of ERK-2, NFkB and COX-2. *Investig. N. Drugs* **2011**, *29*, 207–224. [CrossRef] [PubMed]
22. Zhang, X.; Zhao, W.; Hu, L.; Zhao, L.; Huang, J. Carotenoids inhibit proliferation and regulate expression of peroxisome proliferators-activated receptor gamma (PPAR c) in K562 cancer cells. *Arch. Biochem. Biophys.* **2011**, *512*, 96–106. [CrossRef] [PubMed]
23. Ong, X.S.; Hang, J.Z.; Ang, M.W.; Iu, W.L.; Xin-bin, G.U. Astaxanthin Induces Mitochondria-Mediated Apoptosis in Rat Hepatocellular Carcinoma CBRH-7919 Cells. *Biol. Pharm. Bull.* **2011**, *34*, 839–844.
24. Zhang, L.; Wang, H. Multiple mechanisms of anti-cancer effects exerted by astaxanthin. *Mar. Drugs* **2015**, *13*, 4310–4330. [CrossRef] [PubMed]
25. Mccubrey, J.A.; Steelman, L.S.; Chappell, W.H.; Abrams, S.L.; Wong, W.T.; Chang, F.; Lehmann, B.; Terrian, D.M.; Milella, M.; Stivala, F.; et al. Roles of the RAF/MEK/ERK pathway in cell growth, malignant transformation and drug resistance. *Biochim Biophys Acta.* **2009**, *1773*, 1263–1284. [CrossRef] [PubMed]
26. Wee, P.; Wang, Z. Epidermal growth factor receptor cell proliferation signaling pathways. *Cancers* **2017**, *9*, 52.
27. Wu, W.-S.; Wu, J.-R.; Hu, C.-T. Signal cross talks for sustained MAPK activation and cell migration: The potential role of reactive oxygen species. *Cancer Metastasis Rev.* **2008**, *27*, 303–314. [CrossRef]
28. Jhou, B.; Song, T.; Lee, I.; Hu, M.; Yang, N. Lycopene Inhibits Human liver adenocarcinoma SK-Hep-1 Cells Metastasis by Down Regulation of NADPH Oxidase 4 Protein Expression. *J. Agric. Food Chem.* **2017**, *65*, 6893–6903. [CrossRef]
29. Hayashi, M.; Ishibashi, T.; Maoka, T. Effect of astaxanthin rich extract derived from Paracoccus carotinifaciens on cognitive function in middle aged and older individuals. *J. Clin. Biochem. Nutr.* **2018**, *62*, 195–205. [CrossRef]
30. Zhang, J.; Cao, M.; Yang, W.; Sun, F.; Xu, C.; Yin, L.; Pu, Y. Inhibition of Glucose-6-Phosphate Dehydrogenase Could Enhance 1, 4-Benzoquinone-Induced Oxidative Damage in K562 Cells. *Oxid. Med. Cell. Longev.* **2016**, *2016*, 3912515. [CrossRef]

31. Zhu, W.; Xue, Y.; Liang, C.; Zhang, R.; Zhang, Z.; Li, H.; Su, D.; Liang, X.; Zhang, Y.; Huang, Q.; et al. S100A16 promotes cell proliferation and metastasis via AKT and ERK cell signaling pathways in human prostate cancer. *Tumour Biol. J. Int. Soc. Oncodev. Biol. Med.* **2016**, *37*, 12241–12250. [CrossRef] [PubMed]
32. Peng, X.; Liu, Y.; Zhu, S.; Peng, X.; Li, H.; Jiao, W.; Lin, P.; Zhang, Z.; Qiu, Y.; Jin, M.; et al. Co-targeting PI3K/Akt and MAPK/ERK pathways leads to an enhanced antitumor effect on human hypopharyngeal squamous cell carcinoma. *J. Cancer Res. Clin. Oncol.* **2019**, *145*, 2921–2936. [CrossRef]
33. Bi, T.; Zhu, A.; Yang, X.; Qiao, H.; Tang, J.; Liu, Y.; Lv, R. Metformin synergistically enhances antitumor activity of cisplatin in gallbladder cancer via the PI3K/AKT/ERK pathway. *Cytotechnology* **2018**, *70*, 439–448. [CrossRef] [PubMed]
34. Meco, D.; Servidei, T.; Lamorte, G.; Binda, E.; Arena, V.; Riccardi, R. Ependymoma stem cells are highly sensitive to temozolomide in vitro and in orthotopic models. *Neuro. Oncol.* **2014**, *16*, 1067–1077. [CrossRef] [PubMed]
35. Aggarwal, V.; Tuli, H.S.; Varol, A.; Thakral, F.; Yerer, M.B.; Sak, K.; Varol, M.; Jain, A.; Khan, M.A.; Sethi, G. Role of reactive oxygen species in cancer progression: Molecular mechanisms and recent advancements. *Biomolecules* **2019**, *9*, 735. [CrossRef]
36. Shono, T.; Yokoyama, N.; Uesaka, T.; Kuroda, J.; Takeya, R.; Yamasaki, T.; Amano, T.; Mizoguchi, M.; Suzuki, S.O.; Niiro, H.; et al. Enhanced expression of NADPH oxidase Nox4 in human gliomas and its roles in cell proliferation and survival. *Int. J. Cancer* **2008**, *123*, 787–792. [CrossRef]
37. Zhou, Q.; Xu, J.; Yang, L.; Gu, C.; Xue, C. Thermal stability and oral absorbability of astaxanthin esters from Haematococcus pluvialis in Balb/c mice. *J. Sci. Food Agric.* **2019**, *99*, 3662–3671. [CrossRef]
38. Yang, C.; Zhang, H.; Liu, R.; Zhu, H.; Zhang, L.; Tsao, R. Bioaccessibility, Cellular Uptake, and Transport of Astaxanthin Isomers and their Antioxidative Effects in Human Intestinal Epithelial Caco-2 Cells. *J. Agric. Food Chem.* **2017**, *65*, 10223–10232. [CrossRef]
39. Cuddapah, V.A.; Robel, S.; Watkins, S.; Sontheimer, H. A neurocentric perspective on glioma invasion. *Nat. Rev. Neurosci.* **2014**, *15*, 455–465. [CrossRef]
40. Gao, X.; Yue, Q.; Liu, Y.; Fan, D.; Fan, K.; Li, S.; Qian, J.; Han, L.; Fang, F.; Xu, F.; et al. Image-guided chemotherapy with specifically tuned blood brain barrier permeability in glioma margins. *Theranostics* **2018**, *8*, 3126–3137. [CrossRef]
41. Blanchette, M.; Tremblay, L.; Lepage, M.; Fortin, D. Impact of drug size on brain tumor and brain parenchyma delivery after a blood-brain barrier disruption. *J. Cereb. Blood Flow Metab.* **2014**, *34*, 820–826. [CrossRef] [PubMed]
42. Breitenbach, J. Expression in Escherichia coZi and properties of the carotene ketolase from Haematococcus pluvialis. *FEMS Microbiol. Lett.* **1996**, *140*, 241–246. [CrossRef] [PubMed]
43. Rhodes, A.C.E. Dietary effects on carotenoid composition in the marine harpacticoid copepod Nitokra lacustris. *J. Plankton Res.* **2007**, *29*, i73–i83. [CrossRef]
44. Tsuji, S.; Ohno, Y.; Nakamura, S.; Yamada, T.; Noda, Y. Temozolomide has anti-tumor effects through the phosphorylation of cPLA 2 on glioblastoma cells. *Brain Res.* **2019**, *1723*, 146396. [CrossRef]
45. Zhou, X.-Y.; Zhang, F.; Hu, X.-T.; Chen, J.; Tang, R.-X.; Zheng, K.-Y.; Song, Y.-J. Depression can be prevented by astaxanthin through inhibition of hippocampal inflammation in diabetic mice. *Brain Res.* **2017**, *1657*, 262–268. [CrossRef]
46. Duan, J.; Gao, Y.; Zhang, X.; Wang, X.; Wang, B.; Meng, X. International Immunopharmacology CD30 ligand deficiency accelerates glioma progression by promoting the formation of tumor immune microenvironment. *Int. Immunopharmacol.* **2019**, *71*, 350–360. [CrossRef]
47. Maoka, T. Structural studies of carotenoids in plants, animals, and food products. In *Carotenoids*; Wiley: Hoboken, NJ, USA, 2016; pp. 103–129.

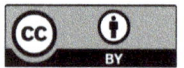

© 2020 by the authors. Licensee MDPI, Basel, Switzerland. This article is an open access article distributed under the terms and conditions of the Creative Commons Attribution (CC BY) license (http://creativecommons.org/licenses/by/4.0/).

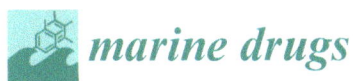

Article

Transcriptome Analysis of the Inhibitory Effect of Astaxanthin on *Helicobacter pylori*-Induced Gastric Carcinoma Cell Motility

Suhn Hyung Kim and Hyeyoung Kim *

Department of Food and Nutrition, Brain Korea 21 PLUS Project, College of Human Ecology, Yonsei University, Seoul 03722, Korea; cigdoli2@naver.com
* Correspondence: kim626@yonsei.ac.kr; Tel.: +82-2-2123-3125

Received: 21 June 2020; Accepted: 14 July 2020; Published: 15 July 2020

Abstract: *Helicobacter pylori* (*H. pylori*) infection promotes the metastasis of gastric carcinoma cells by modulating signal transduction pathways that regulate cell proliferation, motility, and invasion. Astaxanthin (ASTX), a xanthophyll carotenoid, is known to inhibit cancer cell migration and invasion, however the mechanism of action of ASTX in *H. pylori*-infected gastric epithelial cells is not well understood. To gain insight into this process, we carried out a comparative RNA sequencing (RNA-Seq) analysis of human gastric cancer AGS (adenocarcinoma gastric) cells as a function of *H. pylori* infection and ASTX administration. The results were used to identify genes that are differently expressed in response to *H. pylori* and ASTX. Gene ontology (GO) analysis identified differentially expressed genes (DEGs) to be associated with cell cytoskeleton remodeling, motility, and/or migration. Among the 20 genes identified, those encoding c-MET, PI3KC2, PLCγ1, Cdc42, and ROCK1 were selected for verification by real-time PCR analysis. The verified genes were mapped, using signaling networks contained in the KEGG database, to create a signaling pathway through which ASTX might mitigate the effects of *H. pylori*-infection. We propose that *H. pylori*-induced upregulation of the upstream regulator c-MET, and hence, its downstream targets Cdc42 and ROCK1, is suppressed by ASTX. ASTX is also suggested to counteract *H. pylori*-induced activation of PI3K and PLCγ. In conclusion, ASTX can suppress *H. pylori*-induced gastric cancer progression by inhibiting cytoskeleton reorganization and reducing cell motility through downregulation of c-MET, EGFR, PI3KC2, PLCγ1, Cdc42, and ROCK1.

Keywords: *Helicobacter pylori*; gastric carcinoma; astaxanthin; cell motility; cell migration

1. Introduction

Globally, gastric cancer is the fifth most common type of cancer and the third leading cause of death from cancer [1]. *Helicobacter pylori* infection is the major cause of gastric cancer, accounting for more than 60% of the cases [2]. Gastric cancer metastasizes at a high rate, localizing primarily in the liver, peritoneum, lung, and bone [3].

Metastatic cancer occurs as a result of the invasion of the surrounding stroma by primary tumor cells, followed by intravasation of the primary tumor into lymphatic or blood vessels, and finally, by extravasation and colonization of the tumor cells at a distant organ site [4]. Metastasis is initiated when cancer cells acquire specialized behaviors that allow them to breach the basement membrane of the extracellular matrix (ECM). Cancer cells undergo epithelia–mesenchymal transition (EMT), which enables them to lose intercellular junctions and to gain a migratory cell phenotype [5]. Modulation of cell motility is the determinant step in early local invasion. Cell motility requires continuous turnover of the cytoskeleton and modification of cell–cell and cell–substratum adhesions [6].

Cell locomotion involves three major processes. At the leading edge, the cell extends itself via reorganization of the actin cytoskeleton. At the trailing edge, the cell remodels its cytoskeleton to generate a contractile force. During this process, extracellular proteases are secreted to degrade the ECM, and to clear the path ahead [7]. A motile cell elongates itself at the leading edge through the polymerization of actin monomers into sheet-like structures known as lamellipodia. Protruding from the lamellipodial actin network are filopodia, which are spike-like structures formed from bundles of cross-linked actin microfilaments. Filopodia function in environmental sensing, cell migration, and cell–cell interaction. During the course of cell movement, the fliopodia located at the leading edge of the cell makes integrin to contact with the ECM while the cell breaks its surface adhesions at the rear, detaching its trailing edge from the substratum, and moving forward via an actomysin contractile force [8]. Increased filopodia formation and upregulation of filopodia proteins such as fascin and myosin-X promote cell migration, and are characteristic of invasive carcinoma cells [9].

Cell motility and morphology are regulated by small G proteins of the Rho family of the Ras-related GTPases. The Rho GTPases Rho, Rac, and cell division control protein 42 (Cdc42) coordinate the different steps of cell locomotion. Rho regulates formation of stress fibers and generation of the contractile force at the trailing edge of the moving cell. Rac modulates formation of membrane ruffles and lamellipodia, whereas Cdc42 is involved in formation of filopodia and focal adhesions at the leading edge of the cell [10]. Rho acts through its effector protein Rho-associated coiled-coil forming kinase (ROCK) to activate myosin light chain (MLC) for formation of stress fibers. Cdc42 and Rac regulate actin polymerization by activating Wiskott–Aldrich syndrome protein (WASP) and WASP-family verprolin-homologous protein (WAVE), respectively. WAVE and WASP activate the complex of actin-related proteins (ARP)2 and ARP3 to initiate the formation of new actin polymerization sites at lamellipodia. [11]

The cell motility cascade mediated by Rho GTPases is activated by chemokines, cytokines, and growth factors. Chemokines such as chemokine C-X-C motif ligand 12 (CXCL12), and growth factors such as epidermal growth factor (EGF), hepatocyte growth factor (HGF), platelet-derived growth factor (PDGF), or fibroblast growth factor (FGF), bind cell surface receptors which activate signaling pathways that regulate cytoskeleton restructuring and cell migration [6,12]. Receptor tyrosine kinases that are activated upon binding their ligand growth factors, mediate the cell migration pathway. In particular, the EGR receptor (EGFR) and HGF receptor c-MET are highly expressed in many carcinomas [13,14].

In an early study, transcriptional array analysis of AGS cells infected with *H. pylori* indicated that genes associated the innate immune response (including the inflammatory response) and cell motility are the genes most impacted by the *H. pylori* infection [15]. *H. pylori* infection of the stomach lining promotes gastric carcinogenesis through increased inflammatory responses which lead to increased cell proliferation and migration [16–18]. *H. pylori* adhesion to gastric epithelial cells induces tyrosine kinase phosphorylation and results in cytoskeleton rearrangement [19]. *H. pylori*-induced upregulation of pro-inflammatory cytokines has been shown to promote cell motility and cell elongation [20]. In addition, *H. pylori* infection cause EMT by increasing soluble heparin-binding epidermal growth factor (HB-GF) shedding via upregulation of gastrin and matrix metalloprotease (MMP)-7 [21].

Virulent strains of *H. pylori* possess a cytotoxin-associated gene (cag) pathogenicity island (cagPAI) that encodes a type IV secretion system through which the virulence factor CagA is translocated into the host cell. Investigations have demonstrated that cagPAI is responsible for the upregulation of the proinflammatory cytokine interleukin-8 (IL-8), activation of EGFR and c-MET signaling, activation of the transcription factors activator protein-1 (AP-1) and nuclear factor kappa-light-chain-enhancer of activated B cells (NF-κB), activation of mitogen-activated protein (MAP) kinases and cellular stress response kinases, and activation of the small GTPases Rac1 and Cdc42 [22–31].

Astaxanthin (ASTX), a 3,30-dihydroxy-β, β-carotene-4,40-dione, is a xanthophyll carotenoid, produced primarily by marine microalgae/phytoplankton. ASTX gives lobster, salmon, and krill their red color [32]. ASTX's multiple conjugated π-bonds give rise to ASTX's powerful antioxidant properties [33], which underlie its cytoprotective effects [34,35]. Numerous studies have been carried out to identify and delineate the effects of ASTX on inflammation-driven diseases including cancer. Specifically, ASTX has been shown to inhibit the migration, invasion, and/or proliferation of cancerous gastric [36], liver [37], ovarian [38], breast [39], colon [40], and melanoma cells [41]. In addition, ASTX is known to target cancer-related signal transduction pathway proteins and their regulators, namely inflammatory cytokines, membrane receptors (e.g., peroxisome proliferator-activated receptor gamma (PPARγ), transcriptional regulators (e.g., NF-κB, signal transducer and activator of transcription 3 (STAT3), NF-2-related factor 2 (Nf2), and zinc finger E-box binding homeobox (ZEB)), and protein kinases (e.g., janus kinase (JAK), protein kinase B (PKB), phosphoinositide 3-kinase (PI3K) and the MAP kinases c-Jun N-terminal kinase (JNK), extracellular signal-related kinase (ERK), and p38) [35–43].

The present study was carried out to identify the cell signaling pathway(s) through which ASTX acts on gastric carcinoma AGS cells to mitigate *H. pylori*-induced activation of cytoskeleton remodeling, cell motility, and cell migration. RNA-sequencing (RNA-Seq) analysis was performed to determine which genes undergo altered expression in AGS cells in response to ASTX administration and *H-pylori*-infection. Gene ontology (GO) analysis identified differentially expressed genes (DEGs) to be associated with cell cytoskeleton remodeling, motility, and migration. Among these are DEGs encoding c-MET, PI3KC2β, PLCγ1, Cdc42, and ROCK1, which we confirmed by executing real-time PCR analysis. Herein, we propose a signaling-network through which ASTX might act to counter the effects of *H. pylori* infection, and thereby protect against *H. pylori*-induced gastric cancer metastasis.

2. Results

2.1. Gene Expression Profile of H. pylori-Infected and/or ASTX-Treated AGS Cells

Gene expression was compared between uninfected AGS cells (None) vs. *H. pylori*-infected AGS cells (HP), between HP and *H. pylori*-infected AGS cells treated with ASTX (ASTX + HP), and between None and uninfected AGS cells treated with ASTX (ASTX). RNA-Seq analysis identified 1006 DEGs among the four experimental systems. *H. pylori* infection upregulated 191 genes and downregulated 20 genes, whereas ASTX treatment upregulated 190 genes and downregulated 48 genes. ASTX treatment of the AGS cells prior to *H. pylori* infection resulted in upregulation of 112 genes, seven of which are repressed by *H. pylori* infection, and downregulation of 664 genes, 62 of which are upregulated in response to *H. pylori* infection. The DEGs observed for pairs of the four experimental groups are compared in the Venn diagram shown in Figure 1.

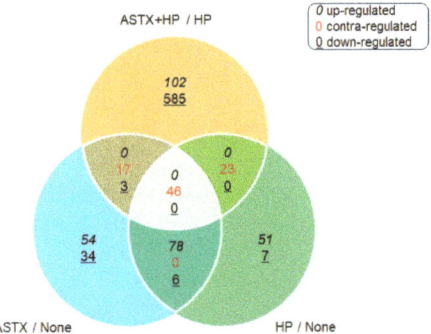

Figure 1. A comparison of the differentially expressed genes (DEG) expression pattern observed between pairs, and between paired-pairs, of the four experimental groups (None, *Helicobacter pylori*-infected AGS cells (HP), Astaxanthin (ASTX), and ASTX + HP). The numbers reported in black italic font correspond to upregulated DEGs, the numbers reported in black underlined font correspond to downregulated genes and the numbers reported in red regular font correspond to genes that are upregulated in one set of experimental groups and downregulated in the other.

2.2. GO Analysis of DEGs

The DEGs identified above were further analyzed using GO annotation to identify and categorize each gene according to the respective biological process with which they are associated, namely aging, angiogenesis, apoptotic process, cell cycle, cell death, cell differentiation, cell migration, cell proliferation, DNA repair, extracellular matrix, immune response, inflammatory response, cell motility, and cell secretion. The GO categories shared between the DEGs observed for the experimental systems None and HP are inflammatory response, aging, cell migration, and cell motility (Figure 2A). The GO annotations of DEGs that are differentially regulated in the ASTX + HP vs. HP experimental systems include immune response, apoptotic process, cell migration, and DNA repair (Figure 2B). Genes differentially expressed by ASTX treatment in the absence of *H. pylori* infection are associated with cell proliferation, cell migration, the apoptotic process, and the cell cycle (Figure 2C). Among the DEGs that are strongly upregulated by ASTX treatment are genes that encode superoxide dismutase 1, superoxide dismutase 2, TNF receptor-associated factor 7, and serine/threonine kinase 17a (which regulates cell death and apoptosis), protein kinase N2, protein lipase C gamma (PLCγ), protein phosphatase 2, and ROCK1 (which regulates cell migration and cell death).

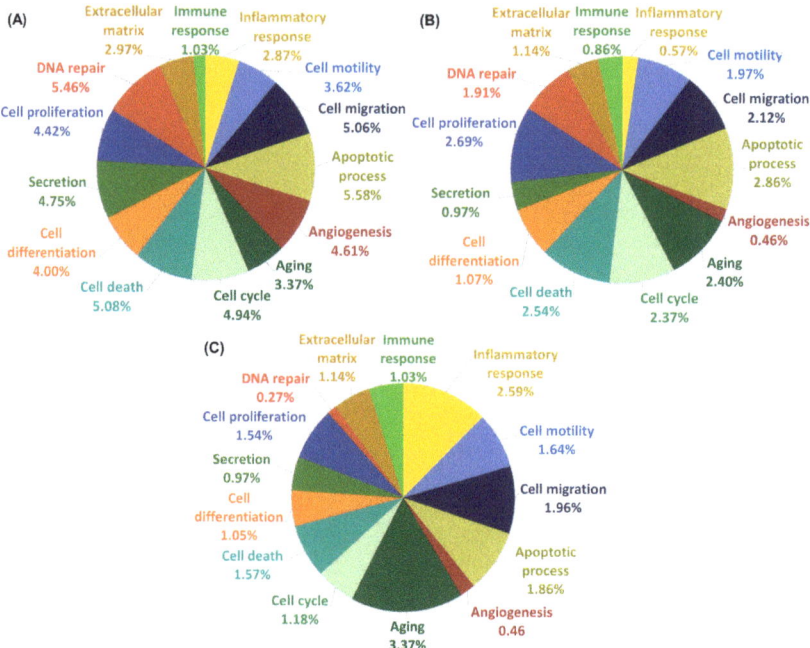

Figure 2. Pie chart representations of the findings from Gene Ontology (GO) biological process annotation analysis of DEGs associated with None vs. HP (**A**), or HP vs. ASTX + HP (**B**), or None vs. ASTX (**C**). The percent fraction of the DEGs annotated with a particular GO biological process is shown for each of the three pairs of experimental systems compared.

The overlap in the biological processes identified by the GO annotation analysis represented in Figure 2 centers on cell proliferation, apoptosis, and migration/motility. As the combined cell migration and cell motility categories make up the largest fraction of shared DEG annotations, we carried out further analysis of the DEGs that fall in these two categories. We were particularly interested in identifying the DEGs within this combined category that are upregulated in AGS cells in response to *H. pylori* infection but are not upregulated in AGS cells treated with ASTX prior to *H. pylori* infection. Accordingly, the normalized (log2) read counts determined for the DEGs of interest are reported in

Table 1, and depicted in the heatmap shown in Figure 3. These results were used to construct a signal transduction pathway that governs cell migration/mobility and that is upregulated in AGS cells in response to *H. pylori* infection but not upregulated or upregulated to a smaller extent in cells treated with ASTX prior to infection. This pathway is presented and discussed in the following section.

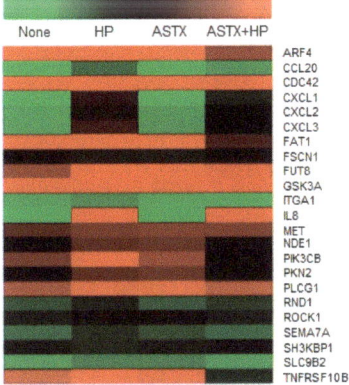

Figure 3. Heatmap representation of the expression levels of DEGs associated with cell migration/motility, which are upregulated in AGS cells in response to *H. pylori* infection but experience less, or no upregulation, in infected cells pretreated with ASTX. The normalized expression levels are reported in Table 1. The color gradient from green to red corresponds to increasing gene expression.

Table 1. Expression levels of DEGs associated with cell migration/motility, which are upregulated in AGS cells in response to *H. pylori* infection but experience less, or no upregulation, in infected cells pretreated with ASTX. The expression level of each gene is reported as the read count normalized to the log2 value.

Gene ID	Normalized (log2) Read Count				Encoded Protein
	None	HP	ASTX	ASTX + HP	
ARF4	7.424	8.152	8.192	6.187	ADP-ribosylation factor 4
CCL20	0.116	2.928	0.000	2.179	Chemokine C-C motif ligand 20
CDC42	9.142	9.921	9.389	6.982	Cell division control protein 42 homolog
CXCL1	1.005	5.432	1.348	4.080	Chemokine C-X-C motif ligand 1
CXCL2	2.008	5.274	2.124	4.697	Chemokine C-X-C motif ligand 2
CXCL3	2.023	5.557	2.193	4.950	Chemokine C-X-C motif ligand 3
FAT1	7.348	8.019	8.158	5.615	FAT atypical cadherin 1
FUT8	6.201	7.140	7.199	6.646	Fucosyltransferase 8 alpha 1,6 fucosyltransferase
GSK3A	7.385	8.294	8.267	8.362	Glycogen synthase kinase 3 alpha
ITGA1	1.946	2.266	1.831	1.728	Integrin alpha 1
IL8	0.704	7.118	0.341	6.954	Interleukin 8
MET	5.712	6.961	6.059	6.022	Met proto-oncogene
NDE1	5.108	5.734	5.819	5.165	Nude neurodevelopment protein 1
PIK3CB	5.937	7.222	6.233	4.757	Phosphatidylinositol-4,5-bisphosphate 3-kinase catalytic subunit beta
PKN2	4.999	5.727	5.828	4.947	Protein kinase N2
PLCG1	6.315	6.806	6.962	6.451	Phospholipase C gamma-1
RND1	3.343	4.082	3.228	3.647	Rho family GTPase 1
ROCK1	4.122	4.820	4.957	4.123	Rho-associated coiled-coil containing protein kinase 1
SEMA7A	2.916	3.803	3.406	2.948	Semaphoring 7A GPI membrane anchor
SLC9B2	2.137	2.614	2.601	2.130	Solute carrier family 9 subfamily B2
TNFRSF10B	6.533	7.260	6.763	3.900	Tumor necrosis factor receptor superfamily member 10b

2.3. Functional Pathway Analysis of DEGs Altered by H. pylori Infection but Normalized by ASTX Pretreatment

Having identified the DEGs associated with cell motility and migration that are protected by ASTX from upregulation by *H. pylori* infection, our next step was to map them onto a signal transduction network, which we generated using the KEGG database and input from published studies of cell motility/migration signaling pathways. As illustrated in Figure 4, signaling is initiated by cytokine CXCL-mediated activation of the chemokine receptor CXCR, or by growth factor-mediated activation of a receptor tyrosine kinase. The cytokines CXCL1, CXCL2, and CXCL3 are among the DEGs through which ASTX mitigates *H. pylori*-induced upregulation (Table 1). In addition, the MET gene, which encodes the receptor tyrosine kinase c-MET (also known as HGF receptor), is also subject to upregulation by *H. pylori* and partially suppressed by AGS cell pretreatment with ASTX.

DEGs listed in Table 1 that impact downstream cell motility/migration signaling are PLCG1 (encodes phospholipase C gamma 1 (PLCγ1)), PIK3CB (encodes phosphatidylinositol-4,5-bisphosphate 3-kinase C2β (PI3KC2β)), CDC42 (encodes cell division control protein homolog 42 (Cdc42)), and ROCK1 (encodes Rho-associated coiled-coil containing protein kinase 1 (ROCK)). PI3KC2β and PLCγ1 have been implicated in the promotion of cytoskeleton rearrangement and cell motility [36]. Cdc42 and ROCK1 serve to transmit signals from PI3K and PLCγ to downstream partners. As is described under Section 2.4, c-MET, PI3KC2β, PLCγ1, Cdc42, and ROCK1 mRNA levels were determined to verify the RNA-seq results, and to compare the effects of *H. pylori* infection, and ASTX pretreatment, on the level of transcription.

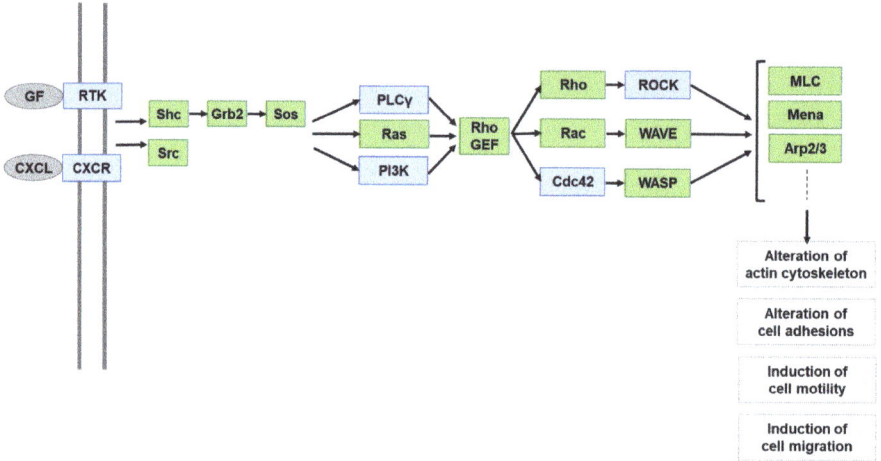

Figure 4. Depiction of a cancer cell motility and migration signaling network model that includes DEGs identified by RNA-seq analysis (Table 1) as displaying upregulated genes in *H. pylori*-infected in AGS cells. The DEG-encoded proteins are colored blue and the suggested pathway mediators are colored green.

2.4. Determinations of c-MET, PI3KC2β, PLCγ1, Cdc42, and ROCK1 mRNA Levels in H. pylori-Infected AGS Cells, with and without ASTX Pretreatment

To compare the transcriptional level of the DEGs encoding c-MET, PI3KC2β, PLCγ1, Cdc42, and ROCK1 in *H. pylori*-infected AGS cells with and without ASTX pretreatment, real-time PCR was carried out. The results reported in Figure 5 show that *H. pylori* infection increases the respective mRNA levels in the absence of ASTX pretreatment, whereas *H. pylori* infection of ASTX-pretreated cells had little or no effect on the mRNA levels.

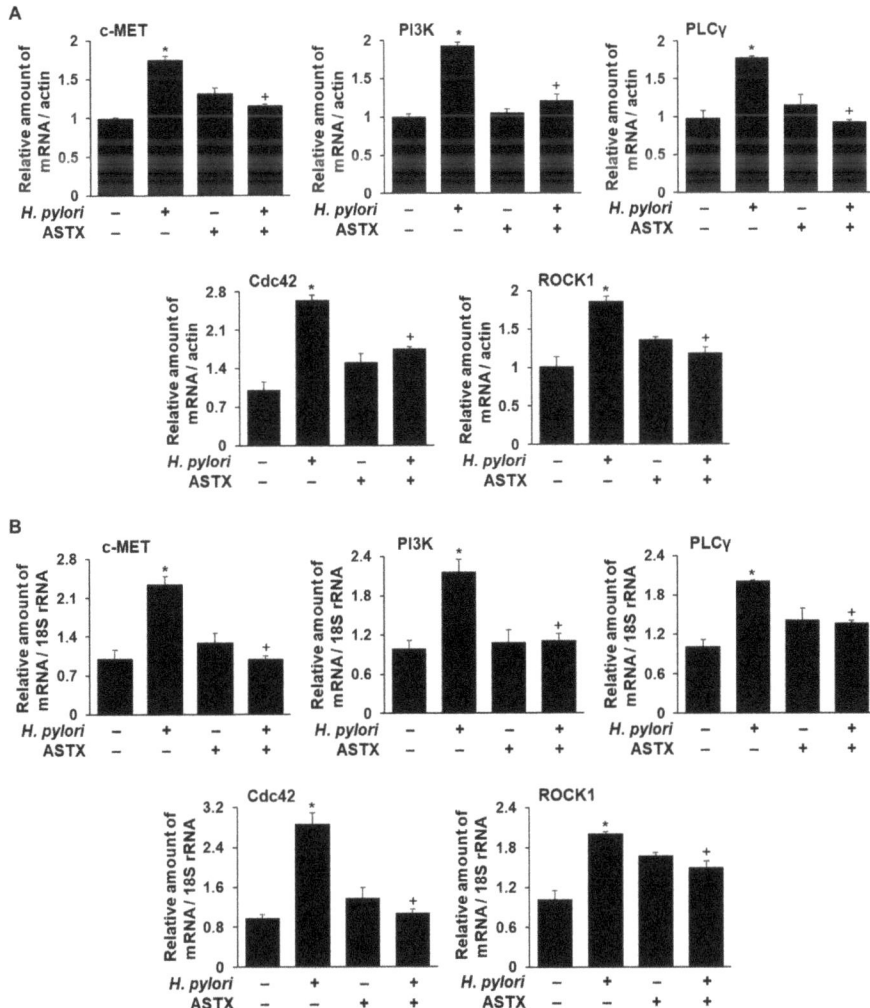

Figure 5. Changes in the levels of mRNAs encoding c-MET, PI3KC2β, PLCγ1, Cdc42, and ROCK1 in *H. pylori*-infected AGS cells, with and without ASTX pretreatment, determined by real-time PCR. AGS cells were pretreated with vehicle (DMSO) or 5 μM ASTX for 3 h and then incubated with *H. pylori* at a 1:50 cell ratio for 1 h. The relative amounts of c-MET, PI3KC2β, PLCγ1, Cdc42, and ROCK1 mRNA in AGS cells were measured by real-time PCR. The mRNA levels were normalized to that of β-actin (**A**) or 18S rRNA (**B**). All values are expressed as the mean ± S.E. For each experiment, the number of each group was three ($n = 3$ per each group). A Student's *t*-test was used for statistical analysis. * $p < 0.05$ vs. uninfected cells; + $p < 0.05$ vs. *H. pylori*-infected cells without ASTX treatment.

3. Discussion

Cell migration, which is essential to cancer metastasis, is triggered by coordinated modulation of the cytoskeleton and cell–cell and cell–substratum adhesions. A moving cell extends itself at the front by creating protrusions in the intended direction and by making new focal adhesions with the substratum. On the rear ends of the cell, the cell contracts itself and releases its adhesions from the substratum. *H. pylori* infection triggers the inflammatory response which directly correlates to higher rate of gastric cancer progression by stimulating cell proliferation, migration, angiogenesis, and invasion [44–46]. Al-Ghoul et al. investigated the association of cagPAI type IV secretion system in cell motility and IL-8 release, and found out that *H. pylori* that induced high secretion of IL-8 in AGS cells were the ones that are capable of triggering cell motility response in the cells [44]. mRNA expression of IL-8 was notably increased starting from 1 h incubation with *H. pylori*, and IL-8 was affecting most of the early phase signal pathways in AGS cells infected with *H. pylori*, especially around 1 h of infection [47,48]. Major signaling pathways leading to migration and invasion, such as PI3K/Akt, PLCγ, and MAPKs such as p38 and ERK, were activated at early time points of *H. pylori* infection around 30–60 min [47,49,50]. The downstream effectors such as c-Met, Rac1, and Cdc42 were detected in AGS cells at 1 h after *H. pylori* infection [22,51,52]. In this study, preliminary data showed marked increase of IL-8 mRNA expression level from 1 h incubation with *H. pylori*, and thus we aimed to find out which signaling networks are turned on during the first phase response of short-term *H. pylori* infection.

GO analysis of the DEGs identified by RNA-Seq analysis of ASTX-pretreated, *H. pylori*-infected AGS cells, identified 23 DEGs that are associated with cytoskeleton-remodeling, cell-motility, and cell-migration signaling pathways (Figure 3, Table 1). We focused our attention on five of these, namely the c-MET, PI3KC2β, PLCγ1, Cdc42, and ROCK1 encoding genes, and demonstrated that their transcription is upregulated by *H. pylori*, but significantly less so in ASTX-pretreated AGS cells (Figure 5).

The HGF receptor c-Met is known to be an upstream regulator of cell migration [53]. It is highly expressed in cancer cells, where it promotes actin cytoskeleton rearrangement and cell motility [54]. It has also been demonstrated that micro-RNA-499a-mediated suppression of non-small cell lung cancer cell migration and invasion occurs via downregulation of c-MET gene expression [55]. In addition, Churin et al. reported that expression of the c-MET gene is activated within 30 min following *H. pylori* infection of AGS cells, and that this activation is required for *H. pylori*-induced cell motility and scattering [49]. We found that ASTX treatment significantly reduces upregulated c-MET gene expression in *H. pylori*-infected AGS cells (Table 1, Figure 3). Thus, ASTX might target c-Met to suppress AGS cell migration.

The downstream regulators PI3K and PLCγ facilitate the cell motility cascade by modulating the level of phosphatidylinositol 4,5-bisphosphate (PIP2) [56–58]. PI3K generates phosphatidylinositol 3,4,5-trisphosphate (PIP3) from PIP2, or generates PIP2 from phosphatidylinositol 4-phosphate (PIP), thereby facilitating Rho GEF activation and membrane targeting. PI3K is an essential mediator of *H. pylori*-induced AGS cell migration [59]. In previous studies, ASTX treatment reduced invasive behavior of breast cancer cells and oral carcinoma cells by inhibiting PI3K signaling [42,43]. In a recent study carried out with oral squamous cell carcinoma models, Kowshik et al. reported that ASTX inhibits hallmarks of cancer by targeting the PI3K/NF-κB/STAT3 signaling axis [43]. PLCγ is also an important mediator of cell migration in response to growth factor receptor activation [60,61]. PLCγ modulates the level of PIP2, which in turn governs the activation of Rho family proteins as well as actin-modifying proteins such as the actin-severing cofilin [62]. In the present study, we showed that ASTX suppresses upregulation of the transcription of PI3KC2 and PLCγ1, and their downstream targets ROCK1 and Cdc42 resulting from *H. pylori* infection of AGS cells.

4. Materials and Methods

4.1. Cell Line and Culture Conditions

The human gastric adenocarcinoma cell line AGS (ATCC CRL 1739) was purchased from the American Type Culture Collection (ATCC; Rockville, MD, USA). AGS cells were grown in RPMI 1640 medium (Gibco, Grand Island, NY, USA) supplemented with 10% fetal bovine serum (FBS) (Gibco, Grand Island, NY, USA), 100 U/mL penicillin, and 100 µg/mL streptomycin. The cells were cultured at 37 °C under a humidified atmosphere consisting of 95% air and 5% CO_2.

4.2. Treatment of AGS Cells with ASTX

ASTX (Sigma-Aldrich, St. Louis, MO, USA) was dissolved in dimethyl sulfoxide (DMSO) (Sigma-Aldrich, St. Louis, MO, USA) and stored under nitrogen at −80 °C. Before use, the ASTX stock solution was thawed at 70 °C and added to FBS to achieve the desired concentration. Prior to their infection with *H. pylori*, AGS cells were preincubated with pure DMSO diluted by FBS at 0.05% final concentration (v/v) (vehicle control) or with 5 μM ASTX for 3 h. The indicated dose and incubation time of ASTX were chosen based on our previous study that demonstrated the inhibitory effect of ASTX on mitochondrial dysfunction and inflammation in *H. pylori*-infected AGS cells [63]. In particular, 5 μM ASTX exhibited antioxidative effects in AGS cells when preincubated for 3 h.

4.3. Bacterial Strain and H. pylori Infection

The *H. pylori* strain NCTC 11637 was obtained from ATCC. The bacterial cells were grown on chocolate agar plates (Becton Dickinson Microbiology Systems, Cockeysville, MD, USA) at 37 °C, under microaerophilic conditions, using an anaerobic chamber (BBL Campy Pouch® System, Becton Dickinson Microbiology Systems, Franklin Lakes, NJ, USA). AGS cells were seeded and cultured overnight to reach 80% confluency. The *H. pylori* was harvested from the plates, suspended in antibiotic-free RPMI 1640 medium supplemented with 10% fetal bovine serum, and then added to the AGS cell culture at a cellular ratio of 50:1. AGS cells (1.5×10^5/mL) were pretreated with 5 μM ASTX or the control vehicle DMSO for 3 h prior to *H. pylori* stimulation. The cells were then incubated with *H. pylori* for 1 h (for preparation of RNA extracts and for determination of mRNA gene expressions).

4.4. Preparation of Total RNA Extracts and Library Construction

Total RNA extract was isolated using TRI reagent (Molecular Research Center, Cincinnati, OH, USA) and then cleaned and concentrated using the RNeasy MinElute Cleanup Kit (Quiagen, Valencia, CA, USA) according to the manufacturer's protocol. Following determination of the total RNA concentration in each extract, the extracts from three replicate experiments were pooled for RNA-Seq library construction.

AmpliSeq libraries were constructed and sequenced using the Ion Torrent S5™ XL next-generation sequencing system (ThermoFisher Scientific, Waltham, MA, USA) in conjunction with the Ion AmpliSeq Transcriptome Human Gene Expression Kit, according to the manufacturer's instructions. For each sample, 30 ng of total RNA was used for cDNA library preparation. Multiple libraries were multiplexed and clonally amplified using the Ion Chef System (Thermo Fisher Scientific, Waltham, MA, USA), and then sequenced. The ampliSeq RNA Plug in (ver 5.6.0.3) by Torrent Suite Software (Thermo Fisher Scientific, Waltham, MA, USA) was used for data analysis.

4.5. RNA-Sequencing and Bioinformatics Analysis

The total RNA library was subjected to transcriptome sequencing carried out by e-Biogen (www.e-biogen.com, Seoul, Korea). ExDEGA (Excel-based Differentially Expressed Gene Analysis) software (e-Biogen, Seoul, Korea) was used for initial data processing and analysis for differentially expressed genes (DEGs).

Differential gene expression analysis was performed with ExDEGA v1.6.8 software and using a cutoff at the normalized gene expression (log2) of 2 and *p*-value of <0.05. DEGs were identified based on >1.5-fold change observed in transcript levels. After filtering the DEGs, Gene Ontology (GO) analysis was performed using the DAVID bioinformatics program (https://david.ncifcrf.gov), for gene identification and annotation. To identify the functional groups and molecular pathways associated with the observed DEGs, RNA-Seq data were further analyzed using the Kyoto Encyclopedia of Genes and Genomes (KEGG) database (www.genome.jp).

4.6. Validation of DEGs by Real-Time Polymerase Chain Reaction (PCR)

Real-time PCR was performed to validate the expression profiles of DEGs identified from RNA-Seq analysis. Candidate genes were selected in relation to the category of function. Total RNA was isolated using TRI reagent (Molecular Research Center, Cincinnati, OH, USA). Conversion of the RNA to cDNA was carried out by incubating the RNA sample with a random nucleotide hexamer and MuLV reverse transcriptase (Promega, Madison, WI, USA) at 23 °C for 10 min, 37 °C for 60 min, and 95 °C for 5 min. The cDNA was used for real-time PCR with primers specific for human. The sequences of the primers used are 5′-TGCACAGTTGGTCCTGCCATGA-3′ (forward) and 5′-CAGCCATAGGACCGTATTTCGG-3′ (reverse) for c-MET, 5′-TTGTCTGTCACACTTCTGTAGTT-3′ (forward) and 5′-AACAGTTCCCATTGGATTCAACA-3′ (reverse) for PI3KC2β, 5′-TCGTATATCAGCCAAGGACC-3′ (forward) and 5′-AGTACTGGCTTCCAAGAAGG-3′ (reverse) for PLCγ1, 5′-GATGGTGCTGTTGGTAAA-3′ (forward) and 5′-TAACTCAGCGGTCGTAAT-3′ (reverse) for Cdc42, 5′-ATGAGTTTATTCCTACACTCTACCACTTTC-3′ (forward) and 5′-TAACATGGCATCTTCGACGACACTCTAG-3′ (reverse) for ROCK1. For PCR amplification, the cDNA was amplified by 45 repeat denaturation cycles at 95 °C for 30 s, annealing at 55 °C for 30 s, and extension at 72 °C for 30 s. During the first cycle, the 95 °C step was extended to 3 min. The β-actin and 18S rRNA gene was amplified in the same reaction to serve as the reference gene. For β-actin and 18S rRNA, the desired PCR product was obtained using the primer 5′-ACCAACTGGGACGACATGGAG-3′ (forward) and 5′-GTGAGGATCTTCATGAGGTAGTC-3′ (reverse), and 5′-GTAACCCGTTGAACCCCATT-3′ (forward) and 5′-CCATCCAATCGGTAGTAGCG-3′ (reverse), respectively. The relative gene expression of c-MET, PI3KC2β, PLCγ1, Cdc42, and ROCK1 mRNA were normalized to that of β-actin or 18S rRNA.

4.7. Statistical Analysis

For the changes in the levels of mRNAs encoding c-MET, PI3KC2β, PLCγ1, Cdc42, and ROCK1 in *H. pylori*-infected AGS cells, all values are expressed as the mean ± S.E. For each experiment, the number of each group was three ($n = 3$ per each group). A Student's *t*-test was used for statistical analysis. A *p*-value of 0.05 or less was considered statistically significant.

5. Conclusions

Transcriptional array profiling by RNA-Seq analysis of *H. pylori*-infected AGS cells, and *H. pylori*-infected AGS cells pretreated with ASTX was carried out to identify potential mediators in the inhibitory mechanism of ASTX on *H. pylori*-induced inflammatory and carcinogenic responses. Our findings indicate that ASTX can suppress *H. pylori*-induced gastric cancer progression by inhibiting cytoskeleton reorganization and reducing cell motility through downregulation of c-MET, EGFR, PI3KC2, PLCγ1, Cdc42, and ROCK1.

Author Contributions: S.H.K. drafted the manuscript and H.K. edited the manuscript. Both authors have read and agreed to the published version of the manuscript.

Funding: This study was supported by a grant from the National Research Foundation (NRF) of Korea, which is funded by the Korean Government (NRF-2018R1A2B2005575).

Conflicts of Interest: The authors declare no conflicts of interest.

References

1. Bray, F.; Ferlay, J.; Soerjomataram, I.; Siegel, R.L.; Torre, L.A.; Jemal, A. Global cancer statistics 2018: GLOBOCAN estimates of incidence and mortality worldwide for 36 cancers in 185 countries. *CA Cancer J. Clin.* **2018**, *68*, 394–424. [CrossRef] [PubMed]
2. Parkin, D.M. The global health burden of infection-associated cancers in the year 2002. *Int. J. Cancer* **2006**, *118*, 3030–3044. [CrossRef] [PubMed]

3. Riihimäki, M.; Hemminki, A.; Sundquist, K.; Sundquist, J.; Hemminki, K. Metastatic spread in patients with gastric cancer. *Oncotarget* **2016**, *7*, 52307–52310. [CrossRef]
4. Gupta, G.P.; Massagué, J. Cancer metastasis: Building a framework. *Cell* **2006**, *127*, 679–695. [CrossRef] [PubMed]
5. Weinberg, R.A. *The Biology of Cancer*, 2nd ed.; Norton & Company: New York, NY, USA, 2013; Chapter 14; ISBN 978-08-1534-528-2.
6. Jouanneau, J.; Thiery, J.P. Tumor cell motility and invasion. In *Encyclopedia of Cancer*, 2nd ed.; Academic Press: Cambridge, MA, USA, 2002; pp. 467–473. ISBN 978-01-2227-555-5.
7. Mitchison, T.J.; Cramer, L.P. Actin-based cell motility and cell locomotion. *Cell* **1996**, *84*, 371–379. [CrossRef]
8. Lauffenburger, D.A.; Horwitz, A.F. Cell migration: A physically integrated molecular process. *Cell* **1996**, *84*, 359–369. [CrossRef]
9. Jacquemet, G.; Hamidi, H.; Ivaska, J. Filopodia in cell adhesion, 3D migration and cancer cell migration. *Curr. Opin. Cell Biol.* **2015**, *36*, 23–31. [CrossRef]
10. Parri, M.; Chiarugi, P. Rac and Rho GTPases in cancer cell motility control. *Cell Commun. Signal.* **2010**, *8*, 23. [CrossRef]
11. Raftopoulou, M.; Hall, A. Cell migration: Rho GTPases lead the way. *Dev. Biol.* **2004**, *265*, 23–32. [CrossRef]
12. Kedrin, D.; van Rheenen, J.; Hernandez, L.; Condeelis, J.; Segall, J.E. Cell motility and cytoskeletal regulation in invasion and metastasis. *J. Mammary Gland Biol.* **2007**, *12*, 143–152. [CrossRef]
13. Normanno, N.; De Luca, A.; Bianco, C.; Strizzi, L.; Mancino, M.; Maiello, M.R.; Carotenuto, A.; De Feo, G.; Caponigro, F.; Salomon, D.S. Epidermal growth factor receptor (EGFR) signaling in cancer. *Gene* **2006**, *366*, 2–16. [CrossRef]
14. Birchmeier, C.; Birchmeier, W.; Gherardi, E.; Woude, G.F.V. Met, metastasis, motility and more. *Nat. Rev. Mol. Cell Biol.* **2003**, *4*, 915–925. [CrossRef]
15. Guillemin, K.; Salama, N.R.; Tompkins, L.S.; Falkow, S. Cag pathogenicity island-specific responses of gastric epithelial cells to *Helicobacter pylori* infection. *Proc. Natl. Acad. Sci. USA* **2002**, *99*, 15136–15141. [CrossRef] [PubMed]
16. Peek, R.M.; Blaser, M.J. *Helicobacter pylori* and gastrointestinal tract adenocarcinomas. *Nat. Rev. Cancer* **2002**, *2*, 28–37. [CrossRef]
17. Wessler, S.; Gimona, M.; Rieder, G. Regulation of the actin cytoskeleton in *Helicobacter pylori*-induced migration and invasive growth of gastric epithelial cells. *Cell Commun. Signal.* **2011**, *9*, 27. [CrossRef] [PubMed]
18. Wu, C.Y.; Wang, C.J.; Tseng, C.C.; Chen, H.P.; Wu, M.S.; Lin, J.T.; Inoue, H.; Chen, G.H. *Helicobacter pylori* promote gastric cancer cells invasion through a NF-kB and COX-2-mediated pathway. *World J. Gastroenterol.* **2005**, *11*, 3197. [CrossRef] [PubMed]
19. Segal, E.D.; Falkow, S.; Tompkins, L.S. *Helicobacter pylori* attachment to gastric cells induces cytoskeletal rearrangements and tyrosine phosphorylation of host cell proteins. *Proc. Natl. Acad. Sci. USA* **1996**, *93*, 1259–1264. [CrossRef]
20. Wessler, S.; Backert, S. Molecular mechanisms of epithelial-barrier disruption by *Helicobacter pylori*. *Trends Microbiol.* **2008**, *16*, 397–405. [CrossRef]
21. Yin, Y.; Grabowska, A.M.; Clarke, P.A.; Whelband, E.; Robinson, K.; Argent, R.H.; Tobias, A.; Kumari, R.; Atherton, J.C.; Watson, S.A. Helicobacter pylori potentiates epithelial: Mesenchymal transition in gastric cancer: Links to soluble HB-EGF, gastrin and matrix metalloproteinase-7. *Gut* **2010**, *59*, 1037–1045. [CrossRef]
22. Churin, Y.; Kardalinou, E.; Meyer, T.F.; Naumann, M. Pathogenicity island-dependent activation of Rho GTPases Rac1 and Cdc42 in *Helicobacter pylori* infection. *Mol. Microbiol.* **2001**, *40*, 815–823. [CrossRef]
23. Higashi, H.; Nakaya, A.; Tsutsumi, R.; Yokoyama, K.; Fujii, Y.; Ishikawa, S.; Higuchi, M.; Takahashi, A.; Kurashima, Y.; Teishikata, Y.; et al. *Helicobacter pylori* CagA induces Ras-independent morphogenetic response through SHP-2 recruitment and activation. *J. Biol. Chem.* **2004**, *279*, 17205–17216. [CrossRef] [PubMed]
24. Suzuki, M.; Mimuro, H.; Suzuki, T.; Park, M.; Yamamoto, T.; Sasakawa, C. Interaction of CagA with Crk plays an important role in *Helicobacter pylori*–induced loss of gastric epithelial cell adhesion. *J. Exp. Med.* **2005**, *202*, 1235–1247. [CrossRef] [PubMed]
25. Bagnoli, F.; Buti, L.; Tompkins, L.; Covacci, A.; Amieva, M.R. *Helicobacter pylori* CagA induces a transition from polarized to invasive phenotypes in MDCK cells. *Proc. Natl. Acad. Sci. USA* **2005**, *102*, 16339–16344. [CrossRef] [PubMed]

26. Segal, E.D.; Cha, J.; Lo, J.; Falkow, S.; Tompkins, L.S. Altered states: Involvement of phosphorylated CagA in the induction of host cellular growth changes by *Helicobacter pylori*. *Proc. Natl. Acad. Sci. USA* **1999**, *96*, 14559–14564. [CrossRef] [PubMed]
27. Keates, S.; Sougioultzis, S.; Keates, A.C.; Zhao, D.; Peek, R.M.; Shaw, L.M.; Kelly, C.P. cag+ *Helicobacter pylori* induce transactivation of the epidermal growth factor receptor in AGS gastric epithelial cells. *J. Biol. Chem.* **2001**, *276*, 48127–48134. [CrossRef] [PubMed]
28. Mimuro, H.; Suzuki, T.; Tanaka, J.; Asahi, M.; Haas, R.; Sasakawa, C. Grb2 is a key mediator of *Helicobacter pylori* CagA protein activities. *Mol. Cell* **2002**, *10*, 745–755. [CrossRef]
29. Tsutsumi, R.; Takahashi, A.; Azuma, T.; Higashi, H.; Hatakeyama, M. Focal adhesion kinase is a substrate and downstream effector of SHP-2 complexed with *Helicobacter pylori* CagA. *Mol. Cell. Biol.* **2006**, *26*, 261–276. [CrossRef] [PubMed]
30. Palovuori, R.; Perttu, A.; Yan, Y.; Karttunen, R.; Eskelinen, S.; Karttunen, T.J. *Helicobacter pylori* induces formation of stress fibers and membrane ruffles in AGS cells by rac activation. *Biochem. Biophys. Res. Commun.* **2001**, *269*, 247–253. [CrossRef] [PubMed]
31. Wroblewski, L.E.; Noble, P.J.; Pagliocca, A.; Pritchard, D.M.; Hart, C.A.; Campbell, F.; Dodson, A.R.; Dockray, G.J.; Varro, A. Stimulation of MMP-7 (matrilysin) by *Helicobacter pylori* in human gastric epithelial cells: Role in epithelial cell migration. *J. Cell Sci.* **2003**, *116*, 3017–3026. [CrossRef]
32. Yuan, J.P.; Peng, J.; Yin, K.; Wang, J.H. Potential health-promoting effects of astaxanthin: A high-value carotenoid mostly from microalgae. *Mol. Nutr. Food Res.* **2001**, *55*, 150–165. [CrossRef]
33. Higuera-Ciapara, I.; Felix-Valenzuela, L.; Goycoolea, F.M. Astaxanthin: A review of its chemistry and applications. *Crit. Rev. Food Sci. Nutr.* **2006**, *46*, 185–196. [CrossRef] [PubMed]
34. Ambati, R.R.; Phang, S.M.; Ravi, S.; Aswathanarayana, R.G. Astaxanthin: Sources, extraction, stability, biological activities and its commercial applications—A review. *Mar. Drugs* **2014**, *12*, 128–152. [CrossRef] [PubMed]
35. Zhang, L.; Wang, H. Multiple mechanisms of anti-cancer effects exerted by astaxanthin. *Mar. Drugs* **2015**, *13*, 4310–4330. [CrossRef]
36. Kim, J.H.; Park, J.J.; Lee, B.J.; Joo, M.K.; Chun, H.J.; Lee, S.W.; Bak, Y.T. Astaxanthin inhibits proliferation of human gastric cancer cell lines by interrupting cell cycle progression. *Gut Liver.* **2016**, *10*, 369. [CrossRef]
37. Kozuki, Y.; Miura, Y.; Yagasaki, K. Inhibitory effects of carotenoids on the invasion of rat ascites hepatoma cells in culture. *Cancer Lett.* **2000**, *151*, 111–115. [CrossRef]
38. Su, X.Z.; Chen, R.; Wang, C.B.; Ouyang, X.L.; Jiang, Y.; Zhu, M.Y. Astaxanthin combine with human serum albumin to abrogate cell proliferation, migration, and drug-resistant in human ovarian carcinoma SKOV3 cells. *Anti-Cancer Agents Med. Chem.* **2019**, *19*, 792–801. [CrossRef]
39. McCall, B.; McPartland, C.K.; Moore, R.; Frank-Kamenetskii, A.; Booth, B.W. Effects of astaxanthin on the proliferation and migration of breast cancer cells in vitro. *Antioxidants* **2018**, *7*, 135. [CrossRef]
40. Kim, H.Y.; Kim, Y.M.; Hong, S. Astaxanthin suppresses the metastasis of colon cancer by inhibiting the MYC-mediated downregulation of microRNA-29a-3p and microRNA-200a. *Sci. Rep.* **2019**, *9*, 1–10. [CrossRef]
41. Chen, Y.T.; Kao, C.J.; Huang, H.Y.; Huang, S.Y.; Chen, C.Y.; Lin, Y.S.; Wen, Z.H.; Wang, H.M.D. Astaxanthin reduces MMP expressions, suppresses cancer cell migrations, and triggers apoptotic caspases of in vitro and in vivo models in melanoma. *J. Funct. Foods* **2017**, *31*, 20–31. [CrossRef]
42. Stadelman, K.M. Astaxanthin Decreases Invasion and MMP Activity in Triple Negative Breast Cancer Cells. Doctoral Dissertation, Wake Forest University, Winston-Salem, NC, USA, 2012.
43. Kowshik, J.; Nivetha, R.; Ranjani, S.; Venkatesan, P.; Selvamuthukumar, S.; Veeravarmal, V.; Nagini, S. Astaxanthin inhibits hallmarks of cancer by targeting the PI3K/NF-κB/STAT3 signalling axis in oral squamous cell carcinoma models. *IUBMB Life* **2019**, *71*, 1595–1610. [CrossRef]
44. Al-Ghoul, L.; Wessler, S.; Hundertmark, T.; Krüger, S.; Fischer, W.; Wunder, C.; Haas, R.; Roessner, A.; Naumann, M. Analysis of the type IV secretion system-dependent cell motility of *Helicobacter pylori*-infected epithelial cells. *Biochem. Biophys. Res. Commun.* **2004**, *322*, 860–866. [CrossRef] [PubMed]
45. Moese, S.; Selbach, M.; Kwok, T.; Brinkmann, V.; König, W.; Meyer, T.F.; Backert, S. *Helicobacter pylori* induces AGS cell motility and elongation via independent signaling pathways. *Infect. Immun.* **2004**, *72*, 3646–3649. [CrossRef] [PubMed]
46. Lee, K.E.; Khoi, P.N.; Xia, Y.; Park, J.S.; Joo, Y.E.; Kim, K.K.; Choi, S.Y.; Jung, Y.D. Helicobacter pylori and interleukin-8 in gastric cancer. *World J. Gastroenterol.* **2013**, *19*, 8192. [CrossRef] [PubMed]

47. Takeshima, E.; Tomimori, K.; Kawakami, H.; Ishikawa, C.; Sawada, S.; Tomita, M.; Senba, M.; Kinjo, F.; Mimuro, H.; Sasakawa, C.; et al. NF-κB activation by Helicobacter pylori requires Akt-mediated phosphorylation of p65. *BMC Microbiol.* **2009**, *9*, 36. [CrossRef] [PubMed]
48. Eftang, L.L.; Esbensen, Y.; Tannæs, T.M.; Bukholm, I.R.; Bukholm, G. Interleukin-8 is the single most up-regulated gene in whole genome profiling of *H. pylori* exposed gastric epithelial cells. *BMC Microbiol.* **2012**, *12*, 9. [CrossRef]
49. Churin, Y.; Al-Ghoul, L.; Kepp, O.; Meyer, T.F.; Birchmeier, W.; Naumann, M. *Helicobacter pylori* CagA protein targets the c-MET receptor and enhances the motogenic response. *J. Cell Biol.* **2003**, *161*, 249–255. [CrossRef]
50. Chang, Y.J.; Wu, M.S.; Lin, J.T.; Chen, C.C. Helicobacter pylori-induced invasion and angiogenesis of gastric cells is mediated by cyclooxygenase-2 induction through TLR2/TLR9 and promoter regulation. *J. Immunol.* **2005**, *175*, 8242–8252. [CrossRef]
51. Xie, C.; Yang, Z.; Hu, Y.; Cao, X.; Chen, J.; Zhu, Y.; Lu, N. Expression of c-Met and hepatocyte growth factor in various gastric pathologies and its association with Helicobacter pylori infection. *Oncol. Lett.* **2017**, *14*, 6151–6155. [CrossRef]
52. Oliveira, M.J.; Costa, A.C.; Costa, A.M.; Henriques, L.; Suriano, G.; Atherton, J.C.; Machado, J.C.; Carneiro, F.; Seruca, R.; Mareel, M.; et al. Helicobacter pylori induces gastric epithelial cell invasion in a c-Met and type IV secretion system-dependent manner. *J. Biol. Chem.* **2006**, *281*, 34888–34896. [CrossRef]
53. Xiang, C.; Chen, J.; Fu, P. HGF/Met signaling in cancer invasion: The impact on cytoskeleton remodeling. *Cancers* **2017**, *9*, 44. [CrossRef]
54. Ma, P.C.; Maulik, G.; Christensen, J.; Salgia, R. c-MET: Structure, functions and potential for therapeutic inhibition. *Cancer Metastasis Rev.* **2003**, *22*, 309–325. [CrossRef] [PubMed]
55. Luo, W.; Huang, B.; Li, Z.; Li, H.; Sun, L.; Zhang, Q.; Qui, X.; Wang, E. MicroRNA-449a is downregulated in non-small cell lung cancer and inhibits migration and invasion by targeting c-MET. *PLoS ONE* **2013**, *8*, e64759. [CrossRef] [PubMed]
56. Yin, H.L.; Janmey, P.A. Phosphoinositide regulation of the actin cytoskeleton. *Annu. Rev. Physiol.* **2003**, *65*, 761–789. [CrossRef] [PubMed]
57. Rei, K.; Nobes, C.D.; Thomas, G.; Hall, A.; Cantrell, D.A. Phosphatidylinositol 3-kinase signals activate a selective subset of Rac/Rho-dependent effector pathways. *Curr. Biol.* **1996**, *6*, 1445–1455. [CrossRef]
58. Rodrigues, G.A.; Falasca, M.; Zhang, Z.; Ong, S.H.; Schlessinger, J. A novel positive feedback loop mediated by the docking protein Gab1 and phosphatidylinositol 3-kinase in epidermal growth factor receptor signaling. *Mol. Cell. Biol.* **2000**, *20*, 1448–1459. [CrossRef]
59. Nagy, T.A.; Frey, M.R.; Yan, F.; Israel, D.A.; Polk, D.B.; Peek, R.M. Helicobacter pylori regulates cellular migration and apoptosis by activation of phosphatidylinositol 3-kinase signaling. *J. Infect. Dis.* **2009**, *199*, 641–651. [CrossRef]
60. Wells, A.; Grandis, J.R. Phospholipase C-γ1 in tumor progression. *Clin. Exp. Metastasis* **2003**, *20*, 285. [CrossRef]
61. Khoshyomn, S.; Penar, P.L.; Rossi, J.; Wellsge, A.; Abramson, D.L.; Bhushan, A. Inhibition of phospholipase C-γ1 activation blocks glioma cell motility and invasion of fetal rat brain aggregates. *Neurosurgery* **1999**, *44*, 568–577. [CrossRef]
62. Mouneimne, G.; Soon, L.; DesMarais, V.; Sidani, M.; Song, X.; Yip, S.C.; Ghosh, M.; Eddy, R.; Backer, J.M.; Condeelis, J. Phospholipase C and cofilin are required for carcinoma cell directionality in response to EGF stimulation. *J. Cell Biol.* **2004**, *166*, 697–708. [CrossRef]
63. Kim, S.H.; Lim, J.W.; Kim, H. Astaxanthin Inhibits Mitochondrial Dysfunction and Interleukin-8 Expression in *Helicobacter pylori*-Infected Gastric Epithelial Cells. *Nutrients* **2018**, *10*, 1320. [CrossRef]

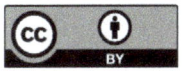 © 2020 by the authors. Licensee MDPI, Basel, Switzerland. This article is an open access article distributed under the terms and conditions of the Creative Commons Attribution (CC BY) license (http://creativecommons.org/licenses/by/4.0/).

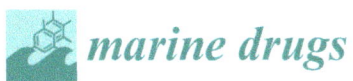

Review

Halophilic Carotenoids and Breast Cancer: From Salt Marshes to Biomedicine

Micaela Giani [1,2,*], Yoel Genaro Montoyo-Pujol [3], Gloria Peiró [4] and Rosa María Martínez-Espinosa [1,2]

[1] Biochemistry and Molecular Biology Division, Agrochemistry and Biochemistry Department, Faculty of Sciences, University of Alicante, Ap. 99, E-03080 Alicante, Spain; rosa.martinez@ua.es

[2] Applied Biochemistry Research Group, Multidisciplinary Institute for Environmental Studies "Ramón Margalef", University of Alicante, Ap. 99, E-03080 Alicante, Spain

[3] Breast Cancer Research Group, Research Unit, Alicante Institute for Health and Biomedical Research (ISABIAL) Hospital General Universitario, Pintor Baeza 12, E-03010 Alicante, Spain; yoelgenaro93@hotmail.com

[4] Department of Pathology, Alicante Institute for Health and Biomedical Research (ISABIAL) Hospital General Universitario, Pintor Baeza 12, E-03010 Alicante, Spain; gloriapeiro@googlemail.com

* Correspondence: micaela.giani@ua.es

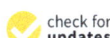

Citation: Giani, M.; Montoyo-Pujol, Y.G.; Peiró, G.; Martínez-Espinosa, R.M. Halophilic Carotenoids and Breast Cancer: From Salt Marshes to Biomedicine. *Mar. Drugs* 2021, *19*, 594. https://doi.org/10.3390/md19110594

Academic Editors: Elena Talero and Javier Ávila-Román

Received: 30 September 2021
Accepted: 20 October 2021
Published: 21 October 2021

Publisher's Note: MDPI stays neutral with regard to jurisdictional claims in published maps and institutional affiliations.

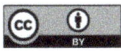

Copyright: © 2021 by the authors. Licensee MDPI, Basel, Switzerland. This article is an open access article distributed under the terms and conditions of the Creative Commons Attribution (CC BY) license (https://creativecommons.org/licenses/by/4.0/).

Abstract: Breast cancer is the leading cause of death among women worldwide. Over the years, oxidative stress has been linked to the onset and progression of cancer. In addition to the classical histological classification, breast carcinomas are classified into phenotypes according to hormone receptors (estrogen receptor—RE—/progesterone receptor—PR) and growth factor receptor (human epidermal growth factor receptor—HER2) expression. Luminal tumors (ER/PR-positive/HER2-negative) are present in older patients with a better outcome. However, patients with HER2-positive or triple-negative breast cancer (TNBC) (ER/PR/HER2-negative) subtypes still represent highly aggressive behavior, metastasis, poor prognosis, and drug resistance. Therefore, new alternative therapies have become an urgent clinical need. In recent years, anticancer agents based on natural products have been receiving huge interest. In particular, carotenoids are natural compounds present in fruits and vegetables, but algae, bacteria, and archaea also produce them. The antioxidant properties of carotenoids have been studied during the last years due to their potential in preventing and treating multiple diseases, including cancer. Although the effect of carotenoids on breast cancer during in vitro and in vivo studies is promising, clinical trials are still inconclusive. The haloarchaeal carotenoid bacterioruberin holds great promise to the future of biomedicine due to its particular structure, and antioxidant activity. However, much work remains to be performed to draw firm conclusions. This review summarizes the current knowledge on pre-clinical and clinical analysis on the use of carotenoids as chemopreventive and chemotherapeutic agents in breast cancer, highlighting the most recent results regarding the use of bacterioruberin from haloarchaea.

Keywords: breast cancer; carotenoids; bacterioruberin; oxidative stress; antioxidant; pro-oxidant

1. Introduction

Reactive nitrogen (RNS) and oxygen (ROS) species are metabolic by-products generated by all biological systems. More specifically, superoxide radicals ($O_2^{\bullet-}$), hydroxyl radicals ($\bullet OH$), singlet oxygen ($^1O_2$), and hydrogen peroxide (H_2O_2) are the most frequent ROS produced [1]. An equilibrium between ROS production and metabolization is required for most biological processes to function. When there is an imbalance in favor of ROS production, most biomolecules and cellular structures are negatively affected. Over the years, it has been repeatedly reported how oxidative stress can be one of the causes behind the onset and progression of many pathologies, including cancer, heart disease, or diabetes [2].

Cancer is considered a multi-stage process in which genetic and epigenetic alterations accumulate. These alterations produce the dominant activation of different oncogenes and the inactivation of tumor suppressor genes, ultimately leading to the malignant transformation of healthy cells [3,4]. Although a small percentage of human cancers are linked to genetic inheritance, the vast majority are caused by infections, chemical exposure and factors regarding lifestyle, such as smoking, diet, and UV radiation [5]. Over the last decades, there has been a constant rise in research focused on oxidative stress, inflammation, and cancer [6,7]. Antioxidants can counteract oxidative stress, thus helping prevent and delay in the development of this neoplasia [8].

Over the last years, there has been an increasing interest in microbes as natural sources for the production of carotenoids due to their remarkable antioxidant properties. The use of microbial species can be very advantageous since they produce high rates of carotenoids which can be isolated using environmentally friendly approaches; thus reducing the cost and the environmental impact compared to the chemical synthesis of carotenoids [9,10]. Extremophilic microorganisms that inhabit solar salterns (halophilic microbes) are usually exposed to high levels of oxidative stress as a consequence of high solar radiation or high temperatures (up to 50 °C in summer). In response to this stress, they have developed several molecular adaptations, such as the synthesis of carotenoids, which are very active against ROS [11]. Thus, it was described that extreme halophilic microorganisms belonging to Archaea domain (haloarchaea) can produce carotenoids, particularly rare carotenoids containing 50 carbon units, being bacterioruberin the most abundant. Haloarchaeal C_{50} carotenoids have caught the attention of many researchers due to their particular structures, which would provide them with higher scavenger activity than their C_{40} counterparts [12]. However, the actual beneficial effect of these natural antioxidants on human health is yet to be determined.

In this review, we summarize the recent advance in the use of carotenoids in preventing and treating breast cancer, highlighting the potential of bacterioruberin.

2. Breast Cancer Epidemiology

Breast cancer is one of the most frequent malignancies worldwide, representing 11.7% of all cancers [13]. This neoplasia is considered genetically and clinically heterogeneous, including various subtypes, with distinct histopathological patterns and molecular characteristics, resulting in different responses to therapies and prognosis [14–16]. Although mortality risk decreases every year in developed countries, breast cancer incidence increases [13]. Even though there are differences between countries, it is still the leading cause of death in women between 20 and 50 years [17]. However, only less than 10% of breast cancers are thought to be hereditary. Most cases are associated with lifestyle choices, dietary habits, and environmental and reproductive factors that increase the risk of breast cancer and other chronic diseases [18,19]. Significant efforts are currently being made to develop new and improved detection strategies, therapeutic targets, and better treatments. About two decades ago, Perou and colleagues proposed an "intrinsic genetic signature" made up of 496 genes [14]. This genetic signature allowed the classification of breast cancer into four molecular subtypes, representing different biological and clinical entities [14]. Subsequent studies have made it possible to redefine these molecular subtypes [20–22]. However, despite different nomenclatures and molecular subtypes, breast cancer is routinely classified by immunohistochemical methods into four well-differentiated phenotypes based on the expression of estrogen and progesterone receptors (RE/RP) and human epidermal growth factor 2 (HER2): Luminal A, Luminal B, HER2-pure, and triple negative (TNBC), the latter being the most heterogeneous [23]:

- Luminal A tumors represent 50–60% of all breast cancer cases. These tumors show ER and PR expression, but HER2 is negative. In general, patients have a good prognosis since these tumors have low histological grade and proliferation rates [24];
- Luminal B tumors are also ER/PR positive, and they can present HER2 overexpression/amplification or not, with higher proliferation rates than Luminal A tumors. In addition, these tumors progress to some extent faster than Luminal A tumors [25];

- HER2-enriched tumors express neither of the two hormone receptors (HR), and they are HER2-positive. Generally, this molecular subtype is associated with a high histological grade, and, from a clinical point of view, it is characterized by having a poor prognosis. Nevertheless, therapies targeting HER2 proteins are usually successful [26];
- TNBC express neither HR nor HER2, and, therefore, they have no specific target for treatment. However, clinically, they behave more aggressively, with higher metastasis rates to the brain and lung [27].

Representative cell lines for each defined breast cancer subtype are available for in vitro assays so that the distinctive effect of antitumor agents can be explored (Figure 1). T47-D (Figure 1A) and MCF-7 (Figure 1B) cell lines present an ER/PR+ phenotype, thus being examples of Luminal A subtype. BT-474 presents Luminal B features such as HER2 overexpression, as well as ER/PR expression (Figure 1C). HER2-enriched subtype can be studied thanks to SK-BR-3 (Figure 1D) and MDA-MB-453 cell lines. Among triple negative tumors, we can distinguish between triple negative/Basal-like and triple negative/Claudin low depending on gene expression characteristics [28], with MDA-MB-468 (Figure 1E) and MDA-MB-231 (Figure 1F) as their representative cell lines, respectively.

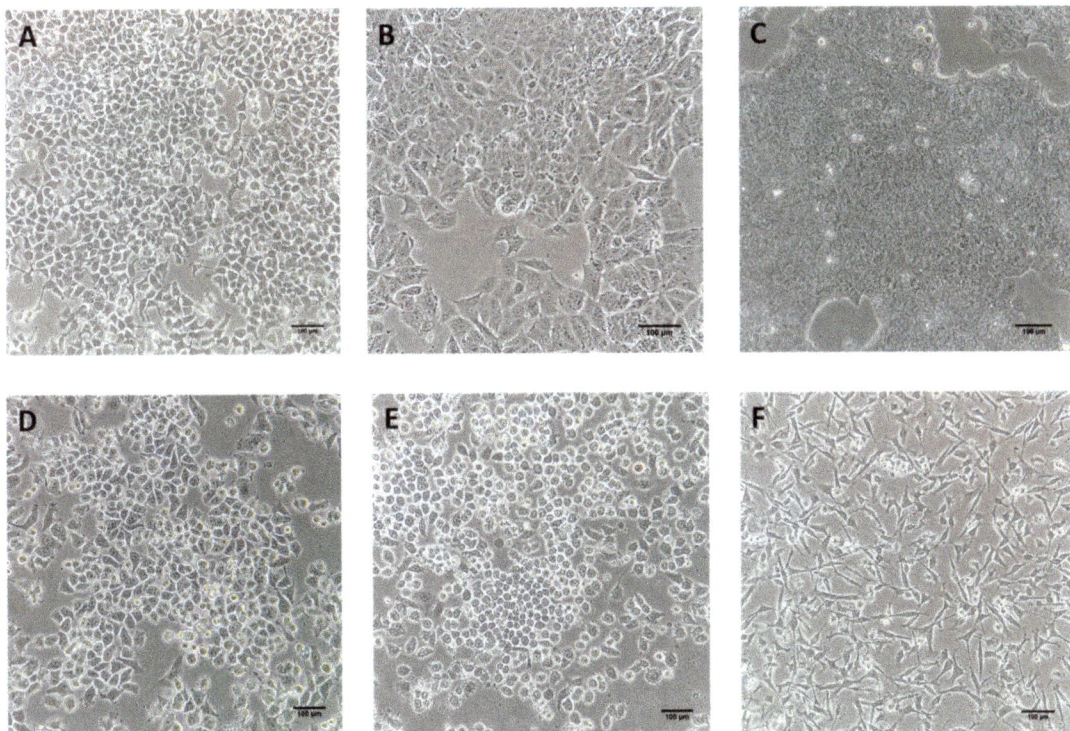

Figure 1. Breast cancer cell lines. (**A**) T47-D and (**B**) MCF-7 cell lines are representative of luminal A (ER/PR+) phenotypes. (**C**) BT-474 cell line represents the Luminal B/HER2+ tumors. (**D**) SK-BR-3 cell line is characterized by the lack of ER and PR expression but it overexpresses the HER2/c-erb-2 gene, thus representing HER2-enriched subtype. (**E**) MDA-MB-468 cell line belongs to the triple negative/Basal-like (ER/PR and HER2 negative) phenotype. (**F**) MDA-MB-231 cell line constitutes the triple negative/Claudin-low subtype. (Image credit: Yoel Genaro Montoyo-Pujol). Scale bars of 100 µm are included in each micrograph.

About 60–70% of breast cancers are of luminal subtype, therefore hormone-sensitive and responsive to endocrine therapy and relatively good prognosis [29]. However, HER2-positivity has been more frequently reported in HR-negative than HR-positive cancers, correlated with aggressive clinical behavior and poor prognosis. Despite the fact that novel HER2-targeted therapies have dramatically improved the outcome in HR-negative/HER2-positive patients, drug-related side effects are yet major obstacles ahead [30].

TNBC represents a specific subtype accounting for approximately 15–20% of breast cancers, characterized by negative ER/PR/HER2 expression. Patients show a highly aggressive clinical outcome, tending to earlier relapses and frequent metastasis to the brain and lungs, and, therefore, poorer survival compared with other subtypes [31].

In addition, neoplastic transformation results from the dysfunction of signal transduction networks that regulate molecular communications and cellular processes. Among them, several signaling pathways have been described to be deregulated in breast carcinoma, including the PI3K/Akt/mTOR pathway, Notch pathway, Hedgehog pathway, ERK/MAPK pathway, NF-kB pathway, FOXO1/JAK/STAT pathway, TP53 pathway, Wnt/β-catenin, as well as apoptotic and cell cycle pathways. These networks are highly adaptable and dynamic [32].

Furthermore, the results of recent retrospective and prospective clinical studies have shown that the molecular classification of breast cancer subtypes and the mechanisms of interaction between tumors and immune cells of different subtypes are significant for predicting therapeutic response and prognosis and developing individualized treatment [33]. Therefore, despite the overall successes in breast cancer therapy, which have improved the prognosis, significant challenges exist in managing and treating patients who recur, develop resistance, or show no responsiveness since they do not have therapeutic targets. Hence, it is urgent to investigate novel and more effective agents without side effects in addition to conventional chemotherapy. In this regard, carotenoids are attracting enormous attention as promising drug candidates in breast cancer treatment.

3. The Role of Oxidative Stress in Cancer

Cancer in humans is a multifactorial pathology triggered by endogenous and exogenous factors [34]. During the development of tumors, nutrient and oxygen concentrations change due to the dynamics of the vasculature. Combining these changes with tissue remodeling events shapes the tumor metabolic landscape, complexly involving both cell-autonomous and non-cell-autonomous mechanisms [35,36]. It is not entirely clear how tumors cope with low nutrient and oxygen concentrations. When such deficits are sensed, suitable cellular responses are elicited, and new vasculature is ultimately established [37]. Changes in mitochondrial metabolism mediate early responses to sharp drops in oxygen tension and, in particular, the generation of reactive oxygen species (ROS) [38].

Although ROS are essential in maintaining the equilibrium between pro-oxidant and antioxidant molecules, an excessive amount of these molecules negatively affects the structure and function of most biomolecules [39]. Oxidative stress can cause DNA damage and mutations, hydrolyzation of DNA bases, oncogene activation, and chromosomal abnormalities [40]. These alterations can promote tumor progression since they modify the transcriptomic profile, thus leading to impaired cell growth [41]. CpG islands can also be affected, causing loss of epigenetic information [42]. Furthermore, the oxidation of DNA by ROS releases 8-hydroxy-2-deoxyguanosine, which can generate DNA mutations [43,44]. Other possible DNA modifications include strand breaks, DNA-protein crosslinks, base-free sites, and base and sugar lesions [45]. However, not only DNA is affected by oxidative stress. ROS can oxidize lipoproteins, and the polyunsaturated lipids in the cell membrane due to lipid peroxidation [46]. In fact, lipid peroxidation is a radical chain reaction that generates cytotoxic and mutagenic compounds, such as malondialdehyde [46]. In addition, protein structure might be damaged, leading to conformational changes or loss of function [47].

ROS release during oxidative stress can be provoked by endogenous or exogenous stimuli [48]. In addition, countless enzymatic reactions in the cell are endogenous sources of oxidative stress as part of the metabolism [49]. For example, the radical $O_2 \bullet^-$ is released by lipoxygenases, cyclooxygenases, and inflammatory cells during cellular respiration [50]. However, it is well established that also lifestyle strongly influences the levels of oxidative stress, thus increasing the risk of cancer development [51,52].

Several oncogenic pathways are activated by high levels of ROS [53], such as the phosphoinositide 3-kinases pathway (PI3K). Phosphatase and tensin homolog (PTEN) can be inactivated by the oxidation of its regulatory Cys 124 residue due to the interaction with ROS, such as H_2O_2 [54]. Furthermore, the formation of a disulfide bond between Cys124 and Cys71 leads to PTEN inactivation, thus inducing the hyperactivation of the PI3K signaling pathway [55,56]. In consequence, protein kinase B (AKT) is constantly upregulated, which results in the continuous expression of genes involved in the activation of the cell cycle, for example, cyclin-dependent kinase 1 (CDK1) [57]. During the initiation of a tumor, blood vessels are poorly developed, creating a hypoxic environment [58]. Hypoxia causes an alteration in the mitochondrial electron transport chain, which releases more ROS that contributes to the activation of hypoxia-inducing factor-1 (HIF-1) [59]. More specifically, prolyl hydroxylase domain (PHD), a HIF-1 inhibitor, is inactivated in ROS. HIF-1 is a transcription factor that induces the expression of vascular endothelial growth factor (VEGF) and aerobic glycolysis [60]. In addition, tumor proliferation is enhanced due to the HIF-1-dependent activation of the c-Myc pathway [61]. High ROS levels also contribute to the invasiveness of a tumor due to the activity of transforming growth factor beta-1 (TGFß1) [62]. TGFß1 induces the epithelial-mesenchymal transition (EMT) and the secretion of various invasiveness biomarkers, such as VEGF and interleukin 6 [63]. Furthermore, ROS activates matrix metalloproteinase (MMP) synthesis via Ras and MAPK signaling pathways or via NF-kB [64].

Tumor cells can tolerate higher ROS levels than normal cells since they modulate the redox environment and use it to proliferate. Nevertheless, if a certain threshold of ROS levels is surpassed, even tumor cells cannot adapt, and, therefore, cell death pathways are activated [53].

In particular, high levels of oxidative stress in breast cancer have been reported in the literature since breast cancer cells also present an enhanced ROS production and low catalase activity. ER-positive tumors show higher levels of 8-hydroxy-2-deoxyguanosine than ER-negative [65]. Gene alterations in breast cancer are thought to be caused by ROS released by estrogen-induced oxidative stress. Breast tissue is sensitive to DNA damage by natural and synthetic estrogens [66,67]. It has been repeatedly stated that elevated ROS levels induce tumor initiation. As a consequence, cancer cells with a robust antioxidant capacity may experience selection pressure. However, cancer cells also present higher ROS concentrations than normal cells. Based on this premise, it has been suggested that cancer cells could be more sensitive than normal cells to a further increase in ROS levels, thus selectively targeting neoplastic cells [22,45]. In theory, these additional ROS would spare their effect on normal cells because ROS would be present at physiological levels [68]. However, there are still no solid results from pre-clinical and clinical studies to support this theory, and much work remains to be performed to draw firm conclusions.

The use of antioxidants holds promises since they would exert their antioxidant activity on non-tumoral cells, whereas pro-oxidant activity would affect cancer cells. This approach is based on the pro-oxidant activity that many antioxidants presents, which will be further discussed in Section 5.1. However, pro-oxidant therapy is an emerging concept that has not been deeply explored yet. In addition, many breast cancer chemotherapeutic drugs, such as taxanes and anthracyclines, can induce oxidative stress in the brain and blood as a side effect [69].

For this reason, the administration of exogenous antioxidants has been studied during the last years to counteract the detrimental effects of neoplastic treatment in healthy tissues to prevent neurotoxicity [70]. Particularly, phytochemicals such as some carotenoids, terpenoids, and polyphenols can modulate various oncogenic pathways. Therefore, they are being investigated as potential therapeutics [71].

4. Antioxidants as a Defense Mechanism against Oxidative Stress

Antioxidants are molecules that can prevent or slow damage to cells caused by free radicals, which are unstable molecules produced during metabolic reactions, not only under "standard metabolic conditions" but also as a response to stressful environmental parameters or other pressures. They are sometimes called "free-radical scavengers". From a functional point of view, antioxidants prevent or delay the oxidation of other molecules through the donation of hydrogen atoms or electrons. They are essential in the protection of the cells against free radicals like reactive oxygen species (ROS) and reactive nitrogen species (RNS), and, therefore, against oxidative stress [72].

Antioxidants can be classified into several groups based on their role, chemical composition, etc. The most used classification establishes two broad divisions, depending on whether they are soluble in water (hydrophilic) or lipids (lipophilic). Water-soluble antioxidants react with oxidants in the cell cytosol and the blood plasma, while lipid-soluble antioxidants protect cell membranes from lipid peroxidation [73].

Cells can use several defense mechanisms against ROS and RNS, which work together to scavenge free radicals. There are endogenous and exogenous antioxidants, the latter being synthetic or natural [74]. Cells synthesize some molecules showing antioxidant activity, such as glutathione, alpha-lipoic acid, coenzyme Q, ferritin, uric acid, bilirubin, metallothionein, L-carnitine, and small proteins such as thioredoxins (TRX). In addition, they act as an efficient reducing agent, scavenging reactive oxygen species and maintaining other proteins in their reduced state [75]. However, among the endogenous antioxidant repertoire of cells, it is worth highlighting the activity of some enzymes commonly named "antioxidant enzymes" [76]. A few of these enzymes are following listed:

- Superoxide dismutase (SOD): catalyze the breakdown of the superoxide anion into oxygen and hydrogen peroxide [77];
- Catalase (CAT): catalyze the conversion of hydrogen peroxide to water and oxygen, using either an iron or manganese cofactor [78];
- Peroxiredoxins (PRXs): peroxidases that catalyze the reduction in hydrogen peroxide, organic hydroperoxides, as well as peroxynitrite [79];
- Glutathione peroxidases (GPXs): these are enzymes involved in a more complex pathway termed "glutathione system", which includes glutathione, glutathione reductase, glutathione peroxidases, and glutathione S-transferases. Within this series of reactions, glutathione peroxidase catalyzes the breakdown of hydrogen peroxide and organic hydroperoxides [80].

Based on the analyzed literature focused on antioxidant enzymes and cancer, the following features can be highlighted: (i) the activity of antioxidant enzymes is important for diagnosing neoplastic diseases such as non-small-cell lung cancer, bladder cancer, ovarian cancer, and colon cancer; (ii) non-small-cell lung cancer is usually characterized by decreased SOD and CAT activity and increased glutathione GST activity. Lowered SOD, CAT, and GPx activity are characteristic of bladder cancer. XOR, CAT, SOD, and GPx expression is decreased in patients with ovarian cancer. Colorectal cancer is characterized by increased MnSOD expression (in vitro studies) and SOD expression while CAT, GPx, and GR are decreased (in vivo study); and finally, (iii) SOD, CAT, and XOR are proposed as prognostic markers in cancer of the lung, bladder, ovarian, and colon [81]. Moreover, antioxidants can also be chemically synthesized, such as N-acetyl cysteine (NAC), pyruvate, selenium, butylated hydroxytoluene (BHT), butylated hydroxyanisole (BHA), and propyl gallate [82]. Some of these synthetic compounds have been tested in neoplastic cells reporting radioprotection, protection against acute toxicity of chemicals, antimutagenic activity, and antitumorigenic action [83]. However, BHT and BHA are not exempt from controversy since contradictory data involves their beneficial effects and their potentially harmful effects on human health [84]. The concerns regarding their biosafety are based on several studies reporting endocrine-disrupting effects [85], reproductive toxicity [86], and carcinogenity [87]. The controversy encourages re-evaluating the use of these synthetic antioxidants and exploring already known and new naturally derived antioxidants that may benefit human health.

Natural antioxidants are incorporated through the diet, including vitamins and carotenoids. Regarding vitamins, Vitamins C, E, and A show significant antioxidant activities. Vitamin C, also named ascorbic acid, is a redox catalyst that can reduce, and thereby neutralize ROS, such as hydrogen peroxide. Vitamin A is not a powerful antioxidant itself, but it has been reported that it plays a key role in inhibiting hepatic stellate cells (an effector of hepatocellular carcinoma) activation via suppressing thioredoxin-interacting protein and reducing oxidative stress levels. Finally, vitamin E (liposoluble) protects membranes from oxidation by reacting with lipid radicals produced in the lipid peroxidation chain reaction [88,89].

In recent decades, the relevance of antioxidants in various biological processes such as aging, cancer, and inflammation has been reported [71,90–92]. Different approaches have been assessed, from prevention to treatment of several pathologies. Antioxidants could also help reduce the side effects of the oxidative stress generated by chemo and radiotherapy [93,94]. Among all antioxidants, carotenoids, many of which have been identified and extracted from marine microorganisms [10,12,95], have attracted a lot of attention due to their remarkable antioxidant properties and their potential as anticancer and immunomodulatory agents.

5. Carotenoids

Carotenoids are isoprenoid polyenes displaying lipophilic properties. In nature, they are pigments ranging from yellow to red which can be found in plants, algae, microorganisms, and some animals [96,97]. There are more than 750 different carotenoid structures identified [98]. Carotenoids can be classified into two main groups: carotenes and xanthophylls. On the one hand, carotenes, such as β-carotene, have a chemical structure composed uniquely of carbon and hydrogen and are all vitamin A precursors (Figure 2A).

On the other hand, xanthophylls present at least one oxygen group in their hydrocarbon chain (Figure 2B) [99]. In contrast, they cannot act as precursors for vitamin A. Since carotenoids are composed of isoprenoid units, they usually contain numerous conjugated double bonds in their structure. This characteristic, combined with cyclic end groups in some cases, generates a series of stereoisomers that differ in their chemical and physical properties, such as solubility, stability, and light absorption [100]. When two parts of the structure linked by a double bond are on opposite sides of the plane, the carotenoid is in E-configuration. On the contrary, if both parts are on the same side of the plane it is called Z-configuration [101].

Fruits and vegetables contain many carotenoids, including α-carotene, β-carotene, lycopene, lutein, and zeaxanthin, among others [100]. Carotenoids are very well known for their remarkable antioxidant properties [102]. However, their relevance is not only subject to their ROS scavenging capacity. They can inhibit tumor growth and invasiveness and are apoptosis inducers, as it will be further discussed in Section 6 with the example of breast cancer [103]. Carotenoids can also modulate gene expression and possess anti-inflammatory and immunomodulatory activities [104] (Figure 3). The anti-inflammation mechanisms of carotenoids include targeting inflammatory biomarkers, such as chemokines and cytokines, a acute-phase proteins. Carotenoids can also promote PI3K/Akt and nuclear factor erythroid 2-like 2 (Nrf2) signaling pathways [105]. In addition, they can inhibit NF-kB, p38 MAPK, and JAK-2/STAT-3 signaling pathways, which are also related to tumorigenesis. Some carotenoids, such as astaxanthin, prevent neuronal death by regulating the Wnt/β-catenin signaling pathway and inducing angiogenesis [106]. However, in the case of tumor cells, carotenoids avoid the development of blood vessels, exerting an anti-angiogenic activity [107,108]. Anti-adiposity activity has also been reported for some carotenoids, such as cantaxanthin, through the differentiation of adipose cells [109]. Carotenoids have been reported to induce the proliferation of immunocompetent cells and might boost host resistance to pathogens. For example, astaxanthin positively influenced the intracellular calcium concentration and enhanced the capacity of neutrophils to eliminate microbes [102]. Furthermore, carotenoids can also increase gap junction formation, which might be related to their anti-carcinogenic properties [110].

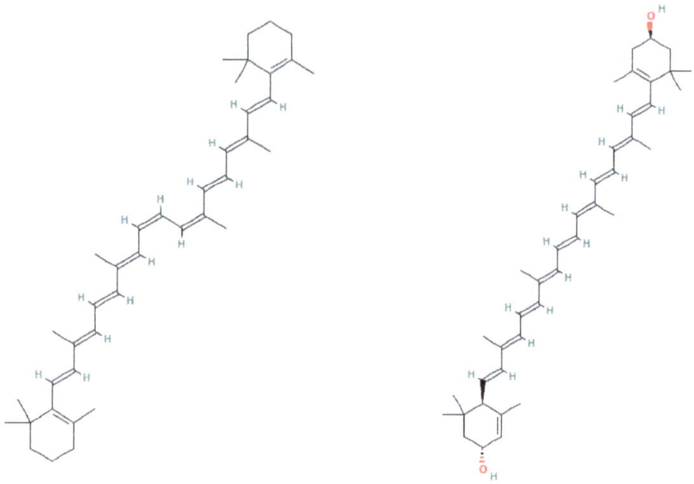

Figure 2. Examples of chemical 2D structures of carotenoids: (**A**) a carotenoid: cis-β,β-carotene (CID: 5927317) and (**B**) a xanthophyll: all-*trans*-lutein (CID: 6433159). The oxygen group is highlighted in red. Chemical 2D structures obtained from PubChem (NIH).

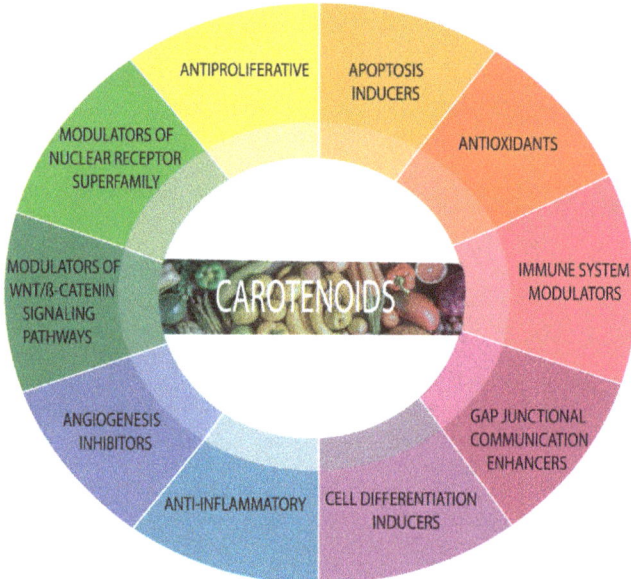

Figure 3. Biological properties of carotenoids. Although they are mainly known by their antioxidant activity, carotenoids can exert various effects on cells.

5.1. Antioxidants or Pro-Oxidants?

Carotenoids' antioxidant activity is attributed to their double-bonded structure and their ability to delocalised unpaired electrons [111]. As a result, carotenoids are capable of quenching free radicals, such as superoxide ($O_2\bullet-$), hydroxyl ($\bullet OH$), and peroxyl ($ROO\bullet$) radicals. Carotenoids can also prevent lipid damage from peroxidation [112]. However, recent studies have provided evidence on the pro-oxidant activity of carotenoids under certain conditions. As a consequence of this pro-oxidant potential, the concentration of ROS might increase. Nevertheless, this property does not disregard the protective role of carotenoids. Still, the conditions determining the antioxidant and pro-oxidant activity must be clarified to ensure the goal [113]. Whether a carotenoid shows pro-oxidant or antioxidant properties depends mainly on the partial pressure of dioxygen (pO_2) and the carotenoid concentration [41]. When pO_2 is high, a carotenoid radical is generated (Car•), reacting with O_2 releasing a carotenoid-peroxyl radical (Car-OO•). This compound can exert pro-oxidant activity through the oxidation of unsaturated lipids [114]. In conclusion, carotenoids usually exhibit antioxidant activity in the presence of low pO_2 whereas, antioxidant behavior is lost or becomes pro-oxidant when pO_2 is high [115]. Elevated concentrations of a carotenoid also give rise to pro-oxidant behavior [41]. When the amount of oxidized anti-oxidant surpass certain levels, the pro-oxidant activity becomes more plausible, leading to an increase in lipid peroxidation and modulating redox-sensitive genes and transcription factors [116,117]. In addition, each type of tumor presents a particular redox status which may influence how the carotenoid interacts with ROS [118]. However, pro-oxidant activity has proven to be helpful in the treatment of some tumor cells.

6. Breast Cancer and Carotenoids

Among the several lifestyle factors that might contribute to cancer development, dietary habits are one of the key ones [119]. However, antioxidant compounds, such as carotenoids, present naturally in food are promising chemopreventive agents [120,121] and have chemotherapeutical properties [122,123]. Several epidemiological studies have revealed how the intake of fruit and vegetables, and more specifically of the carotenoids absorbed from these foods, correlates to a reduced incidence of different types of tumors [124–126]. Furthermore, carotenoids have been frequently reported to suppress the onset and progression of cancer by different mechanisms [102]. In addition, they are capable of counteracting other forms of cellular stress by modulating signaling pathways [127]. Therefore, carotenoids alone or in combination with conventional anticancer drugs might be a promising therapeutic strategy in the treatment of this pathology. Several chemotherapeutic drugs, such as alkylating agents and platinum-based compounds, release free radicals while exerting their cytotoxic activity [128]. Free radicals are partially responsible for tissue and organ injuries, such as cardiotoxicity, nephrotoxicity, and DNA damage. Although endogenous antioxidants contribute to restoring oxidative balance, these natural pigments can also quench ROS activity. For this reason, carotenoids can alleviate the side effects of chemotherapy by protecting healthy tissues with their antioxidant activity [103,129]. The supplementation of carotenoids for cancer prevention is based on several mechanisms, including a role in cell cycle progression, the Wnt/β-catenin signaling pathway, and the modulation of inflammatory cytokines [130–132].

6.1. In Vitro and In Vivo Studies

Several carotenoids have shown antitumor activity in in vitro and in vivo assays. Lycopene delayed insulin-like growth factor 1 (IGF-1)-induced cell cycle progressionand apoptosis [133,134] in the MCF-7 breast cancer cell line. Lycopene and β-carotene were confirmed to induce cell cycle arrest and apoptosis in MCF-7, MDA-MB-231, and MDA-MB-235 cell lines [135]. Although lycopene and β-carotene are classified into different groups, they have many structural similarities that suggest that lycopene could activate retinoid-like receptors. The activation of these nuclear receptors leads to the transcription of several target genes, among which we would like to highlight RARβ given that it is a tumor suppressor gene. It is worth mentioning that most breast cancer tumors and breast cancer cell lines present low levels of RARβ receptor expression, thus potentially serving as a biomarker. Carotenes can work as precursors of (all-*trans*)-retinoic acid, which acts as ligand for RAR. The mechanism of action of β-carotene might be involved with retinoic acid metabolism and the transcriptional activation of antiproliferative and pro-apoptotic genes. Another signaling pathway involved in regulating the activity of breast cancer stem cells is PI3K/Akt, since Akt downregulates glycogen synthetase kinase 3β (GSK3β) by phosphorylation in the Ser9 residue, thus stabilizing β-catenin. Wnt/β-catenin signaling pathway plays a role in modulating stem cell self-renewal, differentiation, and cell proliferation [136]. Crocin and crocetin can negatively impact the viability and the ability of invasion of triple-negative breast cancer cells (4T1) through the Wnt/β-catenin pathway [137]. β-carotene also inhibited the proliferation of MCF-7 cells by decreasing the expression of the anti-apoptotic proteins Bcl-2 and PARP and the survival protein NF-kB. It also downregulated Akt and ERK1/2, and, in consequence, there was a lower expression of superoxide dismutase-2 [122].

Recent studies have reported how lutein can induce cell death in the MCF-7 cell line while protecting normal mammary cells (SV40) from apoptosis induced by chemotherapeutical drugs [123]. Another study confirmed the antineoplastic activity of lutein by inducing apoptosis and cell-cycle arrest in MCF-7 and MDA-MB-468 cell lines. The selective effect on tumor cells seems to be due to the induction of ROS production, therefore, due to its pro-oxidant activity [138]. Mammary tumor growth was inhibited by the intake of lutein in female BALB/c mice [107]. An antiproliferative effect was also detected in fucoxanthin treatment in MDA-MB-231 cells and xenograft model [139]. Another marine carotenoid, astaxanthin, repressed cancer stem cell stemness genes and induced apoptosis in the SKBR3 cell line, indicating that it might be helpful in the improvement of current therapies [140,141]. In addition, lycopene, zeaxanthin, and capsanthin induced apoptosis in MDA-MB-231 and seem to be involved in reversing multidrug resistance [142]. Aside from those, lycophyll, luteoxanthin, and violaxanthin were also highly effective. However, lutein, antheraxanthin, and violaxanthin were moderately successful in reversing multidrug resistance.

Metastasis and cell migration can also be inhibited by carotenoids [143]. The migration of MCF-7 and MDA-MB-231 cell lines was reduced after the treatment with astaxanthin [144]. Lutein was also reported to modulate adherin, vimentin, and N-cadherin levels, which are epithelial-mesenchymal transition (EMT) associated factors [145]. In addition, it inhibited NOTCH signaling pathway which is related to cell invasion and migration [146]. Furthermore, several apocarotenoids inhibited migration and EMT associated factors in BT-549 and MDA-MB-231 [147]. Therefore, carotenoids and apocarotenoids could be helpful preventing metastasis in triple negative tumors. However, there is still lack of evidence supporting this theory and much work remains to be completed.

Combination therapy of carotenoids with chemotherapeutic agents show a lot of promise. Recently, doxorubicin was combined with β-carotene and lutein to induce oxidative stress-mediated apoptosis in MCF-7 and MDA-MB-231 breast cancer cell lines. The pro-oxidant activity selectively affects tumor cells, sparing normal breast epithelial cells (MCF10A) [148] (Figure 4). Co-treatment of astaxanthin with the Phase I anticancer drug carbendazim showed a synergistic effect on the MCF-7 cell lines [149]. In combination with hyperthermia, crocin successfully inhibited the growth of the MDA-MB-468 TNBC cell line, whereas MCF-10A normal cells were not affected [150]. In addition, lutein and taxanes, such as paclitaxel, demonstrated a synergistic effect on MCF-7 and MDA-MB-468 cell lines [138]. Zeaxanthin and violaxanthin were capable of enhancing the antiproliferative effect of epirubicin on MCF-7 cells resistant to anthracycline [151].

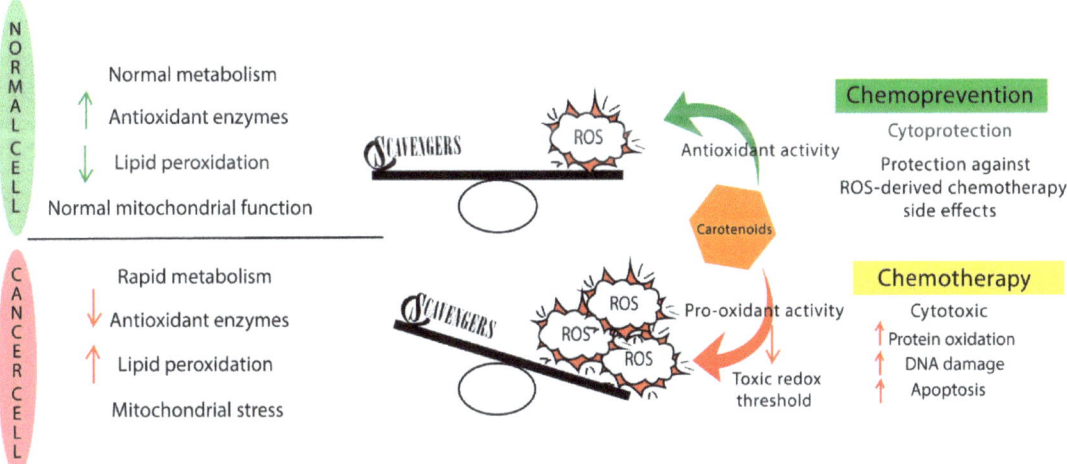

Figure 4. Major differences in cancer and normal cells metabolism. Over a certain ROS threshold, antioxidants present a pro-oxidant activity that leads to the apoptosis of malignant cells. Hence, its potential as chemotherapeutic agent. The antioxidant activity acts as a chemopreventive under homeostatic levels of ROS in normal cells.

6.2. Breast Cancer Antitumor Activity of Carotenoids: Clinical Trials

Most clinical trials start from the premise that high levels of carotenoids in plasma, obtained from carotenoid-rich foods, can prevent the development of breast cancer [152,153]. Table 1 includes all registered clinical trials which are studying the effect of carotenoids on breast cancer patients. Recent studies have associated high levels of β-carotene in plasma with lower ER-breast cancer risk [154] and with reduced systemic inflammation and cognitive improvements in breast cancer survivors [155]. It is worth highlighting the results from the trial NCT00000611, which analyzed serum concentrations of carotenoids, retinol and tocopherols in women to assess a possible association between these values and postmenopausal breast cancer risk. They concluded that indeed, high levels of α-carotene and β-carotene were inversely associated with the risk of developing breast cancer [156], which coincided with other similar studies [152]. Increased levels of carotenoids in plasma were also associated with less oxidative stress in breast cancer survivors, but inflammatory biomarkers were not affected [157]. A correlation between high levels of α-carotene and reduced breast cancer risk was found [139,158], which was consistent with the results obtained from the Nurse Health study [159] and the Women's Health Initiative [156].

Similarly, plasma concentrations of β-carotene and β-cryptoxanthin were inversely correlated with breast cancer risk [160]. In another study, plasma total carotenoid concentration was related to a diminished risk of breast cancer recurrence in patients with an early-stage diagnosis [161]. However, not all clinical trials agree with these results. Although an association between high levels of total plasma carotenoids and reduced oxidative stress was reported in line with previous trials, these authors also concluded that carotenoids were not able to protect against breast cancer relapse in postmenopausal breast cancer survivors [162,163].

In general, most clinical trials related to carotenoids and breast cancer target the effect of carotenoid-rich food intake on breast cancer survivors [164]. However, as previously mentioned, lifestyle is critical in preventing and progressing breast cancers and the levels of oxidative stress. In this matter, oxidative stress plays a significant role in cancer development and is also deeply involved in depression, affecting how patients deal with their pathology [165]. For this reason, a recent clinical trial is assessing the effect of music therapy on different biomarkers of oxidative stress, including carotenoids (NCT04446624).

In summary, there is still not enough evidence to validate the potential benefits of carotenoids in preventing and treating breast cancer. Most clinical trials agree that a high intake of carotenoids may prevent high-risk and aggressive breast cancer, but further studies are required to draw a solid conclusion. Furthermore, no clinical trials assessing the supplementation of carotenoids in breast cancer patients, and, therefore, there is a complete lack of knowledge regarding this topic. Some studies in other types of cancer have reported controversial results [166]. Still, the chemopreventive use of carotenoids and the chemotherapeutical results in in vitro and in vivo studies encourage deepening the potential of carotenoids as part of the treatment of breast cancer patients.

Table 1. Clinical trials involving carotenoids in breast cancer.

NCT Number	Status [1]	Stage	Aim	Outcome	Reference
NCT03625635	Unknown	NA	Effect of a nutritional intervention on body composition, metabolism, and antioxidant activity	Reduced fat mass while preserving skeletal muscle mass	[167]
NCT02067481	Completed	Phase II	Effect of diet and physical activity in breast cancer survivors	Unknown	UP
NCT00000611	Completed	Phase III	Effect on higher fruit and vegetable intake on BC patients	High levels of plasma carotenoids associated with less BC risk	[156]
NCT02109068	Completed	Phase III	Effect of weight loss in BC survivors	Unknown	UP
NCT02110641	Active, no recruiting	NA	Effect of weight loss in BC survivors	Unknown	[168]
NCT04374747	Recruiting	NA	Effect of fruit and vegetable intake to reduce BC risk in lactating women	Not measured	[169]
NCT04446624	Completed	NA	Effect of music therapy in oxidative stress markers, such as carotenoids	Unknown	UP
NCT00120016	Completed	NA	Impact of a Mediterranean diet on BC risk	Plasma carotenoids increase with fruit and vegetable intake	[170]

[1] Data obtained from ClinicalTrials.gov on 30th September 2021; BC: breast cancer NA: not applicable; UP: unpublished.

7. Rare Carotenoids from Halophilic Microorganisms: The Future of Biomedicine?

Bacterioruberin from Haloarchaea

Haloarchaea have been in the spotlight during the last years due to their ability to synthesize compounds of high biotechnological interest, such as bioplastics, thermophilic enzymes, and a particular type of carotenoid [12].

Haloarchaea synthesize mainly a rare C_{50} carotenoid called bacterioruberin (BR) and its derivatives: bisanhydrobacterioruberin (BABR), monoanhydrobacterioruberin (MABR), and 2-isopentenyl-3,4-dehydrorhodopin (IDR) [171–174]. Other derivatives have been detected at lower concentrations, such as haloxanthin and 3,4-dehydromonoanhydrobacterioruberin; and depending on the haloarchaeal species, such as 3,4-epoxymonoanhydrobacterioruberin, which has only been described in *Haloferax volcanii* carotenoid extracts [175]. Although β-carotene, lycopene, and phytoene have also been identified in haloarchaeal extracts, they are present at low concentrations [171,176]. BR, which is the most abundant, presents an interesting chemical structure since its hydrocarbon chain is particularly long, with 50 carbon units (Figure 5). Furthermore, it possesses 13 conjugated double bonds in an all-*trans* conformation. This together with the 4 hydroxyl groups that arise from the terminal ends, provide this carotenoid with a higher scavenging potential than their C_{40} counterparts, lycopene, and β-carotene.

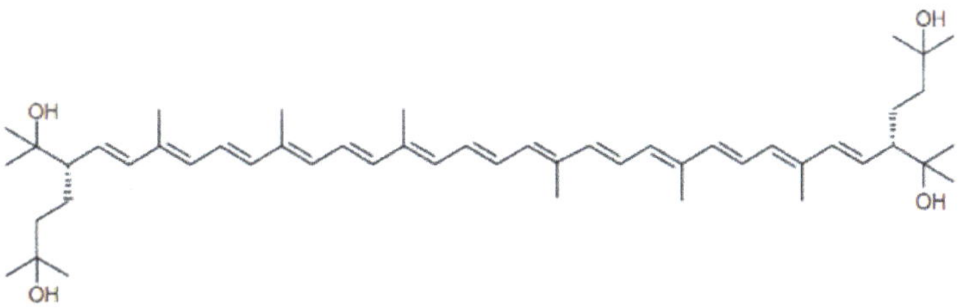

Figure 5. Chemical structure of the haloarchaeal carotenoid bacterioruberin.

A recent study using *Haloferax mediterranei* describes how BR counteracts the oxidative stress generated by high concentrations of the oxidant hydrogen peroxide. BR successfully neutralized hydrogen peroxide, confirming that cells use this carotenoid to keep the oxidative balance and that this compound is indeed very efficient against ROS [176]. This distinct chemical structure has awakened the interest of many researchers during the last years due to the potential biotechnological and biomedical applications that could have [12]. Unfortunately, there is still scarce information about its antiproliferative activity. However, recent studies have reported that BR could selectively inhibit cell growth in cell lines from different cancer types, including breast cancer (MCF-7) BR induced more substantial caspase-mediated apoptosis than that of the chemotherapeutical agent, 5-fluorouracil (5-FU) and showed a higher selectivity index than 5-FU. In addition, BR was a more potent suppressor of matrix metalloprotease 9 (MMP-9) [177]. MMP-9 is one of the key proteases involved in many cancer processes, such as angiogenesis, invasion, and metastasis [178]. However, the nature of the mechanism involved is not currently clear, and therefore, much work remains to be completed. In addition, it is still unknown if it will also exert pro-oxidant activity and under what conditions. However, the successful results obtained in other biomedical areas, such as cryopreservation [179] and anti-viral activity [177] invite us to explore what BR could offer to breast cancer prevention and treatment.

8. Controversy and Setbacks Observed

The fact that the same molecule can exhibit antioxidant and pro-oxidant activity has been subject to controversy and has questioned the efficacy of these compounds in the treatment of tumors [118]. Another debatable point is that no consensus in the doses should be administered in clinical trials. Therefore, it is complicated to make comparisons and draw conclusions. It is also worth mentioning that endogenous factors, such as the genetic variability in antioxidant enzymes in each patient, may compromise the efficacy of these compounds [180].

Breast cancer is a very heterogeneous malignant neoplasia [181] whose different subtypes may differ in the levels of oxidative stress. The redox status of each subtype should be characterized so that the use of antioxidants, such as carotenoids, in the treatment of breast cancer can be refined. Each result contributes to a better understanding of the role of carotenoids in breast cancer patients.

However, most studies concur that consuming a collection of carotenoids is a better anticancer strategy than a high intake of one specific carotenoid. Nowadays, there is particular controversy regarding using antioxidants due to the complexity in recognizing their positive or negative effects on patient outcomes. In addition, most clinical trials have focused on the supplementation of carotenoids to diminish adverse chemotherapy effects or as chemopreventive compounds [154,164]. Although many in vitro and in vivo assays focus on the antitumor effect of carotenoids, trials focused on carotenoids as an actual treatment for breast cancer are nonexistent. Therefore, it is hard to confirm if carotenoids could be helpful in the fight against this common pathology among women. One of the potential changes in the current approach on using carotenoids in clinical trials could be intravenous administration instead of supplementation to reach a higher plasmatic concentration. What is clear is that further research on this topic is required to make a clear conclusion.

9. Conclusions

In closing, for many years, natural compounds have been useful in preventing many diseases. Some of those, such as taxane, was part of the development of current chemotherapeutical drugs [182]. To date, almost half of current anticancer drugs are derivatives of natural compounds or their mimics [183]. Now it is time to evaluate if carotenoids could rise from chemopreventive to chemotherapeutical agents. For this reason, preclinical research should be encouraged to elucidate what is the exact role of carotenoids in the onset and progression of breast cancer.

Moreover, the precise conditions under which a carotenoid shows antioxidant or pro-oxidant activity must be determined. Combined therapy studies are also key to establish any positive or negative interaction with current chemotherapy protocols. Finally, novel carotenoids, such as bacterioruberin, need to be investigated to deepen their potential value in treating malignant neoplasias.

Author Contributions: R.M.M.-E. conceived the global project and managed the funding. M.G. and R.M.M.-E. conceived and designed the study and conducted the bibliographic and bibliometric analysis focused on antioxidants, free radicals, and carotenoids; Y.G.M.-P. and G.P. integrated data from literature related to breast cancer and oxidative stress; all authors analysed the literature and contributed equally to the writing of the original draft and final editing. All authors have read and agreed to the published version of the manuscript.

Funding: This work was funded by a research grant from MINECO Spain (RTI2018-099860-B-I00), Generalitat Valenciana (PROMETEO/2021/055;A) and VIGROB-309 (University of Alicante).

Conflicts of Interest: The authors declare no conflict of interest.

References

1. Bayir, H. Reactive oxygen species. *Crit. Care Med.* **2005**, *33*, S498–S501. [CrossRef] [PubMed]
2. Lenaz, G. Mitochondria and Reactive Oxygen Species. Which Role in Physiology and Pathology? In *Advances in Mitochondrial Medicine*; Scatena, R., Bottoni, P., Giardina, B., Eds.; Advances in Experimental Medicine and Biology; Springer: Dordrecht, The Netherlands, 2012; Volume 942, pp. 93–136. ISBN 978-94-007-2868-4.
3. Hanahan, D.; Weinberg, R.A. Hallmarks of Cancer: The Next Generation. *Cell* **2011**, *144*, 646–674. [CrossRef] [PubMed]
4. Bray, F.; Me, J.F.; Soerjomataram, I.; Siegel, R.L.; Torre, L.A.; Jemal, A. Global cancer statistics 2018: GLOBOCAN estimates of incidence and mortality worldwide for 36 cancers in 185 countries. *CA A Cancer J. Clin.* **2018**, *68*, 394–424. [CrossRef]
5. Martín-Moreno, J.M.; Soerjomataram, I.; Magnusson, G. Cancer causes and prevention: A condensed appraisal in Europe in 2008. *Eur. J. Cancer* **2008**, *44*, 1390–1403. [CrossRef]
6. Hayes, J.D.; Dinkova-Kostova, A.T.; Tew, K.D. Oxidative Stress in Cancer. *Cancer Cell* **2020**, *38*, 167–197. [CrossRef]
7. Sosa, V.; Moline, T.; Somoza, R.; Paciucci, R.; Kondoh, H.; Lleonart, M.E. Oxidative stress and cancer: An overview. *Ageing Res. Rev.* **2013**, *12*, 376–390. [CrossRef]
8. Janciauskiene, S. The Beneficial Effects of Antioxidants in Health and Diseases. *Chronic Obstr. Pulm. Dis. J. COPD Found.* **2020**, *7*, 182–202. [CrossRef]
9. Chandra, P.; Sharma, R.K.; Arora, D.S. Antioxidant compounds from microbial sources: A review. *Food Res. Int.* **2019**, *129*, 108849. [CrossRef]
10. Torregrosa-Crespo, J.; Montero, Z.; Fuentes, J.L.; García-Galbis, M.R.; Garbayo, I.; Vílchez, C.; Martínez-Espinosa, R.M. Exploring the Valuable Carotenoids for the Large-Scale Production by Marine Microorganisms. *Mar. Drugs* **2018**, *16*, 203. [CrossRef]
11. Oren, A. The microbiology of red brines. In *Advances in Applied Microbiology*; Elsevier: Amsterdam, The Netherlands, 2020; Volume 113, pp. 57–110. ISBN 978-0-12-820709-3.
12. Giani, M.; Garbayo, I.; Vílchez, C.; Martínez-Espinosa, R.M. Haloarchaeal Carotenoids: Healthy Novel Compounds from Extreme Environments. *Mar. Drugs* **2019**, *17*, 524. [CrossRef] [PubMed]
13. Sung, H.; Ferlay, J.; Siegel, R.L.; Laversanne, M.; Soerjomataram, I.; Jemal, A.; Bray, F. Global Cancer Statistics 2020: GLOBOCAN Estimates of Incidence and Mortality Worldwide for 36 Cancers in 185 Countries. *CA A Cancer J. Clin.* **2021**, *71*, 209–249. [CrossRef]
14. Perou, C.; Sørlie, T.; Eisen, M.; Van De Rijn, M.; Jeffrey, S.; Rees, C.A.; Pollack, J.R.; Ross, D.T.; Johnsen, H.; Akslen, L.A.; et al. Molecular portraits of human breast tumours. *Nature* **2000**, *406*, 747–752. [CrossRef] [PubMed]

15. Sørlie, T.; Tibshirani, R.; Parker, J.; Hastie, T.; Marron, J.S.; Nobel, A.; Deng, S.; Johnsen, H.; Pesich, R.; Geisler, S.; et al. Repeated observation of breast tumor subtypes in independent gene expression data sets. *Proc. Natl. Acad. Sci. USA* **2003**, *100*, 8418–8423. [CrossRef] [PubMed]
16. Chen, Z.; Xu, L.; Shi, W.; Zeng, F.; Zhuo, R.; Hao, X.; Fan, P. Trends of female and male breast cancer incidence at the global, regional, and national levels, 1990–2017. *Breast Cancer Res. Treat.* **2020**, *180*, 481–490. [CrossRef] [PubMed]
17. Sopik, V. International variation in breast cancer incidence and mortality in young women. *Breast Cancer Res. Treat.* **2020**, *186*, 497–507. [CrossRef] [PubMed]
18. Kamińska, M.; Ciszewski, T.; Łopacka-Szatan, K.; Miotła, P.; Starosławska, E. Breast cancer risk factors. *Menopausal Rev.* **2015**, *3*, 196–202. [CrossRef]
19. Iacoviello, L.; Bonaccio, M.; de Gaetano, G.; Donati, M.B. Epidemiology of breast cancer, a paradigm of the "common soil" hypothesis. *Semin. Cancer Biol.* **2020**, *72*, 4–10. [CrossRef]
20. Goldhirsch, A.; Wood, W.C.; Coates, A.S.; Gelber, R.D.; Thürlimann, B.; Senn, H.-J. Strategies for subtypes—dealing with the diversity of breast cancer: Highlights of the St Gallen International Expert Consensus on the Primary Therapy of Early Breast Cancer 2011. *Ann. Oncol.* **2011**, *22*, 1736–1747. [CrossRef]
21. Lehmann, B.; Bauer, J.A.; Chen, X.; Sanders, M.E.; Chakravarthy, A.B.; Shyr, Y.; Pietenpol, J.A. Identification of human triple-negative breast cancer subtypes and preclinical models for selection of targeted therapies. *J. Clin. Investig.* **2011**, *121*, 2750–2767. [CrossRef]
22. Lehmann, B.D.; Jovanović, B.; Chen, X.; Estrada, M.V.; Johnson, K.N.; Shyr, Y.; Moses, H.L.; Sanders, M.E.; Pietenpol, J.A. Refinement of Triple-Negative Breast Cancer Molecular Subtypes: Implications for Neoadjuvant Chemotherapy Selection. *PLoS ONE* **2016**, *11*, e0157368. [CrossRef]
23. Hecht, F.; Pessoa, C.F.; Gentile, L.B.; Rosenthal, D.; Carvalho, D.; Fortunato, R.S. The role of oxidative stress on breast cancer development and therapy. *Tumor Biol.* **2016**, *37*, 4281–4291. [CrossRef]
24. Gao, J.J.; Swain, S.M. Luminal A Breast Cancer and Molecular Assays: A Review. *Oncologist* **2018**, *23*, 556–565. [CrossRef] [PubMed]
25. Ades, F.; Zardavas, D.; Bozovic-Spasojevic, I.; Pugliano, L.; Fumagalli, D.; de Azambuja, E.; Viale, G.; Sotiriou, C.; Piccart, M. Luminal B Breast Cancer: Molecular Characterization, Clinical Management, and Future Perspectives. *J. Clin. Oncol.* **2014**, *32*, 2794–2803. [CrossRef] [PubMed]
26. Figueroa-Magalhães, M.C.; Jelovac, D.; Connolly, R.M.; Wolff, A.C. Treatment of HER2-positive breast cancer. *Breast* **2013**, *23*, 128–136. [CrossRef] [PubMed]
27. Yin, L.; Duan, J.-J.; Bian, X.-W.; Yu, S.-C. Triple-Negative breast cancer molecular subtyping and treatment progress. *Breast Cancer Res.* **2020**, *22*, 1–13. [CrossRef]
28. Dai, X.; Cheng, H.; Bai, Z.; Li, J. Breast Cancer Cell Line Classification and Its Relevance with Breast Tumor Subtyping. *J. Cancer* **2017**, *8*, 3131–3141. [CrossRef]
29. Harbeck, N.; Penault-Llorca, F.; Cortes, J.; Gnant, M.; Houssami, N.; Poortmans, P.; Ruddy, K.; Tsang, J.; Cardoso, F. Breast cancer. *Nat. Rev. Dis. Prim.* **2019**, *5*, 1–31. [CrossRef]
30. Iqbal, N.; Iqbal, N. Human Epidermal Growth Factor Receptor 2 (HER2) in Cancers: Overexpression and Therapeutic Implications. *Mol. Biol. Int.* **2014**, *2014*, 1–9. [CrossRef]
31. Goldhirsch, A.; Winer, E.P.; Coates, A.S.; Gelber, R.D.; Piccart-Gebhart, M.; Thürlimann, B.; Senn, H.-J.; Albain, K.S.; Andre, F.; Bergh, J.; et al. Personalizing the treatment of women with early breast cancer: Highlights of the St Gallen International Expert Consensus on the Primary Therapy of Early Breast Cancer 2013. *Ann. Oncol.* **2013**, *24*, 2206–2223. [CrossRef]
32. Kolch, W.; Halasz, M.; Granovskaya, M.; Kholodenko, B. The dynamic control of signal transduction networks in cancer cells. *Nat. Rev. Cancer* **2015**, *15*, 515–527. [CrossRef]
33. Waks, A.G.; Winer, E.P. Breast Cancer Treatment. *JAMA* **2019**, *321*, 288–300. [CrossRef] [PubMed]
34. Katzke, V.A.; Kaaks, R.; Kühn, T. Lifestyle and Cancer Risk. *Cancer J.* **2015**, *21*, 104–110. [CrossRef]
35. Junttila, M.R.; de Sauvage, F.J. Influence of tumour micro-environment heterogeneity on therapeutic response. *Nature* **2013**, *501*, 346–354. [CrossRef] [PubMed]
36. Ghesquière, B.; Wong, B.; Kuchnio, A.; Carmeliet, P. Metabolism of stromal and immune cells in health and disease. *Nature* **2014**, *511*, 167–176. [CrossRef] [PubMed]
37. Anastasiou, D. Tumour microenvironment factors shaping the cancer metabolism landscape. *Br. J. Cancer* **2016**, *116*, 277–286. [CrossRef] [PubMed]
38. Chandel, N.S.; Maltepe, E.; Goldwasser, E.; Mathieu, C.E.; Simon, M.C.; Schumacker, P.T. Mitochondrial reactive oxygen species trigger hypoxia-induced transcription. *Proc. Natl. Acad. Sci. USA* **1998**, *95*, 11715–11720. [CrossRef]
39. Rahal, A.; Kumar, A.; Singh, V.; Yadav, B.; Tiwari, R.; Chakraborty, S.; Dhama, K. Oxidative Stress, Prooxidants, and Antioxidants: The Interplay. *BioMed Res. Int.* **2014**, *2014*, 1–19. [CrossRef]
40. Kryston, T.B.; Georgiev, A.B.; Pissis, P.; Georgakilas, A.G. Role of oxidative stress and DNA damage in human carcinogenesis. *Mutat. Res. Mol. Mech. Mutagen.* **2011**, *711*, 193–201. [CrossRef]
41. Valko, M.; Rhodes, C.; Moncol, J.; Izakovic, M.; Mazur, M. Free radicals, metals and antioxidants in oxidative stress-induced cancer. *Chem. Interact.* **2006**, *160*, 1–40. [CrossRef]

42. Gào, X.; Zhang, Y.; Burwinkel, B.; Xuan, Y.; Holleczek, B.; Brenner, H.; Schöttker, B. The associations of DNA methylation alterations in oxidative stress-related genes with cancer incidence and mortality outcomes: A population-based cohort study. *Clin. Epigenetics* **2019**, *11*, 14. [CrossRef]
43. Sova, H.; Jukkolavuorinen, A.; Puistola, U.; Kauppila, S.; Karihtala, P. 8-Hydroxydeoxyguanosine: A new potential independent prognostic factor in breast cancer. *Br. J. Cancer* **2010**, *102*, 1018–1023. [CrossRef] [PubMed]
44. Nishida, N.; Arizumi, T.; Takita, M.; Kitai, S.; Yada, N.; Hagiwara, S.; Inoue, T.; Minami, Y.; Ueshima, K.; Sakurai, T.; et al. Reactive Oxygen Species Induce Epigenetic Instability through the Formation of 8-Hydroxydeoxyguanosine in Human Hepatocarcinogenesis. *Dig. Dis.* **2013**, *31*, 459–466. [CrossRef] [PubMed]
45. Cooke, M.S.; Evans, M.D.; Dizdaroglu, M.; Lunec, J. Oxidative DNA damage: Mechanisms, mutation, and disease. *FASEB J.* **2003**, *17*, 1195–1214. [CrossRef] [PubMed]
46. Ayala, A.; Muñoz, M.F.; Argüelles, S. Lipid Peroxidation: Production, Metabolism, and Signaling Mechanisms of Malondialdehyde and 4-Hydroxy-2-Nonenal. *Oxidative Med. Cell. Longev.* **2014**, *2014*, 1–31. [CrossRef] [PubMed]
47. Brieger, K.; Schiavone, S.; Miller, J.; Krause, K.-H. Reactive oxygen species: From health to disease. *Swiss Med. Wkly.* **2012**, *142*, w13659. [CrossRef]
48. Sarniak, A.; Lipińska, J.; Tytman, K.; Lipińska, S. Endogenous mechanisms of reactive oxygen species (ROS) generation. *Postepy Hig. Med. Dosw. (Online)* **2016**, *70*, 1150–1165. [CrossRef] [PubMed]
49. Forrester, S.J.; Kikuchi, D.S.; Hernandes, M.S.; Xu, Q.; Griendling, K.K. Reactive Oxygen Species in Metabolic and Inflammatory Signaling. *Circ. Res.* **2018**, *122*, 877–902. [CrossRef] [PubMed]
50. Chiste, R.C.; Freitas, M.; Mercadante, A.Z.; Fernandes, E. Superoxide Anion Radical: Generation and Detection in Cellular and Non-Cellular Systems. *Curr. Med. Chem.* **2015**, *22*, 4234–4256. [CrossRef]
51. Klaunig, J.E. Oxidative Stress and Cancer. *Curr. Pharm. Des.* **2019**, *24*, 4771–4778. [CrossRef]
52. Poljšak, B.; Jamnik, P.; Raspor, P.; Pesti, M. Oxidation-Antioxidation-Reduction Processes in the Cell: Impacts of Environmental Pollution. In *Encyclopedia of Environmental Health*; Elsevier: Amsterdam, The Netherlands, 2011; pp. 300–306, ISBN 978-0-444-52272-6.
53. Shin, J.; Song, M.-H.; Oh, J.-W.; Keum, Y.-S.; Saini, R.K. Pro-Oxidant Actions of Carotenoids in Triggering Apoptosis of Cancer Cells: A Review of Emerging Evidence. *Antioxidants* **2020**, *9*, 532. [CrossRef]
54. Huu, T.N.; Park, J.; Zhang, Y.; Park, I.; Yoon, H.; Woo, H.; Lee, S.-R. Redox Regulation of PTEN by Peroxiredoxins. *Antioxidants* **2021**, *10*, 302. [CrossRef]
55. Noorolyai, S.; Shajari, N.; Baghbani, E.; Sadreddini, S.; Baradaran, B. The relation between PI3K/AKT signalling pathway and cancer. *Gene* **2019**, *698*, 120–128. [CrossRef] [PubMed]
56. Ersahin, T.; Tuncbag, N.; Cetin-Atalay, R. The PI3K/AKT/mTOR interactive pathway. *Mol. BioSyst.* **2015**, *11*, 1946–1954. [CrossRef] [PubMed]
57. Li, Q.; Zhu, G.-D. Targeting serine/threonine protein kinase B/Akt and cell-cycle checkpoint kinases for treating cancer. *Curr. Top. Med. Chem.* **2002**, *2*, 939–971. [CrossRef]
58. Tafani, M.; Sansone, L.; Limana, F.; Arcangeli, T.; De Santis, E.; Polese, M.; Fini, M.; Russo, M.A. The Interplay of Reactive Oxygen Species, Hypoxia, Inflammation, and Sirtuins in Cancer Initiation and Progression. *Oxidative Med. Cell. Longev.* **2015**, *2016*, 1–18. [CrossRef]
59. Pezzuto, A.; Carico, E. Role of HIF-1 in Cancer Progression: Novel Insights. A Review. *Curr. Mol. Med.* **2019**, *18*, 343–351. [CrossRef]
60. Jiang, B.-H.; Agani, F.; Passaniti, A.; Semenza, G.L. V-SRC induces expression of hypoxia-inducible factor 1 (HIF-1) and transcription of genes encoding vascular endothelial growth factor and enolase 1: Involvement of HIF-1 in tumor progression. *Cancer Res.* **1997**, *57*, 5328–5335.
61. Moldogazieva, N.T.; Mokhosoev, I.M.; Terentiev, A.A. Metabolic Heterogeneity of Cancer Cells: An Interplay between HIF-1, GLUTs, and AMPK. *Cancers* **2020**, *12*, 862. [CrossRef]
62. Gu, H.; Huang, T.; Shen, Y.; Liu, Y.; Zhou, F.; Jin, Y.; Sattar, H.; Wei, Y. Reactive Oxygen Species-Mediated Tumor Microenvironment Transformation: The Mechanism of Radioresistant Gastric Cancer. *Oxidative Med. Cell. Longev.* **2018**, *2018*, 1–8. [CrossRef]
63. Wang, J.; Xiang, H.; Lu, Y.; Wu, T. Role and clinical significance of TGF-β1 and TGF-βR1 in malignant tumors (Review). *Int. J. Mol. Med.* **2021**, *47*, 55. [CrossRef]
64. Hsieh, C.-L.; Liu, C.-M.; Chen, H.-A.; Yang, S.-T.; Shigemura, K.; Kitagawa, K.; Yamamichi, F.; Fujisawa, M.; Liu, Y.-R.; Lee, W.-H.; et al. Reactive oxygen species–mediated switching expression of MMP-3 in stromal fibroblasts and cancer cells during prostate cancer progression. *Sci. Rep.* **2017**, *7*, 1–14. [CrossRef]
65. Musarrat, J.; Arezina-Wilson, J.; Wani, A. Prognostic and aetiological relevance of 8-hydroxyguanosine in human breast carcinogenesis. *Eur. J. Cancer* **1996**, *32*, 1209–1214. [CrossRef]
66. Cavalieri, E.; Frenkel, K.; Liehr, J.G.; Rogan, E.; Roy, D. Chapter 4: Estrogens as Endogenous Genotoxic Agents–DNA Adducts and Mutations. *J. Natl. Cancer Inst. Monogr.* **2000**, *2000*, 75–94. [CrossRef] [PubMed]
67. Okoh, V.; Deoraj, A.; Roy, D. Estrogen-Induced reactive oxygen species-mediated signalings contribute to breast cancer. *Biochim. Biophys. Acta (BBA) Bioenerg.* **2011**, *1815*, 115–133. [CrossRef] [PubMed]
68. Gorrini, C.; Harris, I.; Mak, T.W. Modulation of oxidative stress as an anticancer strategy. *Nat. Rev. Drug Discov.* **2013**, *12*, 931–947. [CrossRef]

69. Theriault, R.L.; Carlson, R.W.; Allred, C.; Anderson, B.O.; Burstein, H.J.; Edge, S.B.; Farrar, W.B.; Forero, A.; Giordano, S.H.; Goldstein, L.J.; et al. Breast Cancer, Version 3.2013. *J. Natl. Compr. Cancer Netw.* **2013**, *11*, 753–761. [CrossRef] [PubMed]
70. Cauli, O. Oxidative Stress and Cognitive Alterations Induced by Cancer Chemotherapy Drugs: A Scoping Review. *Antioxidants* **2021**, *10*, 1116. [CrossRef]
71. Athreya, K.; Xavier, M.F. Antioxidants in the Treatment of Cancer. *Nutr. Cancer* **2017**, *69*, 1099–1104. [CrossRef]
72. Ji, L.L.; Yeo, D. Oxidative stress: An evolving definition. *Fac. Rev.* **2021**, *10*, 13. [CrossRef]
73. Sies, H. Oxidative stress: Oxidants and antioxidants. *Exp. Physiol.* **1997**, *82*, 291–295. [CrossRef]
74. Flieger, J.; Flieger, W.; Baj, J.; Maciejewski, R. Antioxidants: Classification, Natural Sources, Activity/Capacity Measurements, and Usefulness for the Synthesis of Nanoparticles. *Materials* **2021**, *14*, 4135. [CrossRef]
75. Nordberg, J.; Arnér, E.S. Reactive oxygen species, antioxidants, and the mammalian thioredoxin system. *Free. Radic. Biol. Med.* **2001**, *31*, 1287–1312. [CrossRef]
76. Pisoschi, A.M.; Pop, A. The role of antioxidants in the chemistry of oxidative stress: A review. *Eur. J. Med. Chem.* **2015**, *97*, 55–74. [CrossRef] [PubMed]
77. Johnson, F.; Giulivi, C. Superoxide dismutases and their impact upon human health. *Mol. Asp. Med.* **2005**, *26*, 340–352. [CrossRef] [PubMed]
78. Chelikani, P.; Fita, I.; Loewen, P.C. Diversity of structures and properties among catalases. *Experientia* **2004**, *61*, 192–208. [CrossRef] [PubMed]
79. Rhee, S.G.; Chae, H.Z.; Kim, K. Peroxiredoxins: A historical overview and speculative preview of novel mechanisms and emerging concepts in cell signaling. *Free. Radic. Biol. Med.* **2005**, *38*, 1543–1552. [CrossRef] [PubMed]
80. Matés, J.M.; Campos-Sandoval, J.A.; Santos-Jiménez, J.D.L.; Márquez, J. Glutaminases regulate glutathione and oxidative stress in cancer. *Arch. Toxicol.* **2020**, *94*, 2603–2623. [CrossRef]
81. Cecerska-Heryć, E.; Surowska, O.; Heryć, R.; Serwin, N.; Napiontek-Balińska, S.; Dołęgowska, B. Are antioxidant enzymes essential markers in the diagnosis and monitoring of cancer patients—A review. *Clin. Biochem.* **2021**, *93*, 1–8. [CrossRef]
82. Shahidi, F. Antioxidants. In *Handbook of Antioxidants for Food Preservation*; Elsevier: Amsterdam, The Netherlands, 2015; pp. 1–14, ISBN 978-1-78242-089-7.
83. Hawash, M.; Eid, A.M.; Jaradat, N.; Abualhasan, M.; Amer, J.; Zaid, A.N.; Draghmeh, S.; Daraghmeh, D.; Daraghmeh, H.; Shtayeh, T.; et al. Synthesis and Biological Evaluation of Benzodioxole Derivatives as Potential Anticancer and Antioxidant agents. *Heterocycl. Commun.* **2020**, *26*, 157–167. [CrossRef]
84. Carocho, M.; Ferreira, I. A review on antioxidants, prooxidants and related controversy: Natural and synthetic compounds, screening and analysis methodologies and future perspectives. *Food Chem. Toxicol.* **2013**, *51*, 15–25. [CrossRef]
85. Yang, X.; Song, W.; Liu, N.; Sun, Z.; Liu, R.; Liu, Q.S.; Zhou, Q.; Jiang, G. Synthetic Phenolic Antioxidants Cause Perturbation in Steroidogenesis In Vitro and In Vivo. *Environ. Sci. Technol.* **2017**, *52*, 850–858. [CrossRef] [PubMed]
86. Braver-Sewradj, S.P.D.; Van Spronsen, R.; Hessel, V. Substitution of bisphenol A: A review of the carcinogenicity, reproductive toxicity, and endocrine disruption potential of alternative substances. *Crit. Rev. Toxicol.* **2020**, *50*, 128–147. [CrossRef] [PubMed]
87. Meier, B.W.; Gomez, J.D.; Kirichenko, O.V.; Thompson, J.A. Mechanistic Basis for Inflammation and Tumor Promotion in Lungs of 2,6-Di-tert-butyl-4-methylphenol-Treated Mice: Electrophilic Metabolites Alkylate and Inactivate Antioxidant Enzymes. *Chem. Res. Toxicol.* **2007**, *20*, 199–207. [CrossRef] [PubMed]
88. Jayedi, A.; Rashidy-Pour, A.; Parohan, M.; Zargar, M.S.; Shab-Bidar, S. Dietary Antioxidants, Circulating Antioxidant Concentrations, Total Antioxidant Capacity, and Risk of All-Cause Mortality: A Systematic Review and Dose-Response Meta-Analysis of Prospective Observational Studies. *Adv. Nutr.* **2018**, *9*, 701–716. [CrossRef]
89. Shimizu, H.; Tsubota, T.; Kanki, K.; Shiota, G. All-Trans retinoic acid ameliorates hepatic stellate cell activation via suppression of thioredoxin interacting protein expression. *J. Cell. Physiol.* **2017**, *233*, 607–616. [CrossRef]
90. Sadowska-Bartosz, I.; Bartosz, G. Effect of Antioxidants Supplementation on Aging and Longevity. *BioMed Res. Int.* **2014**, *2014*, 1–17. [CrossRef]
91. Liguori, I.; Russo, G.; Curcio, F.; Bulli, G.; Aran, L.; DELLA Morte, D.; Gargiulo, G.; Testa, G.; Cacciatore, F.; Bonaduce, D.; et al. Oxidative stress, aging, and diseases. *Clin. Interv. Aging* **2018**, *13*, 757–772. [CrossRef]
92. Siti, H.N.; Kamisah, Y.; Kamsiah, J. The role of oxidative stress, antioxidants and vascular inflammation in cardiovascular disease (a review). *Vasc. Pharmacol.* **2015**, *71*, 40–56. [CrossRef]
93. Sahin, K.; Sahin, N.; Kucuk, O. Lycopene and Chemotherapy Toxicity. *Nutr. Cancer* **2010**, *62*, 988–995. [CrossRef] [PubMed]
94. Ilghami, R.; Barzegari, A.; Mashayekhi, M.R.; Letourneur, D.; Crepin, M.; Pavon-Djavid, G. The conundrum of dietary antioxidants in cancer chemotherapy. *Nutr. Rev.* **2019**, *78*, 65–76. [CrossRef]
95. Van Chuyen, H.; Eun, J.-B. Marine carotenoids: Bioactivities and potential benefits to human health. *Crit. Rev. Food Sci. Nutr.* **2017**, *57*, 2600–2610. [CrossRef] [PubMed]
96. Langi, P.; Kiokias, S.; Varzakas, T.; Proestos, C. Carotenoids: From Plants to Food and Feed Industries. In *Microbial Carotenoids*; Barreiro, C., Barredo, J.-L., Eds.; Methods in Molecular Biology; Springer: New York, NY, USA, 2018; Volume 1852, pp. 57–71. ISBN 978-1-4939-8741-2.
97. Hammond, B.R.; Renzi, L.M. Carotenoids. *Adv. Nutr.* **2013**, *4*, 474–476. [CrossRef] [PubMed]
98. Britton, G.; Liaaen-Jensen, S.; Pfander, H. (Eds.) *Carotenoids Handbook*; Birkhäuser Verlag: Basel, Switzerland; Boston, MA, USA, 2004; ISBN 978-3-7643-6180-8.

99. Maoka, T. Carotenoids as natural functional pigments. *J. Nat. Med.* **2019**, *74*, 1–16. [CrossRef]
100. Tanaka, T.; Shnimizu, M.; Moriwaki, H. Cancer Chemoprevention by Carotenoids. *Molecules* **2012**, *17*, 3202–3242. [CrossRef]
101. Liaaen-Jensen, S. Stereochemical aspects of carotenoids. *Pure Appl. Chem.* **1997**, *69*, 2027–2038. [CrossRef]
102. Milani, A.; Basirnejad, M.; Shahbazi, S.; Bolhassani, A. Carotenoids: Biochemistry, pharmacology and treatment. *Br. J. Pharmacol.* **2016**, *174*, 1290–1324. [CrossRef]
103. Saini, R.K.; Keum, Y.-S.; Daglia, M.; Rengasamy, K.R. Dietary carotenoids in cancer chemoprevention and chemotherapy: A review of emerging evidence. *Pharmacol. Res.* **2020**, *157*, 104830. [CrossRef]
104. Koklesova, L.; Liskova, A.; Samec, M.; Buhrmann, C.; Samuel, S.; Varghese, E.; Ashrafizadeh, M.; Najafi, M.; Shakibaei, M.; Büsselberg, D.; et al. Carotenoids in Cancer Apoptosis—The Road from Bench to Bedside and Back. *Cancers* **2020**, *12*, 2425. [CrossRef]
105. Chang, M.X.; Xiong, F. Astaxanthin and its Effects in Inflammatory Responses and Inflammation-Associated Diseases: Recent Advances and Future Directions. *Molecules* **2020**, *25*, 5342. [CrossRef]
106. Xu, Y.; Zhang, J.; Jiang, W.; Zhang, S. Astaxanthin induces angiogenesis through Wnt/β-catenin signaling pathway. *Phytomedicine* **2015**, *22*, 744–751. [CrossRef] [PubMed]
107. Chew, B.P.; Brown, C.M.; Park, J.S.; Mixter, P.F. Dietary lutein inhibits mouse mammary tumor growth by regulating angiogenesis and apoptosis. *Anticancer. Res.* **2003**, *23*, 3333–3339.
108. Wang, J.; Ma, Y.; Yang, J.; Jin, L.; Gao, Z.; Xue, L.; Hou, L.; Sui, L.; Liu, J.; Zou, X. Fucoxanthin inhibits tumour-related lymphangiogenesis and growth of breast cancer. *J. Cell. Mol. Med.* **2019**, *23*, 2219–2229. [CrossRef] [PubMed]
109. Bonet, M.L.; Ribot, J.; Galmés, S.; Serra, F.; Palou, A. Carotenoids and carotenoid conversion products in adipose tissue biology and obesity: Pre-clinical and human studies. *Biochim. Biophys. Acta (BBA) Mol. Cell Biol. Lipids* **2020**, *1865*, 158676. [CrossRef] [PubMed]
110. Esatbeyoglu, T.; Rimbach, G. Canthaxanthin: From molecule to function. *Mol. Nutr. Food Res.* **2016**, *61*. [CrossRef]
111. Mortensen, A.; Skibsted, L.; Truscott, T. The Interaction of Dietary Carotenoids with Radical Species. *Arch. Biochem. Biophys.* **2001**, *385*, 13–19. [CrossRef] [PubMed]
112. Jomova, K.; Valko, M. Health protective effects of carotenoids and their interactions with other biological antioxidants. *Eur. J. Med. Chem.* **2013**, *70*, 102–110. [CrossRef]
113. Ribeiro, D.; Freitas, M.; Silva, A.M.; Carvalho, F.; Fernandes, E. Antioxidant and pro-oxidant activities of carotenoids and their oxidation products. *Food Chem. Toxicol.* **2018**, *120*, 681–699. [CrossRef]
114. Young, A.; Lowe, G.M. Antioxidant and Prooxidant Properties of Carotenoids. *Arch. Biochem. Biophys.* **2001**, *385*, 20–27. [CrossRef]
115. El-Agamey, A.; Lowe, G.M.; McGarvey, D.J.; Mortensen, A.; Phillip, D.M.; Truscott, T.; Young, A. Carotenoid radical chemistry and antioxidant/pro-oxidant properties. *Arch. Biochem. Biophys.* **2004**, *430*, 37–48. [CrossRef]
116. Palozza, P. Prooxidant Actions of Carotenoids in Biologic Systems. *Nutr. Rev.* **1998**, *56*, 257–265. [CrossRef]
117. Yeum, K.-J.; Aldini, G.; Russell, R.M.; Krinsky, N.I. Antioxidant/Pro-oxidant Actions of Carotenoids. In *Carotenoids*; Britton, G., Pfander, H., Liaaen-Jensen, S., Eds.; Birkhäuser Basel: Basel, Switzerland, 2009; pp. 235–268. ISBN 978-3-7643-7500-3.
118. Singh, K.; Bhori, M.; Kasu, Y.A.; Bhat, G.; Marar, T. Antioxidants as precision weapons in war against cancer chemotherapy induced toxicity—Exploring the armoury of obscurity. *Saudi Pharm. J.* **2017**, *26*, 177–190. [CrossRef]
119. Chesson, A.; Collins, A. Assessment of the role of diet in cancer prevention. *Cancer Lett.* **1997**, *114*, 237–245. [CrossRef]
120. Wargovich, M.J. Experimental evidence for cancer preventive elements in foods. *Cancer Lett.* **1997**, *114*, 11–17. [CrossRef]
121. Sporn, M.B.; Suh, N. Chemoprevention: An essential approach to controlling cancer. *Nat. Rev. Cancer* **2002**, *2*, 537–543. [CrossRef] [PubMed]
122. Shree, G.S.; Prasad, K.Y.; Arpitha, H.S.; Deepika, U.R.; Kumar, K.N.; Mondal, P.; Ganesan, P. β-Carotene at physiologically attainable concentration induces apoptosis and down-regulates cell survival and antioxidant markers in human breast cancer (MCF-7) cells. *Mol. Cell. Biochem.* **2017**, *436*, 1–12. [CrossRef] [PubMed]
123. Sumantran, V.N.; Zhang, R.; Lee, D.S.; Wicha, M.S. Differential regulation of apoptosis in normal versus transformed mammary epithelium by lutein and retinoic acid. *Cancer Epidemiol. Biomark. Prev.* **2000**, *9*, 257–263.
124. Zhang, S.; Hunter, D.J.; Forman, M.R.; Rosner, B.A.; Speizer, F.E.; Colditz, G.; Manson, J.E.; Hankinson, S.E.; Willett, W.C. Dietary Carotenoids and Vitamins A, C, and E and Risk of Breast Cancer. *J. Natl. Cancer Inst.* **1999**, *91*, 547–556. [CrossRef] [PubMed]
125. Eastwood, M. Interaction of dietary antioxidants in vivo: How fruit and vegetables prevent disease? *Qjm Int. J. Med.* **1999**, *92*, 527–530. [CrossRef] [PubMed]
126. Holick, C.N.; Michaud, D.S.; Stolzenberg-Solomon, R.; Mayne, S.T.; Pietinen, P.; Taylor, P.R.; Virtamo, J.; Albanes, D. Dietary Carotenoids, Serum beta-Carotene, and Retinol and Risk of Lung Cancer in the Alpha-Tocopherol, Beta-Carotene Cohort Study. *Am. J. Epidemiol.* **2002**, *156*, 536–547. [CrossRef]
127. Palozza, P.; Serini, S.; Di Nicuolo, F.; Calviello, G. Modulation of apoptotic signalling by carotenoids in cancer cells. *Arch. Biochem. Biophys.* **2004**, *430*, 104–109. [CrossRef]
128. Yasueda, A.; Urushima, H.; Ito, T. Efficacy and Interaction of Antioxidant Supplements as Adjuvant Therapy in Cancer Treatment. *Integr. Cancer Ther.* **2015**, *15*, 17–39. [CrossRef]
129. Lamson, D.W.; Brignall, M.S. Antioxidants in cancer therapy; their actions and interactions with oncologic therapies. *Altern Med Rev.* **1999**, *4*, 304–329.

130. Al-Ishaq, R.K.; Overy, A.J.; Büsselberg, D. Phytochemicals and Gastrointestinal Cancer: Cellular Mechanisms and Effects to Change Cancer Progression. *Biomolecules* **2020**, *10*, 105. [CrossRef]
131. Kavitha, K.; Kowshik, J.; Kishore, T.K.K.; Baba, A.B.; Nagini, S. Astaxanthin inhibits NF-κB and Wnt/β-catenin signaling pathways via inactivation of Erk/MAPK and PI3K/Akt to induce intrinsic apoptosis in a hamster model of oral cancer. *Biochim. Biophys. Acta (BBA) Gen. Subj.* **2013**, *1830*, 4433–4444. [CrossRef]
132. Preet, R.; Mohapatra, P.; Das, D.; Satapathy, S.R.; Choudhuri, T.; Wyatt, M.D.; Kundu, C.N. Lycopene synergistically enhances quinacrine action to inhibit Wnt-TCF signaling in breast cancer cells through APC. *Carcinogenesis* **2012**, *34*, 277–286. [CrossRef]
133. Karas, M.; Amir, H.; Fishman, D.; Danilenko, M.; Segal, S.; Nahum, A.; Koifmann, A.; Giat, Y.; Levy, J.; Sharoni, Y. Lycopene Interferes With Cell Cycle Progression and Insulin-Like Growth Factor I Signaling in Mammary Cancer Cells. *Nutr. Cancer* **2000**, *36*, 101–111. [CrossRef]
134. Peng, S.; Li, J.; Zhou, Y.; Tuo, M.; Qin, X.; Yu, Q.; Cheng, H.; Li, Y. In Vitro effects and mechanisms of lycopene in MCF-7 human breast cancer cells. *Genet. Mol. Res.* **2017**, *16*, 1–8. [CrossRef]
135. Gloria, N.F.; Soares, N.; Brand, C.; de Oliveira, F.L.; Borojevic, R.; Teodoro, A.J. Lycopene and beta-carotene induce cell-cycle arrest and apoptosis in human breast cancer cell lines. *Anticancer Res.* **2014**, *34*, 1377–1386. [PubMed]
136. Xu, X.; Zhang, M.; Xu, F.; Jiang, S. Wnt signaling in breast cancer: Biological mechanisms, challenges and opportunities. *Mol. Cancer* **2020**, *19*, 1–35. [CrossRef] [PubMed]
137. Arzi, L.; Riazi, G.; Sadeghizadeh, M.; Hoshyar, R.; Jafarzadeh, N. A Comparative Study on Anti-Invasion, Antimigration, and Antiadhesion Effects of the Bioactive Carotenoids of Saffron on 4T1 Breast Cancer Cells Through Their Effects on Wnt/β-Catenin Pathway Genes. *DNA Cell Biol.* **2018**, *37*, 697–707. [CrossRef] [PubMed]
138. Gong, X.; Smith, J.R.; Swanson, H.M.; Rubin, L.P. Carotenoid Lutein Selectively Inhibits Breast Cancer Cell Growth and Potentiates the Effect of Chemotherapeutic Agents through ROS-Mediated Mechanisms. *Molecules* **2018**, *23*, 905. [CrossRef] [PubMed]
139. Wang, Y.; Gapstur, S.M.; Gaudet, M.M.; Furtado, J.D.; Campos, H.; McCullough, M.L. Plasma carotenoids and breast cancer risk in the Cancer Prevention Study II Nutrition Cohort. *Cancer Causes Control.* **2015**, *26*, 1233–1244. [CrossRef] [PubMed]
140. Ahn, Y.T.; Kim, M.S.; Kim, Y.S.; An, W.G. Astaxanthin Reduces Stemness Markers in BT20 and T47D Breast Cancer Stem Cells by Inhibiting Expression of Pontin and Mutant p53. *Mar. Drugs* **2020**, *18*, 577. [CrossRef]
141. Kim, M.S.; Ahn, Y.T.; Lee, C.W.; Kim, H.; An, W.G. Astaxanthin Modulates Apoptotic Molecules to Induce Death of SKBR3 Breast Cancer Cells. *Mar. Drugs* **2020**, *18*, 266. [CrossRef]
142. Molnár, J.; Gyémánt, N.; Mucsi, I.; Molnár, A.; Szabó, M.; Körtvélyesi, T.; Varga, A.; Molnár, P.; Tóth, G. Modulation of multidrug resistance and apoptosis of cancer cells by selected carotenoids. *In Vivo* **2004**, *18*, 237–244.
143. Koklesova, L.; Liskova, A.; Samec, M.; Zhai, K.; Abotaleb, M.; Ashrafizadeh, M.; Brockmueller, A.; Shakibaei, M.; Biringer, K.; Bugos, O.; et al. Carotenoids in Cancer Metastasis—Status Quo and Outlook. *Biomolecules* **2020**, *10*, 1653. [CrossRef]
144. McCall, B.; McPartland, C.K.; Moore, R.; Frank-Kamenetskii, A.; Booth, B.W. Effects of Astaxanthin on the Proliferation and Migration of Breast Cancer Cells In Vitro. *Antioxidants* **2018**, *7*, 135. [CrossRef]
145. Chen, T.; You, Y.; Jiang, H.; Wang, Z.Z. Epithelial-Mesenchymal transition (EMT): A biological process in the development, stem cell differentiation, and tumorigenesis. *J. Cell. Physiol.* **2017**, *232*, 3261–3272. [CrossRef]
146. Li, Y.; Zhang, Y.; Liu, X.; Wang, M.; Wang, P.; Yang, J.; Zhang, S. Lutein inhibits proliferation, invasion and migration of hypoxic breast cancer cells via downregulation of HES1. *Int. J. Oncol.* **2018**, *52*, 2119–2129. [CrossRef] [PubMed]
147. Chen, L.; Long, C.; Nguyen, J.; Kumar, D.; Lee, J. Discovering alkylamide derivatives of bexarotene as new therapeutic agents against triple-negative breast cancer. *Bioorganic Med. Chem. Lett.* **2018**, *28*, 420–424. [CrossRef] [PubMed]
148. Vijay, K.; Sowmya, P.R.-R.; Arathi, B.P.; Shilpa, S.; Shwetha, H.J.; Raju, M.; Baskaran, V.; Lakshminarayana, R. Low-Dose doxorubicin with carotenoids selectively alters redox status and upregulates oxidative stress-mediated apoptosis in breast cancer cells. *Food Chem. Toxicol.* **2018**, *118*, 675–690. [CrossRef] [PubMed]
149. Atalay, P.B.; Kuku, G.; Tuna, B.G. Effects of carbendazim and astaxanthin co-treatment on the proliferation of MCF-7 breast cancer cells. *Vitr. Cell. Dev. Biol. Anim.* **2018**, *55*, 113–119. [CrossRef] [PubMed]
150. Mostafavinia, S.E.; Khorashadizadeh, M.; Hoshyar, R. Antiproliferative and Proapoptotic Effects of Crocin Combined with Hyperthermia on Human Breast Cancer Cells. *DNA Cell Biol.* **2016**, *35*, 340–347. [CrossRef]
151. Gyémánt, N.; Tanaka, M.; Molnár, P.; Deli, J.; Mándoky, L.; Molnár, J. Reversal of multidrug resistance of cancer cells in vitro: Modification of drug resistance by selected carotenoids. *Anticancer Res.* **2006**, *26*, 367–374. [PubMed]
152. Eliassen, A.H.; Liao, X.; Rosner, B.; Tamimi, R.M.; Tworoger, S.S.; Hankinson, S.E. Plasma carotenoids and risk of breast cancer over 20 y of follow-up. *Am. J. Clin. Nutr.* **2015**, *101*, 1197–1205. [CrossRef] [PubMed]
153. Sato, R.; Helzlsouer, K.J.; Alberg, A.J.; Hoffman, S.C.; Norkus, E.P.; Comstock, G.W. Prospective study of carotenoids, tocopherols, and retinoid concentrations and the risk of breast cancer. *Cancer Epidemiol. Biomark. Prev.* **2002**, *11*, 451–457.
154. Bakker, M.F.; Peeters, P.H.; Klaasen, V.M.; Bueno-De-Mesquita, H.B.; Jansen, E.H.; Ros, M.M.; Travier, N.; Olsen, A.; Tjonneland, A.; Overvad, K.; et al. Plasma carotenoids, vitamin C, tocopherols, and retinol and the risk of breast cancer in the European Prospective Investigation into Cancer and Nutrition cohort1,2. *Am. J. Clin. Nutr.* **2016**, *103*, 454–464. [CrossRef] [PubMed]
155. Zuniga, K.E.; Moran, N.E. Low Serum Carotenoids Are Associated with Self-Reported Cognitive Dysfunction and Inflammatory Markers in Breast Cancer Survivors. *Nutrients* **2018**, *10*, 1111. [CrossRef]

156. Kabat, G.C.; Kim, M.; Adams-Campbell, L.L.; Caan, B.J.; Chlebowski, R.T.; Neuhouser, M.L.; Shikany, J.M.; Rohan, T.E. Longitudinal study of serum carotenoid, retinol, and tocopherol concentrations in relation to breast cancer risk among postmenopausal women. *Am. J. Clin. Nutr.* **2009**, *90*, 162–169. [CrossRef]
157. Butalla, A.C.; Crane, T.E.; Patil, B.; Wertheim, B.C.; Thompson, P.; Thomson, C.A. Effects of a Carrot Juice Intervention on Plasma Carotenoids, Oxidative Stress, and Inflammation in Overweight Breast Cancer Survivors. *Nutr. Cancer* **2012**, *64*, 331–341. [CrossRef]
158. Hu, F.; Yi, B.W.; Zhang, W.; Liang, J.; Lin, C.; Li, D.; Wang, F.; Pang, D.; Zhao, Y. Carotenoids and breast cancer risk: A meta-analysis and meta-regression. *Breast Cancer Res. Treat.* **2011**, *131*, 239–253. [CrossRef] [PubMed]
159. Tamimi, R.M.; Hankinson, S.E.; Campos, H.; Spiegelman, D.; Zhang, S.; Colditz, G.; Willett, W.C.; Hunter, D.J. Plasma Carotenoids, Retinol, and Tocopherols and Risk of Breast Cancer. *Am. J. Epidemiol.* **2005**, *161*, 153–160. [CrossRef] [PubMed]
160. Pouchieu, C.; Galán, P.; Ducros, V.; Latino-Martel, P.; Hercberg, S.; Touvier, M. Plasma Carotenoids and Retinol and Overall and Breast Cancer Risk: A Nested Case-Control Study. *Nutr. Cancer* **2014**, *66*, 980–988. [CrossRef] [PubMed]
161. Rock, C.L.; Flatt, S.W.; Natarajan, L.; Thomson, C.A.; Bardwell, W.A.; Newman, V.A.; Hollenbach, K.A.; Jones, L.; Caan, B.J.; Pierce, J.P. Plasma Carotenoids and Recurrence-Free Survival in Women With a History of Breast Cancer. *J. Clin. Oncol.* **2005**, *23*, 6631–6638. [CrossRef] [PubMed]
162. Thomson, C.A.; Stendell-Hollis, N.R.; Rock, C.L.; Cussler, E.C.; Flatt, S.W.; Pierce, J.P. Plasma and Dietary Carotenoids Are Associated with Reduced Oxidative Stress in Women Previously Treated for Breast Cancer. *Cancer Epidemiol. Biomark. Prev.* **2007**, *16*, 2008–2015. [CrossRef]
163. Mignone, L.I.; Giovannucci, E.; Newcomb, P.A.; Titus-Ernstoff, L.; Trentham-Dietz, A.; Hampton, J.M.; Willett, W.C.; Egan, K.M. Dietary carotenoids and the risk of invasive breast cancer. *Int. J. Cancer* **2009**, *124*, 2929–2937. [CrossRef]
164. Buckland, G.; Travier, N.; Arribas, L.; Del Barco, S.; Pernas, S.; Zamora, E.; Bellet, M.; Cirauqui, B.; Margelí, M.; Munoz, M.; et al. Changes in dietary intake, plasma carotenoids and erythrocyte membrane fatty acids in breast cancer survivors after a lifestyle intervention: Results from a single-arm trial. *J. Hum. Nutr. Diet.* **2019**, *32*, 468–479. [CrossRef]
165. Kapinova, A.; Kubatka, P.; Golubnitschaja, O.; Kello, M.; Zubor, P.; Solar, P.; Pec, M. Dietary phytochemicals in breast cancer research: Anticancer effects and potential utility for effective chemoprevention. *Environ. Health Prev. Med.* **2018**, *23*, 36. [CrossRef]
166. Yu, N.; Su, X.; Wang, Z.; Dai, B.; Kang, J. Association of Dietary Vitamin A and β-Carotene Intake with the Risk of Lung Cancer: A Meta-Analysis of 19 Publications. *Nutrients* **2015**, *7*, 9309–9324. [CrossRef]
167. Limon-Miro, A.T.; Valencia, M.E.; Lopez-Teros, V.; Alemán-Mateo, H.; Méndez-Estrada, R.O.; Pacheco-Moreno, B.I.; Astiazaran-Garcia, H. An individualized food-based nutrition intervention reduces visceral and total body fat while preserving skeletal muscle mass in breast cancer patients under antineoplastic treatment. *Clin. Nutr.* **2021**, *40*, 4394–4403. [CrossRef]
168. Nguyen, T.; Irwin, M.L.; Dewan, A.T.; Cartmel, B.; Harrigan, M.; Ferrucci, L.M.; Sanft, T.; Li, F.; Lu, L.; Salinas, Y.D. Examining the effect of obesity-associated gene variants on breast cancer survivors in a randomized weight loss intervention. *Breast Cancer Res. Treat.* **2021**, *187*, 487–497. [CrossRef]
169. Essa, A.R.; Browne, E.P.; Punska, E.C.; Perkins, K.; Boudreau, E.; Wiggins, H.; Anderton, D.L.; Sibeko, L.; Sturgeon, S.R.; Arcaro, K.F. Dietary Intervention to Increase Fruit and Vegetable Consumption in Breastfeeding Women: A Pilot Randomized Trial Measuring Inflammatory Markers in Breast Milk. *J. Acad. Nutr. Diet.* **2018**, *118*, 2287–2295. [CrossRef]
170. Djuric, Z.; Ren, J.; Blythe, J.; VanLoon, G.; Sen, A. A Mediterranean dietary intervention in healthy American women changes plasma carotenoids and fatty acids in distinct clusters. *Nutr. Res.* **2009**, *29*, 156–163. [CrossRef] [PubMed]
171. Rodrigo-Baños, M.; Garbayo, I.; Vílchez, C.; Bonete, M.-J.; Martínez-Espinosa, R.M. Carotenoids from Haloarchaea and Their Potential in Biotechnology. *Mar. Drugs* **2015**, *13*, 5508–5532. [CrossRef]
172. Rodrigo-Baños, M.; Montero, Z.; Torregrosa-Crespo, J.; Garbayo, I.; Vílchez, C.; Martínez-Espinosa, R.M. Haloarchaea: A Promising Biosource for Carotenoid Production. In *Carotenoids: Biosynthetic and Biofunctional Approaches*; Misawa, N., Ed.; Advances in Experimental Medicine and Biology; Springer: Singapore, 2021; Volume 1261, pp. 165–174. ISBN 9789811573590.
173. Montero-Lobato, Z.; Ramos-Merchante, A.; Fuentes, J.L.; Sayago, A.; Fernández-Recamales, Á.; Martínez-Espinosa, R.M.; Vega, J.M.; Vílchez, C.; Garbayo, I. Optimization of Growth and Carotenoid Production by Haloferax mediterranei Using Response Surface Methodology. *Mar. Drugs* **2018**, *16*, 372. [CrossRef]
174. Kelly, M.; Jensen, S.L.; Theander, O.; Cyvin, S.J.; Hagen, G. Bacterial Carotenoids. XXVI. C50-Carotenoids. 2. Bacterioruberin. *Acta Chem. Scand.* **1967**, *21*, 2578–2580. [CrossRef] [PubMed]
175. Ronnekleiv, M. Bacterial carotenoids 53∗ C50-carotenoids 23; carotenoids of Haloferax volcanii versus other halophilic bacteria. *Biochem. Syst. Ecol.* **1995**, *23*, 627–634. [CrossRef]
176. Giani, M.; Martínez-Espinosa, R. Carotenoids as a Protection Mechanism against Oxidative Stress in Haloferax mediterranei. *Antioxidants* **2020**, *9*, 1060. [CrossRef] [PubMed]
177. Hegazy, G.; Abu-Serie, M.M.; Abo-Elela, G.M.; Ghozlan, H.; Sabry, S.A.; Soliman, N.A.; Abdel-Fattah, Y.R. In Vitro dual (anticancer and antiviral) activity of the carotenoids produced by haloalkaliphilic archaeon Natrialba sp. M6. *Sci. Rep.* **2020**, *10*, 5986. [CrossRef]
178. Huang, H. Matrix Metalloproteinase-9 (MMP-9) as a Cancer Biomarker and MMP-9 Biosensors: Recent Advances. *Sensors* **2018**, *18*, 3249. [CrossRef]

179. Zalazar, L.; Pagola, P.; Miró, M.V.; Churio, M.S.; Cerletti, M.; Martínez, C.; Iniesta-Cuerda, M.; Soler, A.; Cesari, A.; De Castro, R.; et al. Bacterioruberin extracts from a genetically modified hyperpigmented Haloferax volcanii strain: Antioxidant activity and bioactive properties on sperm cells. *J. Appl. Microbiol.* **2018**, *126*, 796–810. [CrossRef] [PubMed]
180. Griñan-Lison, C.; Blaya-Cánovas, J.; López-Tejada, A.; Ávalos-Moreno, M.; Navarro-Ocón, A.; Cara, F.; González-González, A.; Lorente, J.; Marchal, J.; Granados-Principal, S. Antioxidants for the Treatment of Breast Cancer: Are We There Yet? *Antioxidants* **2021**, *10*, 205. [CrossRef] [PubMed]
181. Roulot, A.; Héquet, D.; Guinebretière, J.-M.; Vincent-Salomon, A.; Lerebours, F.; Dubot, C.; Rouzier, R. Tumoral heterogeneity of breast cancer. *Ann. Biol. Clin.* **2016**, *74*, 653–660. [CrossRef] [PubMed]
182. Yassine, F.; Salibi, E.; Gali-Muhtasib, H. Overview of the Formulations and Analogs in the Taxanes' Story. *Curr. Med. Chem.* **2016**, *23*, 4540–4558. [CrossRef] [PubMed]
183. Newman, D.J.; Cragg, G.M. Natural Products as Sources of New Drugs over the Last 25 Years. *J. Nat. Prod.* **2007**, *70*, 461–477. [CrossRef]

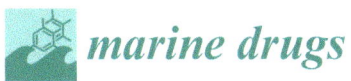

Review

Anti-Inflammatory and Anticancer Effects of Microalgal Carotenoids

Javier Ávila-Román [1,*,†], Sara García-Gil [2], Azahara Rodríguez-Luna [2], Virginia Motilva [2] and Elena Talero [2,*,†]

1. Department of Biochemistry and Biotechnology, Universitat Rovira i Virgili, 43007 Tarragona, Spain
2. Department of Pharmacology, Universidad de Sevilla, 41012 Seville, Spain; sargargil@alum.us.es (S.G.-G.); arodriguez53@us.es (A.R.-L.); motilva@us.es (V.M.)
* Correspondence: franciscojavier.avila@urv.cat (J.Á.-R.); etalero@us.es (E.T.)
† These authors contributed equally to the work.

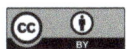

Abstract: Acute inflammation is a key component of the immune system's response to pathogens, toxic agents, or tissue injury, involving the stimulation of defense mechanisms aimed to removing pathogenic factors and restoring tissue homeostasis. However, uncontrolled acute inflammatory response may lead to chronic inflammation, which is involved in the development of many diseases, including cancer. Nowadays, the need to find new potential therapeutic compounds has raised the worldwide scientific interest to study the marine environment. Specifically, microalgae are considered rich sources of bioactive molecules, such as carotenoids, which are natural isoprenoid pigments with important beneficial effects for health due to their biological activities. Carotenoids are essential nutrients for mammals, but they are unable to synthesize them; instead, a dietary intake of these compounds is required. Carotenoids are classified as carotenes (hydrocarbon carotenoids), such as α- and β-carotene, and xanthophylls (oxygenate derivatives) including zeaxanthin, astaxanthin, fucoxanthin, lutein, α- and β-cryptoxanthin, and canthaxanthin. This review summarizes the present up-to-date knowledge of the anti-inflammatory and anticancer activities of microalgal carotenoids both in vitro and in vivo, as well as the latest status of human studies for their potential use in prevention and treatment of inflammatory diseases and cancer.

Keywords: microalgae; carotenoids; inflammation; cancer; oxidative stress

1. Introduction

Microalgae are a vast group of prokaryotic and eukaryotic, mainly photoautotrophic, microorganisms that can be found individually or forming colonies. Moreover, these photosynthetic microorganisms make up the major group of living organisms in terms of species diversity on Earth, having colonized every type of ecological niche in both marine and terrestrial waters [1]. Currently, 50,000 species of microalgae have been described, but the number of new species is increasing yearly, being estimated up to 800,000. In this regard, although only a few of these aquatic microorganisms are able to grow in large-scale settings, microalgae have become an economically promising feedstock for bulk chemicals [2,3]. Moreover, the emergence of biotechnology in the 1960s led to the development of new laboratory and industrial methodologies to grow different species of microalgae. Since then, the worldwide research trends in the microalgal field have increased. In the last 20 years, a multitude of scientific publications have emerged around these aquatic microorganisms since they are a tremendously important source of bioactive molecules, being more diverse than those found in the terrestrial environment.

Firstly, microalga studies showed their potential to be considered by the biodiesel/bioethanol industry due to their high lipid content [4,5], besides promoting an ecological and socio-economic impact [6–8]. Although microalgae have been less studied than macroalgae, their advantages are associated with simple requirements, rapid generation times, and a higher capacity to modulate their metabolism in response to changing environmental conditions. Currently, microalgae remain attractive for the biodiesel industry but also for other sectors such as food, pharmaceuticals, or cosmetics. In this regard, many important drugs have traditionally been provided by terrestrial plants, fungi, and bacteria, but microalgae have become a sustainable resource for these biocomponents. Indeed, there is a current need to find new potential chemical structures for therapeutic use. Additionally, microalgae have raised the worldwide scientific interest since their capacity to synthetize new molecular structures according to seawater composition is widely known [9].

Many studies support microalgae as excellent sources of metabolites such as lipids, carbohydrates, proteins, phenolic compounds, vitamins, and carotenoids, which play physiological roles for themselves and their environment, with real applications in pharmaceutical and nutraceutical industries [10–12]. In this regard, only a few of these compounds, such as n-3 polyunsaturated fatty acids (PUFAs), phycobilins (phycoerythrin and phycocyanin), and carotenoids, including β-carotene, astaxanthin (ATX), zeaxanthin (ZX), and lutein (LUT), have been produced at an industrial scale. However, their low production yield in native microalgae and the difficulty in isolating by economically feasible means may be considered a production problem [2]. Nowadays, biotechnology considers microalgae as producers for a wide range of novel high-value products that have good market opportunities. However, the main challenges to obtain potential microalgal components are the high cost of operation, infrastructure and maintenance, selection of strains, dewatering, and commercial-scale harvesting. The manufacture and commercialization of microalgal products depend on market and financial affairs, among others. Furthermore, the study of their actual potential is limited by the lack of reliable statistical data of the microalga market. For this reason, the current scientific efforts are focused on basic technologies controlling several abiotic conditions to produce microalgal biomass, including different production methods such as open water, greenhouse ponds, and closed photobioreactors. Additionally, chemicals or certain culture conditions such as ultrasonic use by sonication [13–15] and genomic technologies [16] are currently being used in microalga cultivation to obtain high-value-added products [17]. These conditions are aimed in many cases at the food sector as nutritional supplements for vegetarian type diets but also as nutraceuticals. Hence, long-term research is needed to develop systems to create sustainable microalga-based products, since sustainability is a key concern, especially in today's industrial environment. In this way, a multitude of recent international patent licenses [18] are focused on the optimization of microalga growth conditions as well as the system-level optimal yield to produce different bioproducts such as lipids for fuel, proteins for animal feed, or recombinant proteins for purposes of basic research, as well as biotechnological or dermatological/cosmeceutical use [19–23].

Carotenoids, which are one of the most abundant components in microalgae, have shown significant therapeutic potential due to their biological activities. In this context, the advances in biotechnology of microalgae have led to development of methods to increase their production. For example, the outdoor cultivation of *Muriellopsis* sp. (Chlorophyta) has been developed in order to produce high LUT and low metal content, to provide a product with antioxidant properties that may be used for animal feed and human consumption as a dietetic ingredient [24]. More recently, a method was carried out to efficiently extract eicosapaentanoic acid (EPA) and fucoxanthin (FX) from the microalga *Phaeodactylum tricornutum* (Bacillariophyta) [25]. Furthermore, in the last few years, a multitude of studies have shown the industry and academic interest in the potential of carotenoids from microalgae in different industrial sectors. In this regard, a variety of patents and scientific publications in which microalgae, or part of them, are used as functional food or nutraceuticals providing therapeutical potential have been developed. Recently, a patent has been licensed for a microalga-derived carotenoid mixture, which contains diatoxanthin from the microalga Euglena (Euglenozoa) as the main component, besides ZX and alloxanthin. This diatoxanthin-rich product prevents diabetes by suppressing the increment in blood glucose through ingestion along with a high-glycemic index food [26]. In addition, *Chlorella sorokiniana* (Chlorophyta), a microalga rich in glutathione, α-tocopherol, and carotenoids, was reported to have beneficial effects in counteracting oxidative stress preserving mitochondrial liver function in an experimental model of hyperthyroidism in rats [27]. Additionally, anti-inflammatory, antioxidant, and anticancer properties of microalgal carotenoids have been widely demonstrated in different experimental models, but to date there are only a few studies in humans.

The present review summarizes the major findings on microalgal carotenoids with a potential role in inflammation, oxidative stress, and cancer since carotenoids are one of the most abundant compounds in microalgae and they can represent an important commercial outlet.

2. Microalgal Carotenoids

Carotenoids are tetraterpenes obtained from dimerization of geranylgeranyl pyrophosphate in photosynthetic organisms such as plants, including macro- and microalgae, bacteria, some fungi, or some invertebrates [28]. They make up the most abundant lipid-soluble pigments in nature, being responsible for the white, yellow, orange, or red range of colors. There are two types of carotenoids: carotenes, which are hydrocarbon carotenoids such as α- and β-carotene, and xanthophylls, which are oxygenate derivatives, including ZX, ATX, FX, LUT, α- and β-cryptoxanthin (BCX), and canthaxanthin (CX). Carotenoids are essential nutrients for mammals, since they are unable to synthesize them. For this reason, a dietary intake of these compounds is required. The major dietary sources of carotenoids are fruits and vegetables, legumes, cereals, egg yolk, and mammals' milk, as well as micro- and macroalgae [29].

Currently, lycopene, β-carotene, CX, ZX, ATX, and LUT are the main carotenoids produced on a large scale for food products, animal feeds, cosmetics, and pharmaceutical sectors. Their increasing commercial applications have led to a growing market demand of these bioactives. Thus, microalgae have emerged as a rich biosustainable source of carotenoids, with *Arthrospira* (formerly *Spirulina*) (Cyanobacteria), *Chlorella*, *Dunaliella*, and *Haematococcus* (Chlorophyta) being the most common producers of β-carotene, LUT, ATX, FX, ZX, and violaxanthin, among others [30].

2.1. β-Carotene

β,β-carotene, or more commonly named β-carotene (Figure 1A), is the most well-known carotenoid found in many fruits and vegetables [29]. This tetraterpenoid is a vitamin A precursor when consumed and digested. Currently, β-carotene is used as a natural colorant and antioxidant in the food industry [31]. The main microalgal source of β-carotene for the market is *Dunaliella salina* (Chlorophyta), which is able to accumulate up to 8% of dry weight [32]. In addition, the microalgae *Arthrospira platensis* (formerly *Spirulina platensis*) (Cyanobacteria) [33], *Chlamydomonas reinhardtii* (Chlorophyta) [34], *Isochrysis galbana* (Haptophyta), *Phaeodactylum tricornutum* (Bacillariophyta), and *Tetraselmis suecica* (Chlorophyta) have also shown high levels of this carotenoid in large-scale systems [35].

2.2. Lutein

$3R,3'R,6'R$-β,ε-carotene-3,3'-diol or LUT (Figure 1B) is a natural carotenoid synthetized in plants as well as algae. It is an orange-yellow xanthophyll widely used as a feed additive and a food coloration agent in industry [36]. Despite being present in a multitude of vegetables and fruits, its low content has led to the search for new sources of this carotenoid such as in microalgae [37]. In this regard, LUT is accumulated on a large scale in several species of *Chlorella* such as *C. sorokiniana*, *Chromochloris zoofingiensis* (formerly *Chlorella zoofingiensis*), and *Auxenochlorella prothecoides* (formerly *Chlorella protothecoides*) [38], as well as in *Dunaliella salina* [39], the strain *Chlamydomonas* sp. JSC4 [40], and *Tetraselmis suecica* [41].

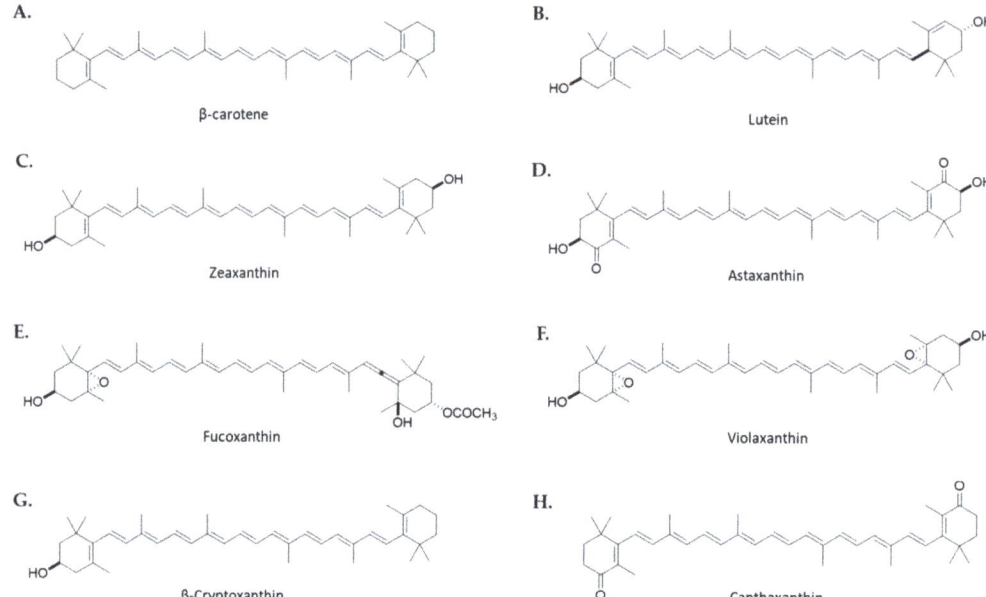

Figure 1. Chemical structures of the main functional carotenoids found in microalgae. Carotenes: β-Carotene (**A**) and xanthophylls: Lutein (**B**), Zeaxanthin (**C**), Astaxanthin (**D**), Fucoxanthin (**E**), Violaxanthin (**F**), β-Cryptoxanthin (**G**) and Canthaxanthin (**H**).

2.3. Zeaxanthin

β,β-carotene-3,3′-diol or ZX (Figure 1C) is a yellow-orange xanthophyll found mainly in dark green leafy vegetables and egg yolks. It has been reported that, like LUT, ZX is accumulated in the central retina and has photoprotective effects against damage by intense light. Regarding microalgae, this xanthophyll has been obtained from the cyanobacteria *Synechocystis* sp. and *Microcystis aeruginosa* [42], as well as the microalgae *Nannochloropsis oculata* (Ochrophyta, Eustigmatophyceae) [43], *Chloroidium saccharophilum* (formerly *Chlorella saccharophila*) [44], and *Dunaliella* sp. [45], and red algae such as *Porphyridium purpureum* (formerly *Porphyridium cruentum*) (Rhodophyta) [35], *Phaeodactylum tricornutum* (Bacillariophyta) [46], or *Heterosigma akashiwo* (Ochrophyta, Raphidophyceae) [47].

2.4. Astaxanthin

3,3′-dihydroxy-β,β′-carotene-4,4′-dione or ATX (Figure 1D) is a xantophyll mainly found in microalgae, marine invertebrates, some fishes like salmon and trout, and even in the feathers of some birds, contributing to their red-orange pigmentation [48]. However, the main source of AXT is *Haematococcus lacustris* (formerly *Haematococcus pluvialis*) (Chlorophyta), whose content may represent up to 3% of dry weight [49], but this xantophyll can also be found in other microalgae such a *Chromochloris zofingiensis* [50], *Chlorococcum* sp. [51], *Dunaliella salina*, *Tetraselmis suecica* [41], *Scenedesmus quadricauda* PUMCC 4.1.40. (Chlorophyta) [52], and *Asterarcys quadricellulare* PUMCC 5.1.1 (Chlorophyta) [53].

2.5. Fucoxanthin

(3S,3′S,5R,5′R,6S,6′R,8′R)-3,5′-dihydroxy-8-oxo-6′,7′-didehydro-5,5′,6,6′,7,8-hexahydro-5,6-epoxy-β,β-caroten-3′-yl acetate, also named FX (Figure 1E), is an orange-colored xanthophyll mainly found in marine environments. This carotenoid is present in a variety of macroalgae, but also in a multitude of species of microalgae such as *Isochrysis* sp. (Haptophyta), *Odontella aurita* [54,55], *Nitzschia laevis* (formerly *Nitzschia amabilis*) [56], and

Chaetoceros neogracili (formerly *Chaetoceros gracilis*) (Bacillariophyta), the coccolithophore *Pleurochrysis carterae* (Haptophyta, Coccolithophyceae) [57], *Phaeodactylum tricornutum* (Bacillariophyta) [46], and the microalga strain *Pavlova* sp. OPMS 30543 (Haprophyta) [58].

2.6. Violaxanthin

5,6,5′,6′-diepoxy-5,6,5′,6′-tetrahydro-β,β-carotene-3,3′-diol, also called violaxanthin (Figure 1F), is a natural orange xanthophyll, which may enzymatically be transformed into ZX when the light energy absorbed by plants exceeds the photosynthesis capacity [59]. It is a pigment found in different plants as well as macro- and microalgae such as *Nannochloropsis oceanica* (Ochrophyta, Eustigmatophyceae) [60], *Jaagichlorella luteoviridis* (formerly *Chlorella luteoviridis*) [61], the strain *Tetraselmis striata* CTP4 (Chlorophyta) [62], and Eustigmatophyte strains such as *Chlorobotrys gloeothece*, *Chlorobotrys regularis*, and *Munda aquilonaris* (formerly *Characiopsis aquilonaris*) [63].

2.7. β-Cryptoxanthin

(1R)-3,5,5-trimethyl-4-[(1E,3E,5E,7E,9E,11E,13E,15E,17E)-3,7,12,16-tetramethyl-18-(2,6,6-trimethylcyclohexen-1-yl)octadeca-1,3,5,7,9,11,13,15,17-nonaenyl]cyclohex-3-en-1-ol, also called BCX (Figure 1G), is a natural orange xanthophyll mainly found in fruits of plants, including in orange rind, papaya, or apples, besides egg yolk and butter. This carotenoid is also found, but in a lower concentration than other carotenoids, in different species of microalgae such as *Phaeodactylum tricornutum* (Bacillariophyta) [64], *Auxenochlorella pyrenoidosa* (formerly *Chlorella pyrenoidosa*) (Chlorophyta) [65], and *Porphyridium purpureum* (Rhodophyta) [66,67].

2.8. Canthaxanthin

β,β-carotene-4,4′-dione or CX (Figure 1H) is a red-orange xanthophyl widely used as a cosmetic and food colorant as well as in poultry as a feed additive. This carotenoid was firstly isolated from the edible mushroom *Cantharellus cinnabarinus*. Moreover, this pigment is present in bacteria, algae, crustacea, some fungi, and various species of fish including carp and golden mullet [68]. Regarding microalgae, this xanthophyll has been found in *Haematococcus lacustris* [69], *Chromochloris zoofingiensis* [70], *Chlorococcum* sp. [51], *Dunaliella salina* [71], *Chlorella vulgaris* (Chlorophyta) [72], *Scenedesmus quadricauda* PUMCC 4.1.40. [52], *Asterarcys quadricellulare* PUMCC 5.1.1 [53], *Picochlorum* sp. SBL2. [73], and *Dactylococcus dissociatus* MT1 (Chlorophyta) [74].

3. Inflammation and Cancer

Acute inflammation is a key component of the response of the immune system to injury and infection that involves the stimulation of defense systems against foreign components and organisms, and the healing and/or repair of damaged tissue. This process is recognized by some cardinal signs, including heat, redness, pain, or swelling. It is characterized by the activation of immune cells, synthesis of proinflammatory mediators, is usually localized and self-limited, and normally returns to homeostasis [75]. Acute inflammation requires suppression of proinflammatory mediators and induction of anti-inflammatory/proresolution mediators as well as the disappearance of leukocytes from the damage area, and the restoration of tissue functionality [76]. However, if the acute inflammatory process is excessive and is not resolved, it may lead to tissue damage, resulting in chronic inflammation, and ultimately fibrosis, with loss of tissue functionality. Consequently, the failure of the resolution of inflammation is strongly associated with the development of many chronic disease states of complex evolution: arthritis, neurodegenerative diseases, metabolic syndrome and associated pathologies, allergy, and periodontal diseases, as well as tumoral processes, among others [77–79]. It has been reported that an adequate diet, a healthy lifestyle, or the establishment of certain preventive strategies, including drugs, nutraceuticals, or components of functional foods, may contribute to the control of inflammatory processes. This section summarizes the main mediators and cells involved in acute and chronic inflammatory responses, as well as describes the link between inflammation and cancer and the main molecular pathways implicated in these processes.

The defense systems of the body are mediated by sequential and coordinated responses called innate and adaptive immunity. The innate immune system is the first line of defense against microbes; it is mediated by cellular elements, including macrophages, neutrophils, dendritic cells, natural cytolytic lymphocytes, or mast cells, as well as by biochemical mechanisms involving agglutinins, the complement system, and many types of lectins, which circulate and provide rapid responses [80]. Macrophages play a pivotal role in all phases of inflammation: in the initiation, help to neutralize and remove pathogens and damaged cells through phagocytosis, and later lead to the termination of inflammation by tissue repair and remodeling responses [81]. Based on responses to different in vitro stimuli appears the macrophage polarization concept of M1/M2 differentiation [82]. M1 macrophages are induced by proinflammatory factors, such as lipopolysaccharide (LPS), cytokines through granulocyte–macrophage colony-stimulating factor, and tumor necrosis factor-α (TNF-α), among others. Later, interleukins (IL), such as IL-1β and IL-6, reactive oxygen species (ROS), and nitric oxide (NO) are released, acting as inducers of a polarized Th1 response. M2 macrophages present a characteristic phagocytic ability of scavenging molecules, as well as produce suppressive mediators, including mannose or galactose receptors and polyamines [83]; they are activated by exposure to Th2-related cytokines (IL-13, IL-4), or anti-inflammatory mediators, including IL-10 and transforming growth factor beta (TGF-β). Accumulating data indicate that M2 macrophages play an important role in microorganism clearance, tissue repair, and inflammation resolution. Nevertheless, some evidence has also shown that M2 macrophages may enhance tumor growth depending on the microenvironmental conditions of this cell population [84].

Adaptative immunity is a response that increases in magnitude and capabilities with each successive exposure to an antigenic stimulus; it is mediated by lymphocytes T and B (cellular immunity and humoral immunity, respectively) and their products. Several types of T cells are detected in the blood, at different stages: effector T lymphocytes can differentiate into T helper (Th) and cytotoxic effector lymphocytes (Tc), which act against cells infected by cytoplasmic intracellular pathogens. Th lymphocytes are differentiated into Th1, which are involved in the elimination of intracellular pathogens (viruses) or phagocytable extracellular organisms (bacteria and fungi), and into Th2, which characteristically act against helminths. In addition, Th cells can differentiate into Th17, T follicular helper cells (Tfh), and T regulatory (Treg) lymphocytes, which exert their activity against commensal bacteria. Regarding B lymphocytes, unmatured cells migrate from bone marrow to spleen and are transformed into B T1 and B T2 lymphocytes; B T2 could be transformed into follicular B cells depending on the signals received through their receptors. In any case, B lymphocytes are T cell-dependent antigen-presenting cells [85].

From a different point of view but complementary to the previous classification, the activation of immune cells regulates two basic effector systems aimed to eliminate potential offending agents: phagocytosis (cellular response) and cytotoxicity [86,87]. Phagocytosis is an effective mechanism of elimination of infectious agents. Although most immune cells are capable of phagocytosis, the most characteristic phagocytes are macrophages and polymorphonuclear neutrophils, which provide a powerful oxidative system and a wide variety of proteolytic enzymes to degrade the phagocytosed material. On the other hand, cytotoxicity is cell-mediated toxicity, and an alternative defense mechanism when phagocytosis cannot resolve the problem: tumor cells, response to viruses, infections by intracellular or large pathogens. These functions are performed by different cell types: (1) eosinophilic and basophilic polymorphonuclear cells that actively participate in the defense against helminths and protozoa by using a receptor for immunoglobulin IgE, which recognizes the pathogen. These cells produce substances with high cytotoxic activity (neurotoxin, cationic protein, or histamine) capable of blocking or killing microorganisms much larger than them. Mast cells also perform this function, as well as participate in the activation of the inflammatory reaction and in allergic processes [88]. (2) Natural cytotoxic cells (NK) that are especially active against tumor cells and cells infected by viruses. These cells are of lymphoid lineage, but do not possess a variable antigen receptor like lymphocytes. They recognize their targets through non-polymorphic receptors, or by using receptors for immunoglobulin–Fc fragment, a process known as antibody-dependent cell cytotoxicity. NK cells kill their targets by activating apoptosis programs [89]. (3) -CD8+, or cytotoxic lymphocytes (T-CTL): when a T-CTL lymphocyte recognizes an antigen–major histocompatibility complex (Ag-MHC), it kills the cell that presents it in a similar way to the NK cell, secreting cytotoxic factors (perforins and granzymes), or interacting with membrane proteins of the target cell. Regarding CD8+ cells, they attack virus-infected cells, where they activate pathways of apoptosis (TNFR1 or Fas, among others). (4) T-CD4 + or Th lymphocytes: although their cytotoxic capacity is much lower than that of T-CTL, and their main function is the activation of other cell types of the immunity response, Th lymphocytes can kill other cells by secreting granzymes or by expressing proapoptotic ligands, including Fas-L or TNF-related apoptosis-inducing ligand, which activate apoptosis programs. (5) Finally, the complement system, which is particularly capable of opsonizing particles to be removed by phagocytes but can also damage membranes and cause cell necrosis [86].

As mentioned above, after the active phase of inflammation, coordinated resolution responses are initiated to prevent chronic inflammation establishment and restore homeostasis [76]. During the initial phase of the acute inflammatory response, the well-known proinflammatory mediators comprising prostaglandins (PGs) and leukotrienes are synthesized from arachidonic acid (ARA) by cyclooxygenases (COXs) and lipoxygenases. Later, in the resolution phase of inflammation, another pathway involving ARA metabolization, via cytochrome P450, is initiated, leading to the production of epoxyeicosatrienoic acids (EETs). These partially oxidized lipidic compounds, oxylipins, may participate in the activation of anti-inflammatory processes and the clearance of cellular debris as well as inhibit numerous proinflammatory cytokines [90]. Additionally, EET, and other epoxy fatty acids, stimulate the production of specialized proresolving mediators (SPMs), such as lipoxins, by shifting ARA metabolism, to support inflammation resolution [91]. In addition to omega-6 arachidonic acid-derived lipoxins, n-3 PUFA-derived SPMs are synthesized from EPA and docosahexaenoic acid and encompass resolvins, protectins, and maresins [76,92]. These lipid autacoids are involved in down-regulation of proinflammatory cytokines/chemokines, inhibition of neutrophil infiltration, and induction of macrophage phagocytosis [93]. Dietary sources of PUFA include fish and algae, and more recently, microalgae [94].

It has been reported that chronic non-resolving inflammation increases the risk of developing cancer. Epidemiological data have evidenced that more than 20% of detected tumors have in their origin, or in their evolution, an important inflammatory component [95]. Inflammation-associated cancer is a long-term process that requires the transformation of normal cells to tumor cells through premalignant lesions. In the inflammation–cancer connection, extrinsic and intrinsic pathways are involved; the extrinsic pathway comprises microbial infections, such as *Helicobacter pylori* and its relationship with gastric cancer, tobacco and lung cancer development, or ultraviolet exposure and its association with skin tumors. Intrinsic factors include mutations in oncogenes and suppressor/repair genes and epigenetic defects, as well as modifications in the immune system [28,96].

Nevertheless, it has also been described that in a previously detected tumor, not linked to a previous inflammatory process, inflammation is present in the surrounding area of the tumor, promoting cancer progression to achieve the malignant phenotype, tissue remodeling, metastasis, and angiogenesis, or the suppression of immune response [97]. Regarding microenvironmental components, it has been reported that macrophages are the most abundant cells in tumor environments and their function in cancer is contradictory. In some types of cancer, these cells have a crucial role in cancer progression and evasion of immune response, which has been correlated to poor prognosis. However, in some gastrointestinal cancers, a large number of macrophages has been related to good prognosis [98]. These findings may be explained by the presence of different macrophage populations in tumor tissues and suggest that macrophage assessment could be used as an innovative prognostic marker.

Given the tumor-promoting effects of macrophages, the development of compounds to target these cells may be a promising strategy for cancer treatment. In this line, different approaches are being considered to inhibit their recruitment, such as inhibition of chemoattractants (C-C chemokine receptor type 2/CCL2 signaling) [99], reduction in macrophages number with bisphosphonates, and inhibition of differentiation and survival (colony stimulating factor 1 (CSF-1)/CSF-1R axis) [100]. However, these types of strategies that focus on general selection have shown limited clinical success [101]. Interestingly, new approaches are being directed to reprogramming macrophages towards an anticancer phenotype. In this line, it has been reported that CD40 agonist antibodies activate antitumor macrophages [102] and other antibodies inhibit the CD47 surface molecule in tumor cells, leading to macrophage-mediated tumor cell phagocytosis [103]. Ongoing studies will let to know the diversity of macrophages in cancer tissues and their clinical interest for cancer prognostic and treatment.

From a molecular and intracellular point of view, during the inflammatory process, a coordinated activation of several signaling pathways is triggered, including phosphatidylinositol 3-kinase/protein kinase B (PI3K/Akt), mitogen-activated protein kinase (MAPK), Janus kinase/signal transduction and activator of transcription (JAK/STAT), or the key transcriptional element nuclear factor-kappa B (NF-κB) that interacts with different nuclear or cytoplasmic elements, including PPAR-γ, which is capable of inhibiting NF-κB activation and the consequent production of numerous cytokines [104–106]. The activation through the innate immune system occurs by pattern recognition receptors (PRRs) and NOD-like receptors (NLRs). Some of these receptors are associated with a multiprotein complex, called the inflammasome, with NOD-LRR and pyrin domain-containing 3 (NLRP3) being the best characterized and involved in the activation of caspase-1 and proteolytic maturation of IL-1β and IL-18 [107]. It has been reported that ROS, produced primarily at the mitochondrial level, are involved in NLRP3 activation [108,109]. Furthermore, exposure to ROS can also activate nuclear factor erythroid 2-related factor 2 (Nrf2), which migrates into the nucleus and induces the expression of genes with antioxidant response element-like sequences in their promoter, such as heme oxygenase-1 (HO-1), peroxiredoxins, and glutamate-cysteine ligase [110,111]. Nrf2 protects normal cells against ROS-induced DNA damage as well as malignant cells against chemotherapy [112]. Nrf2 also stimulates several oncogenes unconnected to antioxidant activity, including matrix metalloproteinase-9 (MMP-9), TNF-α, and vascular endothelial growth factor A (VEGF-A) [113]. Additionally, the aryl hydrocarbon receptor (AHR) is a ubiquitously expressed ligand-activated transcription factor with remarkable physiological roles; it is a key component that can integrate infective or environmental signals into innate and adaptive responses. AHR activity seems to regulate barrier organs, such as the skin, lung, or gut. The liver is exposed to gut-derived alimentary or microbial AHR ligands and, additionally, generates AHR ligands, including metabolic enzymes, such as cytochrome P450, which produces toxic metabolites and increases ROS production [114]. In contrast, AHR ligands from intestinal microbiota are involved in the maintenance of epithelial integrity as well as the generation of the anti-inflammatory IL-22 [115].

On the other hand, necroptosis has been described as programmed necrotic cell death induced by cytokines, Toll-like receptors (TLR), or ROS. After a necroptotic stimulus, the receptor-interacting protein kinase 1 (RIP1)/RIP3 complex phosphorylates and activates the mixed lineage kinase domain-like protein (MLKL), which oligomerizes and translocates to the plasma membrane, forming pores and leading to cell lysis [116]. Additionally, it is interesting to highlight the sirtuin (SIRT) family in the inflammation context. Many of them are histone deacetylases involved in cellular pathways related to the structure and function of tissues, and with capacity to control processes, including inflammation or cancer. Between them, the SIRT1 isoform has a special role in ROS-induced cell death, and SIRT6 has an interesting function in cancer and autophagy. Moreover, SIRT3 shows a potential therapeutic role in different pathologies, including cardiovascular diseases, where a SIRT3 deficiency has been associated with necroptosis, and NLRP3 activation in a diabetic cardiomyopathy [117].

Regarding the role of ROS in the inflammatory response, it has been reported that minimal ROS concentrations may be essential in many intracellular signal processes connected with cell proliferation, apoptosis, or defense against microorganisms. However, high doses or inadequate removal of ROS generate oxidative stress, which cause macromolecular damage and metabolic dysfunctions [118]. Lipid peroxidation is a serious consequence of oxidative stress since the derived products, epoxides, can interact with nucleophilic structures of the cell or with nucleic acids and cause structural damage and mutations. Consequently, an adequate equilibrium between antioxidants and oxidants to maintain cellular homeostasis is necessary [119]. In aerobic organisms, there are a variety of antioxidant, enzymatic, and non-enzymatic systems with protective properties; enzymes include glutathione peroxidase, superoxide dismutase (SOD), and catalase, which are present in various cell sites, such as the cytosol, endoplasmic reticulum, peroxisomes, and mitochondria. This latter organelle is able to generate almost 90% of ROS, mainly through coenzyme Q [120]. In addition, there are substances capable of neutralizing ROS, such as alpha-tocopherol (vitamin E), ascorbic acid (vitamin C), vitamin A, glutathione (GSH), flavonoids, phenolic acids, and carotenes.

As regards cancer, it is known that malignant cells can maintain elevated intracellular ROS levels due to different causes, including mitochondrial damage, rapid metabolism, lipid peroxidation, or metal ion formation, such as copper and iron, as well as reduction in endogenous antioxidants [121]. In cancer cells, the role of ROS is controversial since they have been shown to have both pro- and antitumorigenic functions, depending on the concentrations. In this line, moderate ROS levels can induce cell survival, angiogenesis, and metastasis through activation of the MAPK pathway, which in turn stimulates NF-κB and the subsequent up-regulation of MMPs and VEGF [118]. Nevertheless, regarding its antitumorigenic role, high intracellular ROS levels can induce apoptosis of cancer cells by activation of the proapoptotic proteins Bax, p21, and p27, among others, and a decrease in the antiapoptotic Bcl-2 and Bcl-xL [121]. Therefore, these proapoptotic properties of ROS can serve as a crucial therapeutic strategy to destroy tumor cells. In this line, it is interesting to highlight the role of carotenoids in cancer since these compounds can serve as pro-oxidants in cancerous cells, leading to ROS-induced apoptosis. Furthermore, when they are administered with ROS-stimulating cytotoxic drugs, carotenoids can decrease the dangerous effects of these drugs on normal cells by their antioxidant properties, as well as increase cytotoxicity of drugs towards cancer cells by a pro-oxidant mechanism. Therefore, this synergistic effect of carotenoids with anticancer drugs may be an innovative strategy for cancer treatment [121,122]. Figure 2 shows a diagram of the main targets and signaling pathways in which microalgal carotenoids have shown a direct or indirect ability to modify different signaling pathways.

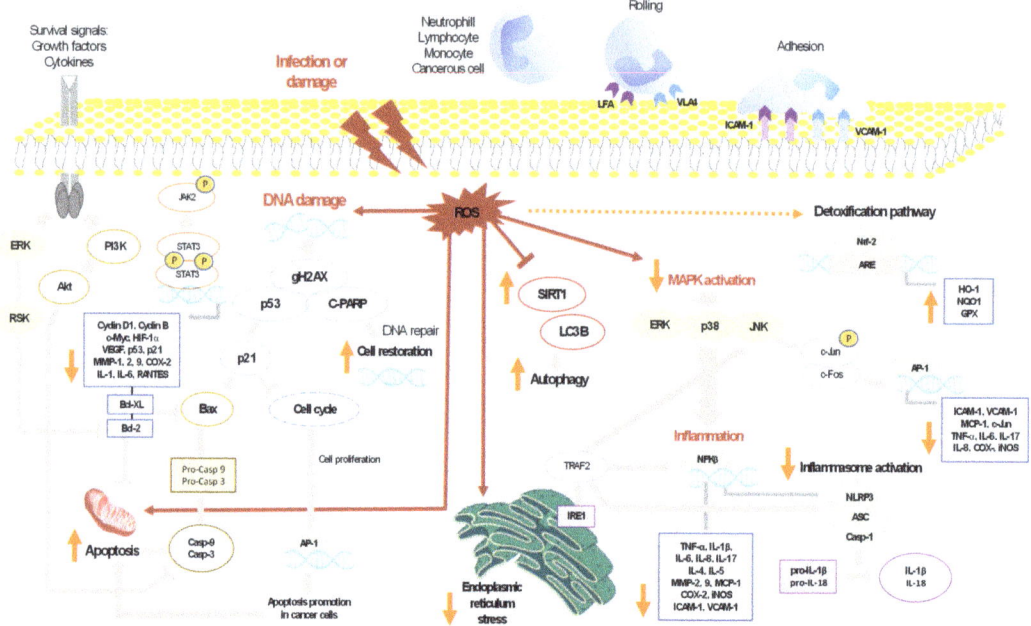

Figure 2. Carotenoids' interaction on major signaling pathways implicated in inflammation or cancer. The figure shows the bioactivity of the carotenoids for different type of cells. Red arrows show the effect of the presence of ROS on several activities in the cell; dashed orange arrow refers to the detoxification pathway that is triggered when ROS are produced; pink arrows show the interconnections of different mediators; orange arrows refer to the bioactivities produced by the different microalgal carotenoids.

4. Anti-Inflammatory Activity of Carotenoids

Sections 4 and 5 summarize the recent up-to-date studies (since 2010 up to June 2021) reporting the anti-inflammatory and anticancer activities of microalgal carotenoids both in vitro and in vivo, as well as the latest status of human studies for their potential use in the prevention and treatment of different inflammatory diseases and cancer. In addition, the molecular mechanisms underlying these effects are described. The most relevant anti-inflammatory and anticancer activities of carotenoids, as well as the main microalgal sources, are summarized in Table 1.

4.1. β-Carotene

4.1.1. In Vitro Studies

Different preclinical in vitro studies have evidenced that β-carotene can prevent and reduce diabetes, which is a chronic low-grade inflammatory disease associated with common complications. In this respect, this compound was evaluated in human endothelial cells isolated from umbilical cord veins (HUVECs) of women suffering from gestational diabetes. The results evidenced that β-carotene prevented vascular inflammation and reduced the nitro-oxidative state induced by TNF-α in HUVECs. These effects were related to an attenuation of vascular cell adhesion molecule 1 and intercellular adhesion molecule 1 (ICAM-1) expression, reduction in NF-κB activation, and suppression of peroxynitrite levels. These findings suggest that a carotenoid-rich diet could play an important role in the prevention of cardiovascular complications of diabetes [123]. Similar findings were obtained in TNF-α-stimulated HUVECs of healthy women after treatment with β-carotene [124]. It has been reported that oxidative stress produced in adipose tissue results in dysregulated production of proinflammatory adipokines by adipocytes, which is related to the pathogenesis of diabetes and obesity. β-Carotene attenuated oxidative stress-induced inflammation via a decrease in the adipokines monocyte chemoattractant protein-1 (MCP-1) and RANTES and an increase in adiponectin in 3T3-L1 adipocytes. The mechanisms underlying these effects were linked to the inhibition of the activation of NF-κB, activator protein-1 (AP-1), and signal transducer and activator of transcription 3 (STAT3) transcription factors [125]. In the same line, the cardioprotective role of a low dose of β-carotene in the prevention of ROS-induced atherosclerosis has been reported in cardiomyoblasts through up-regulation of Nrf2, activation of autophagy, and inhibition of NF-κB and apoptosis [126].

In addition, it has been demonstrated that β-carotene suppressed NLRP3 inflammasome activation in mouse bone marrow macrophages [127] as well as inhibited JAK2/STAT3 and c-Jun N-terminal kinase (JNK)/p38 MAPK signaling pathways in LPS-stimulated macrophages [128]. Similarly, this compound suppressed the pseudorabies virus-induced inflammatory response, which mimics human herpes simplex virus inflammation, in RAW 264.7 macrophages, via reductions in NF-κB and MAPK activation [129].

4.1.2. In Vivo Studies

A number of in vivo models have evidenced the anti-inflammatory effects of β-carotene. Regarding gastrointestinal disorders, oral treatment with this carotenoid at the doses of 5, 10, and 20 mg/kg for 28 days suppressed dextran sodium sulfate (DSS)-induced experimental colitis in mice. Its anti-inflammatory actions were related to a decrease in the transcription factors NF-κB and STAT3 and the subsequent release of IL-17, IL-6, TNF-α, and COX-2. Moreover, β-carotene exerted an antioxidant activity through an increase in Nrf2 and NADPH:quinone oxidoreductase-1 in the colon tissue [130]. Likewise, the attenuations of NF-κB and STAT3 pathways as well as autophagy inhibition were reported after oral administration of this carotenoid (50mg/kg) in a rat model of LPS-induced intestinal inflammation [131]. In addition, it has been reported that intake of β-carotene (40 and 80 mg/kg) for two weeks inhibited NF-κB pathway activation in a model of weaning-induced intestinal inflammation. The authors proposed a new anti-inflammatory mechanism for this carotenoid involving the modulation of microbiota imbalance as a consequence of weaning in piglets [132]. Regarding liver diseases, β-carotene exhibited a hepatoprotective effect in chemically induced hepatic fibrosis by down-regulating NF-κB and its target gene inducible nitric oxide synthase (iNOS) [133]. In the same line, this carotenoid, administered at a dose of 70 mg/kg every other day or combined with rosuvastatin, attenuated hepatic steatosis and the inflammatory response as well as enhanced the lipid profile in a model of non-alcoholic fatty liver induced by a high-fat diet in rats [134].

In relation to cardiovascular disorders, the role of a powder of the microalga *Dunaliella bardawil*, containing 6% β-carotene isomers, was examined in a model of atherosclerosis in apolipoprotein E (apo E)-deficient mice, and fed with a vitamin A-deficient diet. These findings evidenced the formation of atheromas due to lack of vitamin A; nevertheless, β-carotene supplementation decreased levels of plasma cholesterol and prevented atherogenesis [135]. Apo E-/-mice were also used for investigating the actions of dietary β-carotene (800 mg/kg of feed, for 150 days) on angiotensin II-induced chronic renal damage. The results reported a protective effect of this carotenoid by down-regulating the expression of proinflammatory genes related to kidney diseases, including renin 1 and peroxisome proliferator-activated receptor gamma (PPAR-γ) [136].

The beneficial role of β-carotene against skin inflammation has been demonstrated in different animal models. Oral administration of this carotenoid at 0.6 mg/day for 4 weeks attenuated skin inflammatory response in a model of low zinc/magnesium diet-induced atopic dermatitis (AD) in hairless mice. These effects were associated with a down-regulation of the cytokines IL-6, IL-1β, IL-4, and IL-5, a suppression of MMP-9 activity, and an up-regulation of filaggrin levels, a protein involved in skin barrier function [137]. Likewise, the anti-inflammatory activity of β-carotene administered orally (20 mg/kg) for 8 weeks was also reported in a mouse model of oxazolone-induced AD [138]. Furthermore, β-carotene and LUT were evaluated in a mouse model of acute neurogenic inflammation in the ear induced by capsaicin or mustard oil. These carotenoids administered topically at the dose of 100 mg/kg attenuated edema formation; nevertheless, a reduction in myeloperoxidase (MPO) activity and neutrophilic infiltration in the mouse ear was only demonstrated after LUT treatment [139].

In relation to central nervous system disorders, the neuroprotective role of this carotenoid was evaluated for the first time in a rat model of acute spinal cord injury. β-Carotene administered intraperitoneally at different doses (10, 20, 40, and 80 mg/kg) suppressed NF-κB pathway activation and exerted a marked antioxidative effect by decreasing ROS, NO, and malondialdehyde (MDA) levels and up-regulating SOD, Nrf2, and HO-1 [140]. In addition, β-carotene has been demonstrated to have protective effects in other inflammatory diseases such gouty arthritis or asthma. In this line, β-carotene administered orally (30 mg/kg) inhibited NLRP3 inflammasome activation in a model of gouty arthritis in mice, as well as suppressed levels of IL-1β in synovial fluid cells isolated from gout patients [127]. Oral treatment with this carotenoid at 30 mg/kg demonstrated a therapeutic effect in a rat model of ovalbumin-induced asthma via reduction in the proinflammatory cytokines IL-β, IL-6, and TNF-α and an increase in the anti-inflammatory cytokines IL-4 and IL-13 [141].

4.1.3. Human Studies

Regarding clinical studies, a randomized, double-blind, and placebo-controlled clinical trial evaluated the role of *Lactobacillus brevis* KB290 and β-carotene in diarrhea-predominant irritable bowel syndrome-like symptoms in healthy people. The intake of this combination for 12 weeks improved the abdominal pain, reduced stool frequency, and decreased colon inflammation through up-regulation of the cytokine IL-10 [142]. Likewise, a double-blind controlled crossover clinical trial in type 2 diabetes mellitus (T2DM) patients demonstrated that supplementation with a β-carotene-fortified symbiotic food (containing *Lactobacillus sporogenes* as probiotic, 0.1 g inulin as prebiotic, and 0.05 g β-carotene) for 6 weeks enhanced insulin metabolism and lipid profile as well as augmented the antioxidant GSH plasma levels [143]. Another study investigated the effects of β-carotene at the doses of 30 and 90 mg/day for 90 days on wrinkles, elasticity, and ultraviolet (UV)-induced DNA damage in healthy females over the age of 50 years. Interestingly, only the lowest dose was effective in preventing and repairing skin photoaging [144]. These data are consistent with previous studies demonstrating the pro-oxidant effects of β-carotene at high doses as it can produce radical ions that themselves may contribute to cell injury [145].

Finally, previous studies have reported that reduced levels of β-carotene can be detected in patients with different inflammatory disorders, including non-alcoholic fatty liver disease [146], chronic obstructive pulmonary disease [147], acute myocardial infarction [148], infection by *H. pylori* [149], and advanced coronary artery disease [150]. These findings support the protective effects of β-carotene through inhibition of the inflammatory processes.

4.2. Lutein

4.2.1. In Vitro Studies

The beneficial effects of LUT in ocular disorders have been demonstrated in numerous in vitro studies. Along this line, LUT exhibited a protective role in human retinal pigment epithelial cells (ARPE-19 cells) exposed to different stimuli implicated in age-related macular degeneration pathogenesis (AMD), a severe disease that causes vision loss. The mechanisms underlying these actions were associated with an inhibition of apoptosis, VEGF levels, and oxidative stress markers, as well as prevention of autophagy flux alteration [151]. Similarly, a LUT nanoemulsion improved penetration into ARPE-19 cells and protected cells from H_2O_2-induced damage [152]. It has been reported that retinal photo-oxidative damage may lead to inflammation of eyes and AMD-associated lesions. A previous study reported a reduction in proteasome activity in ARPE-19 cells exposed to blue light and that LUT and ZX were able to reverse this effect and regulate inflammation-related genes, such as MCP-1 and IL-8 [153].

Retinal ischemia/reperfusion injury occurs in some eye diseases including glaucoma and diabetic retinopathy. The protective effects of LUT have been reported in a rat Müller cell line exposed to cobalt (II) chloride, a model that mimics the hypoxic/ischemic state. This carotenoid exerted anti-inflammatory effects by reducing NF-κB, IL-1β, and COX-2 levels [154] as well as inhibited apoptosis and autophagy in glial cells [155]. It has been reported that hyperosmoticity of tears induces inflammation and ocular surface damage, playing a main role in dry eye development. In this line, LUT has been shown to be a potential agent for the treatment of dry eye since it suppressed the hyperosmoticity-induced increase in IL-6 through inhibition of NF-κB pathway activation in human corneal epithelial cells [156].

Furthermore, LUT protected a human keratinocyte cell line and primary human keratinocytes from foreskins against UVB-induced damage through an increase in cell viability and proliferation, and reduction in apoptosis [157]. Similarly, LUT pretreatment for 48 h before UVA irradiation preserved tissue architecture in a model of three-dimensional human skin equivalent [158]. The photoprotective effects of this carotenoid were also related to the inhibition of MMP-9 expression and ROS production in UV-irradiated HaCaT [159]. Other papers reported the antioxidant effects of LUT via up-regulation of the Nrf2/HO-1 pathway and its anti-inflammatory actions through inhibition of NF-κB activity in monosodium iodoacetate-induced osteoarthritis in primary chondrocyte cells [160] as well as in LPS-activated microglial cells [161]. In addition, this compound reduced LPS-induced production of TNF-α, IL-6, and IL-1β in peripheral blood mononuclear cells from patients with stable angina [162]. Another action mechanism involved in the anti-inflammatory properties of LUT was related to suppression of the transcription factor AP-1 in LPS-activated macrophages [159]. The antioxidant and anti-inflammatory effects of LUT and its combination with six anthocyanidin glucosides were also evaluated chemically and in Caco-2 cells. LUT alone showed better results than the mixture with the other compounds, demonstrating antioxidant activity through inhibition of liposome peroxidation and anti-inflammatory effects via suppression of the in vitro lipoxygenase-1 activity and reduction in IL-8 and NO levels in Caco-2 cells [163].

4.2.2. In Vivo Studies

Like in vitro studies, the protective effects of LUT in eye disorders, such as AMD, diabetic retinopathy, cataract, uveitis, and dry eye syndrome have been previously reported in a number of animal studies. In this respect, LUT and ZX have been evaluated on high-fat diet-induced retinal inflammation in rats since a high-fat intake has been associated with a high incidence of AMD. Data reported that the mix of both carotenoids (100 mg/kg) enhanced metabolic and lipid profile, as well as reduced oxidative stress in the retina by increasing the Nrf2/HO-1 pathway [164]. Light exposure has been reported to be another risk factor for AMD development since it increases the stress in the retinal pigment epithelium. In this line, a LUT-rich marigold extract, composed of 92% LUT and 8% ZX (100 mg/kg), protected the retina from oxidative stress and inflammation in a model of photostressed retina in mice [165]. Regarding diabetic retinopathy, chronic LUT administration (4.2 and 8.4 mg/kg) in the retina of Ins2$^{Akita/+}$ mice, a genetic model of type 1 diabetes, suppressed microglia activation, which is involved in retinal inflammation, and preserved retinal activity [166]. Likewise, LUT supplementation of 0.1% (wt/wt) was reported to have antioxidative effects in the retina in streptozotocin-induced diabetic mice via down-regulation of ROS-mediated extracellular signal-regulated kinase (ERK) activation [167]. In the same experimental model, administration of 0.5 mg/kg LUT or 0.6 and 3 mg/kg ATX exerted antioxidant and anti-inflammatory effects via inhibition of the NF-κB pathway [168]. Furthermore, intraperitoneal administration of micelles containing LUT (1.3 mmol/kg) in combination with three unsaturated fatty acids protected against cataract formation induced by sodium selenite in rat pups. The mechanisms involved in these actions were related to an increase in antioxidant enzymes activity and down-regulation of proinflammatory markers, such as phospholipase A2 (PLA2), COX-2, iNOS, and NF-κB expression [169], as well as regulation of the chaperone function of lens crystallin [170]. The protective effect of LUT at the doses of 125 and 500 mg/kg has also been demonstrated in LPS-induced uveitis in mice through its antioxidant properties, including reduction in NO and MDA levels and an increase in SOD and glutathione peroxidase activities [171]. In the same model, LUT was reported to protect against uveitis via reduction in IL-8 production in uveal melanocytes accompanied by inhibition of JNK1/2 and NF-κB signaling pathways [172]. Furthermore, a recent study has reported the antioxidative and anti-inflammatory effect of a formulation containing LUT/ZX, curcumin, and vitamin D3 in a rat model of benzalkonium chloride-induced dry eye syndrome [173].

Regarding cardiovascular diseases, the preventive effects of chronic administration of LUT (25, 50, and 100 mg/kg) on atherosclerosis have been reported in ApoE-deficient mice fed a high-fat diet via an increase in PPAR-α, a marker related to lipid metabolism [174]. Likewise, dietary LUT (0.01 g/100 g diet) improved the lipid profile and reduced oxidative stress and cytokine production in aortas of guinea pigs fed a hypercholesterolemic diet [175]. Later, these authors showed the protective effect of this carotenoid against a high-fat diet-induced hepatic injury by inhibiting NF-κB activity [176].

In relation to the potential role of this corotenoid for pain treatment, this carotenoid has been recently investigated in acute trigeminal inflammatory pain induced by mustard oil injection and chronic trigeminal pain following complete Freund's adjuvant administration into rat whisker pads. The results in the acute model demonstrated that intraperitoneal administration of LUT (10 mg/kg) suppressed edema thickness and sensitization of nociceptive processing in spinal trigeminal nucleus caudalis (SpVc) and upper cervical (C1) dorsal horn neurons [177]. Similarly, in the chronic model, the carotenoid was able to reduce the hyperalgesia and neuronal hyperexcitability via COX-2 inhibition [178]. Furthermore, LUT attenuated mustard oil-induced acute neurogenic inflammation via suppression of the activation of transient receptor potential ankyrin 1 (TRPA1) on capsaicin-sensitive sensory nerves [139]. This compound has also been reported to have protective effects against thermal injury in remote organs in rats. Oral administration of this compound at the dose of 250 mg/kg for three days attenuated liver and kidney dysfunction and oxidative damage. Moreover, this carotenoid evidenced anti-inflammatory and antiapoptotic properties by reducing TNF-α and caspase-3 expression, respectively, in the liver, kidneys, and lungs [179]. Regarding central nervous system disorders, LUT at the doses of 80 and 160 mg/kg demonstrated anti-inflammatory and antioxidative actions in a model of severe traumatic brain injury via down-regulation of NF-κB and ICAM-1 expression, and up-regulation of Nrf2 and endothelin-1 levels [180]. The antioxidant and anti-inflammatory actions of LUT have been described in other experimental models, such as osteoporosis in ovariectomized rats [181], alcohol-induced hepatic damage [182], and ischemia/reperfusion injury in skeletal muscle [183].

4.2.3. Human Studies

The effects of LUT in AMD have been previously investigated in a variety of clinical studies. One of the largest was the Age-related Eye Disease Study 2 (AREDS2), a double-blind, randomized trial in people at risk of developing late AMD. The results of this study, which evaluated the effects of a formulation of vitamins and zinc, plus LUT/ZX (10mg/2mg), suggest a reduced risk of developing advanced AMD with the consumption of LUT/ZX [184]. These findings were confirmed in a post hoc study evaluating participants enrolled in AREDS 1 and AREDS2 with no late AMD [185]. Likewise, the protective effects of this carotenoid against the development and progression of AMD have been evidenced in other clinical trials by increasing sensitivity of the retina, macular pigment optical density, and visual performance [186–188]. Nevertheless, other studies that evaluated the effects of co-administration of LUT and PUFA reported protective actions of this combination in some studies [189] and non-significant effects in others [190].

Regarding the photoprotective effects of LUT, a randomized, controlled, double-blind clinical trial in people exposed to UVB/A demonstrated that capsules of LUT (10 mg, twice daily) decreased the skin expression of HO-1, MMP-1, and ICAM-1 [191]. Moreover, oral supplementation with omega-6 and omega-3 fatty acids, ZX, LUT, and vitamin D attenuated sunburn risk in patients with Fitzpatrick skin phototypes I, II, or III [192]. Finally, a recent study confirmed the photoprotective and antiphotoaging effects of a nutritional intervention with different antioxidants, including LUT (3 mg/day), in healthy volunteers [193].

4.3. Zeaxanthin

4.3.1. In Vitro Studies

This carotenoid has been shown to have in vitro anti-inflammatory effects in LPS/H_2O_2-stimulated human adipose-derived mesenchymal stem cells by reduction in ROS production via down-regulation of the protein kinase C/MAPK/ERK pathway [194]. In addition, ZX prevented oxidative stress in ARPE-19 cells due to PI3K/Akt activation as well induction of phase II enzyme expression via Nrf2 activation [195].

4.3.2. In Vivo Studies

The protective role of ZX in ocular diseases has been previously demonstrated in animal models including AMD. In this line, this carotenoid induced an antioxidative response in retinal pigment epithelium, protecting its structure and function in a genetic model of oxidative stress-mediated retinal degeneration in mice [196]. Similarly, this compound attenuated intense light-induced retinal damage by activating Nrf2/HO-1 pathways and suppressing NF-κB expression [197]. Likewise, the neuroprotective effects of LUT/ZX isomers via up-regulation of Nrf2 and down-regulation of NF-κB have been recently reported in a mouse model of traumatic brain injury [198]. On the other hand, ZX was effective in reducing colon inflammation acetic acid-induced ulcerative colitis through an increase in antioxidant defense mechanisms and attenuation of NF-κB levels and the consequent iNOS and COX-2 inhibition [199]. Furthermore, the anti-inflammatory activity of ZX has been evidenced in a model of paw edema in mice [200], as well as in a model of alcoholic fatty liver in rats [201]. This carotenoid also ameliorated diabetes-induced neuroinflammation, improving anxiety and depression [202].

4.3.3. Human Studies

As mentioned in the section on LUT, numerous clinical trials have investigated the effects of a combination of LUT and ZX in ocular disorders. In this regard, supplementation with these carotenoids reduced the risk of developing AMD [184,185,203]. Nevertheless, other studies did not report significant changes after LUT and ZX treatment for the prevention of eye diseases or improvement of macular pigments [204]. In relation to dry eye syndrome, a randomized, double-blind, clinical trial reported that oral supplementation with LUT, ZX, curcumin, and vitamin D3 for 8 weeks enhanced dry eye symptoms and attenuated eye inflammation by reducing MMP-9 levels in tears [205].

4.4. Astaxanthin

4.4.1. In Vitro Studies

ATX has been shown to have in vitro anti-inflammatory effects in THP-1 macrophages through inhibition of NF-κB activation with the subsequent down-regulation of the proinflammatory markers IL-1β, IL-6, TNF-α, and MMP-2 and 9 [206]. In the same line, this carotenoid suppressed the MAPK signaling pathway, up-regulated the Nrf2 pathway, and increased SIRT-1 activity in ethanol or LPS-induced macrophages from several sources [207–209]. In addition, ATX microparticles protected macrophages against radiation-induced damage via suppression of transforming growth factor beta [210]. On the other hand, the neuroprotective role of ATX in LPS-activated BV2 cells has been reported in microglia-mediated inflammation following Alzheimer's disease through inhibition of

MAPK and NF-κB pathway activation [211,212], as well as in particulate matter-stimulated microglial cells [213]. In addition, ATX inactivated STAT3 transcription factor, which led to inhibition of β-secretase activity with the subsequent prevention of amyloid beta accumulation [214]. ATX has also been shown to have antiarthritic properties via reduction of NLRP3 inflammasome stimulation in monosodium urate crystal-activated murine macrophages [215]. Furthermore, ATX protected human primary keratinocytes and HaCaT keratinocytes against UVB-induced damage through reduction of the proinflammatory cytokines IL-8, TNF-α, and IL-1β and the enzymes iNOS and COX-2 [216]. Likewise, the beneficial role of this carotenoid in dry eye treatment was confirmed in human corneal epithelial cells via reduction in TNF-α and IL-1β levels [217]. Finally, the anti-inflammatory and antioxidant effects of this carotenoid have been demonstrated in other in vitro models, including bovine endometritis [218], gastric inflammation by *H. pylori* [219], and osteoporosis [220].

4.4.2. In Vivo Studies

A variety of animal studies have revealed the protective role of ATX against liver inflammation and its progression to cirrhosis and cancer. The mechanisms underlying the anti-inflammatory effects of this carotenoid in the model of non-alcoholic fatty liver were associated with a suppression of endoplasmic reticulum stress and NF-κB [221], a reduction in lipogenic regulator genes [222], and PPAR-α activation [223]. Additionally, the hepatoprotective effects of ATX in liver injury were due to suppression of STAT3 activity in ethanol-induced hepatic damage [224], modulation of gut microbiota [225], inhibition of MAPK pathway activation in acetaminophen-induced hepatic injury [226], and suppression of NF-κB and autophagy in carbon tetrachloride-induced hepatic fibrosis [227] or arsenic-stimulated liver damage [228]. Likewise, dietary ATX (1mg/kg) alleviated high-fructose diet-induced liver inflammation via up-regulation of SIRT-1 and inhibition of NF-κB [229]. Another paper demonstrated that ATX liposomes attenuated LPS-induced acute liver injury in rats, reporting a higher antioxidant and anti-inflammatory activity than free ATX due to an enhancement of its oral bioavailability [230]. In the same line, treatment with ATX (5, 10 and 20 mg/kg) dose-dependently protected against burn-induced acute kidney inflammation through suppression of the TLR4/NF-κB pathway and an increase in HO-1 levels [231].

In relation to cardiovascular diseases, it has been recently described that ATX protected mouse heart against LPS-induced cardiac dysfunction by down-regulating MAPK and PI3K/Akt pathways with the consequent apoptosis inhibition [232]. In addition, several animal studies demonstrated the beneficial role of ATX in diabetes mellitus and metabolic syndrome since this carotenoid enhanced the lipid profile and glucose tolerance as well as reduced insulin resistance in a model of chemically induced diabetes [233] and gestational diabetes [234]. Another paper evidenced that PEGylated ATX had a higher antidiabetic effect than free ATX due to an enhancement in oral bioavailability [235]. Additionally, this carotenoid ameliorated diabetic retinopathy in a rat model of streptozotocin-induced diabetes [168,236]. Regarding diabetes-induced brain damage, ATX improved cognitive function through inhibition of NOS activity and up-regulation of the PI3K/Akt pathway [237], as well as activation of the Nrf2/HO-1 pathway in the cerebral cortex and hippocampus [238].

ATX has also demonstrated anti-inflammatory effects in central nervous disorders, such as depression; in this line, this compound alleviated depressive-like symptoms in a mouse model of LPS-induced inflammation via attenuation of NF-κB activation and the subsequent suppression of COX-2 and iNOS in the hippocampus and prefrontal cortex [239]. In the same model, a recent study reported that oral treatment with an ATX emulsion to increase its bioavailability improved cognitive function and exhibited anti-inflammatory activity by down-regulating inflammation-related proteins such as COX-2, iNOS, TNF-α, IL-6, and IL-1β and increasing IL-10 levels [240]. Furthermore, ATX was effective in attenuating status epilepticus-induced neuroinflammation in rats by suppressing extracellular ATP levels and the consequent P2X7R inhibition, a microglial receptor involved in inflammation [241]. The neuroprotective effects of this compound were also evidenced in a model of subarachnoid haemorrhage via inhibition of MMP-9 levels and activity [242] and up-regulation of SIRT1 expression [243]. In addition, ATX reduced neuroinflammation in other animal models, such as chronic neuropathic pain [244], spinal cord injury [245,246], Alzheimer's disease [247], and acute cerebral infarction [248].

Regarding the potential role of ATX for arthritis treatment, this carotenoid protected cartilage against destruction surgically induced by destabilization of the medial meniscus, through Nrf2 activation [249]. In addition, this carotenoid exhibited antiarthritis properties by attenuating chronic inflammatory pain and suppressing proinflammatory and oxidative stress markers in a rat model of arthritis by complete Freund's adjuvant [250], as well as in monosodium iodoacetate-induced osteoarthritis [251]. ATX also attenuated inflammation in a model of gouty arthritis in rats [215] and in different animal models of gastrointestinal inflammation. In this regard, it has been recently demonstrated that dietary ATX (0.005%) ameliorated oxidative stress, interferon gamma (IFN-γ) levels, and the oncogenes c-myc and cyclin D1 in a mouse model of *H. pylori*-associated gastritis, suggesting the chemopreventive role of this carotenoid in *H. pylori*-induced carcinogenesis [252]. Additionally, ATX administered orally (100 mg/kg) attenuated ochratoxin A-induced cecum inflammation due to suppression of TLR4 and its downstream protein Myd88, as well as inhibition of NF-κB and the subsequent release of TNF-α and IFN-γ [253]. Similarly, ATX supplementation revealed a protective role in DSS-induced ulcerative colitis in mice through down-regulation of NF-κB-induced COX-2 and iNOS expression [254]. Similar findings were reported when ATX was administered to obese mice, suppressing the development of azoxymethane-induced colonic premalignant lesions [255]. Additionally, this carotenoid improved acute pancreatitis in mice via suppression of JAK/STAT3 activity [256].

The beneficial role of ATX in pulmonary disorders has also been reported in different in vivo models. At this respect, this compound exhibited antiasthmatic effects in ovalbumin-induced asthma in mice due to modulation of Th1 and Th2 cytokine profiles [257]. Furthermore, ATX inhibited inflammatory and oxidative response in acute lung injury via attenuation of oxidative/nitrosative stress markers, apoptosis, and NF-κB expression [258] as well as an increase in the Nrf2/HO-1 signaling pathway [259]. As regards skin diseases, it has been reported that this carotenoid administered topically on the ear or back skin of mice alleviated hyperkeratosis and inflammatory response in a model of phthalic anhydride-induced atopic dermatitis. These actions were related to a down-regulation of NF-κB and its proinflammatory target genes iNOS and COX-2 [260,261]. In the same model, ATX-loaded liposomes were more effective than free ATX in alleviating skin inflammation due to inhibition of oxidative stress and STAT3 and NF-κB signaling pathways as well as a reduction of IgE, a marker of allergic inflammation [262]. Likewise, oral treatment with ATX enhanced atopic dermatitis-induced pruritus and inflammation, evidenced by an inhibition of proinflammatory cytokines and L-histidine decarboxylase levels [263]. Moreover, ATX protected mouse skin against burn injury as well as corneal epithelium against UV-induced keratitis by suppressing proinflammatory and oxidative markers and apoptosis [264,265]. On the other hand, ATX has been shown to have anti-inflammatory effects in a mouse model of hyperosmoticity-induced dry eye due to suppression of TNF-α and IL-1β, as well as down-regulation of high-mobility group box 1, a proinflammatory marker involved in ocular damage [217].

4.4.3. Human Studies

Regarding human studies, the photoprotective and antiaging effects of ATX have been demonstrated in a randomized and double-blind study in healthy women exposed to UVB and receiving ATX capsules at 6 or 12 mg/day for 16 weeks. At the end of the study, the carotenoid was effective in attenuating wrinkle formation and improving skin elasticity [266]. Similar results were detected in another clinical trial in participants treated with ATX capsules at 4 mg for 9 weeks [267]. Additionally, an ATX supplement (6 mg/day) for 12 weeks increased cognitive function in patients with mild cognitive impairment [268], and this treatment for 4 weeks alleviated mental and physical fatigue in healthy volunteers [269]. Furthermore, administration of ATX at 8 mg/day for 8 weeks improved the lipid profile and reduced blood pressure in patients with T2DM [270]. Likewise, the beneficial effects of the same dose of ATX in T2DM have been recently reported in a randomized, double-masked clinical trial through reduction in IL-6 and MDA levels as well as down-regulation of microRNA 146a, a proinflammatory marker whose deregulation has been implicated in diabetes pathogenesis and complications [271].

4.5. Fucoxanthin

4.5.1. In Vitro Studies

The carotenoid FX has been shown to have marked anti-inflammatory effects in different in vitro experimental models. In this line, FX suppressed COX-2 and iNOS expression and the consequent production of PGE$_2$ and NO, respectively, as well as reduced TNF-α, IL-1β, and IL-6 levels via inhibition of NF-κB and MAPK pathways in LPS-stimulated RAW 264.7 macrophages [272,273]. A recent study reported that this carotenoid attenuated the palmitate-induced inflammatory response in RAW 264.7 macrophages by improving lipid metabolism and mitochondrial dysfunction. Additionally, this compound blocked the expression gene of M1 markers (IL-6, IL-1β, TNF-α, and Nlrp3) and up-regulated the expression of the M2 marker Tgfβ1, thus suppressing macrophage-induced inflammation [274]. Another study by our group confirmed the anti-inflammatory activity of FX due to a reduction in TNF-α levels in LPS-activated THP-1 macrophages and IL-6 and IL-8 production in TNF-α-stimulated HaCaT keratinocytes, an in vitro model of psoriasis [275].

In relation to neurodegenerative diseases, FX has been demonstrated to have neuroprotective effects in amyloid-β_{42}-stimulated BV2 microglia cells [276], as well as in LPS-activated BV2 cells via inhibition of Akt/NF-κB and MAPK/AP-1 pathways and activation of the Nrf2/HO-1 pathway [277]. Likewise, the antifibrotic effect of FX has also been reported in TGF-β1-stimulated human pulmonary fibroblasts via suppression of MAPK, PI3K/Akt, and Smad2/Smad3 pathways [278]. On the other hand, our group has previously shown that FX protected HaCaT cells against UVB irradiation via attenuation of ROS and IL-6 production [275]. Interestingly, the combination of FX and the polyphenol rosmarinic acid down-regulated inflammasome-related proteins such as NLRP3, ASC, and caspase-1 and up-regulated the Nrf2/HO-1 pathway in UVB-irradiated HaCaT keratinocytes [279]. In the same line, a sunscreen containing FX 0.5 (w/v) revealed photoprotective properties in UVA-stimulated reconstructed human skin (RHS) via reduction in ROS production [280]. These authors also reported that this carotenoid administered topically in RHS attenuated ethanol-induced skin inflammation through an increase in filaggrin expression [281]. As regards ocular diseases, FX protected ARPE-19 cells against high glucose-induced diabetes retinopathy in ARPE-19 cells via up-regulation of Nrf2 and reduction in apoptosis [282].

Furthermore, the potential therapeutic effect of FX has been reported in LPS-stimulated Caco-2 cells, an in vitro intestinal inflammation model. This carotenoid improved the intestinal epithelial barrier and reduced IL-1β and TNF-α levels and increased the anti-inflammatory cytokine IL-10 [283]. In relation to metabolic disorders, FX inhibited lipid accumulation and ROS production by modulating adipogenic and lipogenic mediators and increasing antioxidant enzymes in adipocytes, demonstrating interesting antiobesity properties [284–286]. According with these findings, FX stimulated lipolysis and supressed lipogenesis in oleic acid-induced hepatocytes, a fatty liver cell model, through activation of the SIRT1/AMP-activated protein kinase (AMPK) pathway [287]. In the same line, antiobesity activity has also been reported after fucoxanthinol treatment, a metabolite of FX, in TNF-α-stimulated adipocytes by reducing the levels of adipocytokines, such as IL-6 and MCP-1, and in palmitic acid-stimulated RAW264.7 cells by inhibiting TNF-α production [286]. These effects were confirmed in a model of low-grade chronic inflammation, consisting of a co-culture of adipocytes and macrophages, demonstrating that this compound ameliorated inflammation in adipose tissue [284].

4.5.2. In Vivo Studies

The anti-inflammatory effects of FX have been demonstrated in a variety of animal models. In terms of skin disorders, a study by our group in the 12-O-tetradecanoylphorbol-13-acetate (TPA) model, which mimics psoriatic markers in mouse dorsal skin, evidenced that topical administration of an FX cream improved hyperplasia via suppression of MPO activity and COX-2 expression. Additionally, this preparation protected mouse skin against UVB-induced acute erythema due to inhibition of COX-2 and iNOS expression and up-regulation of the Nrf2/HO-1 pathway [275]. Furthermore, FX-containing Vaseline improved AD skin symptoms in the Nc/Nga mouse model through an increase in regulatory innate lymphoid cell-released IL-2 and IL-10 [288]. This carotenoid (4 and 8mg/kg) also suppressed inflammation in the mouse model of carrageenan-induced paw edema due to inhibition of MAPK, NF-κB, and protein kinase B/Akt pathways [289]. Regarding colon inflammation, treatment with FX at 50 and 100 mg/kg ameliorated DSS-induced acute colitis in mice by down-regulation of the NF-κB/COX-2/PGE2 pathway [290]. Similar results were reported after FX administration in a rat model of carrageenan/kaolin-induced arthritis [291]. According to these findings, this carotenoid (200 mg/kg) improved LPS-induced depressive and anxiety-like behaviors via suppression of NF-κB and its proinflammatory target genes iNOS, COX-2, IL-1β, IL-6, and TNF-α, as well as activation of AMPK [292]. In addition, FX treatment demonstrated antifibrotic actions in bleomycin-induced pulmonary fibrosis in mice [293], as well as antiasthmatic effects in an ovalbumin-induced asthma mouse model [294,295].

The therapeutic effects of FX in metabolic diseases have been demonstrated in different animal models of obesity. In this respect, oral administration of FX (0.2, 0.4, and 0.6 %) was effective in reducing inflammation through reduction in IL-1β, TNF-α, iNOS, and COX-2 in a model of high-fat diet-induced obesity [296]. Later, this effect was confirmed in the same model after administration of FX at the dose of 1 mg/kg, showing that this carotenoid improved the lipid profile and insulin resistance and decreased blood pressure. Furthermore, FX up-regulated the anti-inflammatory cytokine adiponectin and inhibited leptin expression, a hormone associated with obesity [297,298]. In the same model, FX demonstrated antiobesity properties via modulation of gut microbiota composition [297,298] and stimulation of the Nrf2/NQO1 pathway [299]. Likewise, FX supplementation (0.1 and 0.2%) prevented obesity development and reduced hyperglycemia in diabetic/obese KK-Ay mice, by supressing MCP-1 and TNF-α, which are involved in insulin resistance [286]. Moreover, an extract from *Laminaria japonica* with a high FX content enhanced insulin sensitivity and reduced lipidic peroxidation in a model of streptozotocin- and nicotinamide-induced diabetes [300]. In relation to hepatic disorders, the protective effect of dietary FX (0.2%) has been reported in a mouse model of non-alcoholic fatty liver induced by a high-fat diet via suppression of hepatic fat accumulation and MCP-1 expression [301]. In the same line, FX treatment (10, 20 or 40mg/kg) protected against alcohol-induced liver damage via up-regulation of Nrf2 and suppression of the TLR4-mediated NF-κB pathway [302].

4.5.3. Human Studies

Regarding human studies, a randomized controlled clinical trial has recently reported the protective effect of a combination of fucoidan, a polysaccharide mainly derived from brown seaweed (825 mg), and FX (825 mg), twice a day for 24 weeks in non-alcoholic fatty liver disease patients. The results demonstrated that this treatment improved the lipid profile and reduced hepatic steatosis and inflammation by inhibiting plasma levels of IL-6 and IFN-γ [303].

4.6. β-Cryptoxanthin
4.6.1. In Vivo Studies

The beneficial role of BCX has been reported in different animal studies. In this line, this carotenoid administered orally (2 and 4 mg/kg) protected the retina against light-induced damage through an increase in antioxidant status as well as a reduction in NF-κB levels and the subsequent production of IL-1β and IL-6 [304]. As regards metabolic disorders, the antiobesity properties of dietary BCX for 12 weeks have been reported in a mouse model of high-fat diet-induced insulin resistance. The mechanisms underlying this effect were associated with a down-regulation of NF-κB expression and up-regulation of the Nrf2/HO-1 pathway [305], as well as modulation of the M1/M2 status, resulting in an increase in the M2 macrophage population [306]. Likewise, the cardioprotective effect of this carotenoid has been recently reported in a rat model of ischemia/reperfusion-induced myocardial injury by down-regulating the NF-κB pathway [307]. In addition, BCX attenuated the development of surgically induced osteoarthritis by inhibiting proinflammatory cytokine levels [308] as well as ameliorated cigarette smoke-induced lung inflammatory response and squamous metaplasia via reduction in the NF-κB/TNF-α pathway [309].

4.6.2. Human Studies

Regarding human studies, a randomized, double-masked, and placebo-controlled clinical trial enrolling subjects suffering non-alcoholic fatty liver disease demonstrated that a BCX capsule for 12 weeks attenuated oxidative stress and inflammatory processes via reduction in MDA and IL-6 serum levels, respectively [310].

Table 1. Microalgal carotenoids and their described activities in inflammation and cancer.

Carotenoid	Source	Bioactivity	References
β-Carotene	*Dunaliella salina* *Chlamydomonas reinhardtii* *Isochrysis galbana* *Tetraselmis suecica*	**Inflammation**	
		Colitis	[130–132]
		Hepatic fibrosis	[133]
		Non-alcoholic fatty liver	[134]
		Atherosclerosis	[135,136]
		Atopic dermatitis	[137,138]
		Neurogenic inflammation	[139]
		Acute spinal cord injury	[140]
		Arthritis	[127]
		Asthma	[141]
		Irritable bowel syndrome	[142]
		Type 2 diabetes mellitus	[143]
		Skin photoaging	[144,145]
		Cancer	
		Colon cancer	[311,312]
		Liver cancer	[313,314]
		Gastric cancer	[315,316]
		Esophageal squamous cell carcinoma	[317,318]
		Prostate cancer	[319]
		Neuroblastoma	[320]
		Breast cancer	[321–323]
		Pancreatic cancer	[324]
		Non-Hodgkin lymphoma	[325]
Lutein	*Chlorella sorokiniana* *Chromochloris zoofingiensis* *Auxenochlorella protothecoides* *Dunaliella salina* *Chlamydomonas* sp. *Tetraselmis suecica*	**Inflammation**	
		Age-related macular degeneration	[165,184–188]
		Diabetic retinopathy	[166–168]
		Uveitis	[171,172]
		Dry eye syndrome	[173]
		Atherosclerosis	[174,175]

Table 1. *Cont.*

Carotenoid	Source	Bioactivity	References
Lutein	*Chlorella sorokiniana* *Chromochloris zoofingiensis* *Auxenochlorella protothecoides* *Dunaliella salina* *Chlamydomonas* sp. *Tetraselmis suecica*	**Inflammation**	
		Hepatic injury	[176]
		Pain	[139,177–179]
		Osteoporosis	[181]
		Alcohol-induced hepatic damage	[182]
		Ischemia/Reperfusion	[183]
		Photoprotective/Antiaging effects	[191–193]
		Cancer	
		Colon cancer	[326,327]
		Hepatocellular carcinoma	[328]
		Breast cancer	[329,330]
		Bladder cancer	[331]
		Renal cell carcinoma	[332]
		Neck cancer	[333]
		Non-Hodgkin lymphoma	[325]
		Pharyngeal cancer	[334]
		Esophageal cancer	[318]
		Pancreatic cancer	[335]
Zeaxanthin	*Synechocystis* sp. *Microcystis aeruginosa* *Nannochloropsis oculata* *Chloroidium saccharophilum* *Dunaliella* sp. *Porphyridium purpureum* *Heterosigma akashiwo*	**Inflammation**	
		Age-related macular degeneration	[184,185,196,336]
		Traumatic brain injury	[198]
		Colitis	[199]
		Edema	[200]
		Alcoholic fatty liver	[201]
		Depression/Anxiety	[202]
		Eye dry syndrome	[205]
		Cancer	
		Uveal melanoma	[337]
		Pancreatic cancer	[338]
		Ovarian cancer	[339]
		Bladder cancer	[331]
		Breast cancer	[330]
		Non-Hodgkin lymphoma	[325]
		Pharyngeal cancer	[334]
		Esophageal cancer	[318]
		Colon cancer	[340]
		Pancreatic cancer	[335]
Astaxanthin	*Haematococcus lacustris* *Chromochloris zofingiensis* *Chlorococcum* sp. *Dunaliella salina* *Tetraselmis suecica*	**Inflammation**	
		Non-alcoholic fatty liver	[221–223]
		Liver inflammation	[224–230]
		Kidney inflammation	[231]
		Cardiac dysfunction	[232]
		Diabetes mellitus	[233–235,270,271]
		Diabetes-related disorders	[168,236–238]
		Depression	[239,240,341]
		Epilepsy-induced neuroinflammation	[241–243]
		Acute cerebral infarction	[248]
		Arthritis	[215,249–251,342]
		Colitis	[254,255]
		Asthma	[257]
		Acute lung injury	[258,259,343]
		Contact dermatitis	[344]
		Atopic dermatitis	[260–263]

Table 1. Cont.

Carotenoid	Source	Bioactivity	References
Astaxanthin	Haematococcus lacustris Chromochloris zofingiensis Chlorococcum sp. Dunaliella salina Tetraselmis suecica	**Inflammation**	
		Dry eye	[217]
		Photoprotective/ Antiaging effects	[266]
		Cognitive function	[268]
		Cancer	
		Hepatocellular carcinoma	[345–347]
		Mammary tumor	[348]
		Colon cancer	[349]
		Esophageal cancer	[350]
		Oral cancer	[351,352]
		Prostate cancer	[353]
		Lung metastatic melanoma	[354]
Fucoxanthin	Isochrysis sp. Odontella aurita Chaetoceros neogracilis Chrysotila carterae Phaeodactylum tricornutum Pavlova sp.	**Inflammation**	
		Psoriasis/Acute erythema	[275]
		Atopic dermatitis	[288]
		Edema	[289]
		Colitis	[290]
		Arthritis	[291]
		Depression/Anxiety	[292]
		Lung injury	[278,293]
		Asthma	[294,295]
		Obesity	[296–299]
		Diabetes	[300]
		Non-alcoholic fatty liver	[301–303]
		Cancer	
		Colon cancer	[355–359]
		Lung cancer	[360–362]
		Hepatocellular carcinoma	[363]
		Glioblastoma	[364]
		Cervical cancer	[365]
		Melanoma	[366]
		Sarcoma	[367]
β-Cryptoxanthin	Phaeodactylum tricornutum Auxenochlorella pyrenoidosa Porphyridium purpureum	**Inflammation**	
		Obesity	[305,306]
		Ischemia/Reperfusion	[307]
		Osteoarthritis	[308]
		Lung inflammation	[309]
		Non-alcoholic fatty liver	[310]
		Cancer	
		Gastric cancer	[368,369]
		Hepatocellular carcinoma	[370]
		Lung cancer	[371–373]
		Non-Hodgkin lymphoma	[374]
		Colon cancer	[375]
		Head/Neck cancer	[333]
		Breast cancer	[376]
		Renal cell carcinoma	[377]

5. Anticancer Activity of Carotenoids

5.1. β-Carotene

5.1.1. In Vitro Studies

Numerous in vitro studies have reported the anticancer activity of β-carotene in gastrointestinal cancers. In this line, this carotenoid inhibited the cell growth of the colorectal cancer cells HT-29 [378] and Caco-2 [379]. In addition, β-carotene exhibited anticancer properties via suppression of M2 macrophage polarization, which has a main role in promoting tumor progression and metastasis, as well as reduction in the migration and invasion of HCT116 colon cancer cells [311]. Another paper demonstrated that the molecular mechanisms underlying the anti-colon cancer effects of β-carotene were related to regulation of epigenetic modifications, including an increase in histone acetylation and reduction in DNA methylation [340].

Moreover, β-carotene was reported to act as a proapoptotic agent in gastric cancer cells through reduction in the expression and activity of Ku proteins, which are involved in the repair process of damaged DNA [380]. Furthermore, this carotenoid inhibited proliferation of *H. pylori*-infected gastric adenocarcinoma cells through suppression of NF-κB activation, which in turn down-regulated tumor necrosis factor receptor-associated factor 1 (TRAF1) and TRAF2 expression [381], as well as inhibition of β-catenin signaling and oncogene expression [382]. As regards esophagus cancer, β-carotene has been reported to suppress the growth of a human esophageal squamous cell carcinoma cell line and induce apoptosis via down-regulation of NF-κB/Akt pathway activation and caveolin-1 protein expression [383]. Later, these authors demonstrated a greater antiproliferative effect of β-carotene when it was combined with 5-fluorouracil [317]. Other mechanisms underlying the anticancer effects of this carotenoid in esophageal squamous carcinoma cells include up-regulation of PPAR-γ and down-regulation of cyclin D1 and COX-2 expression [384]. Likewise, β-carotene, in combination with α-carotene, demonstrated a strong antiproliferative activity as well as a reduction in DNA synthesis in esophageal cancer cells [385]. In relation to hepatic cancer, a mixture of different carotenoids, including α- and β-carotene, lycopene, LUT, and BCX, evidenced a higher antimetastatic activity than individual carotenoids in human hepatocarcinoma SK-Hep-1 cells [386]. In addition, β-carotene at a plasma peak concentration exhibited genotoxic and cytotoxic antitumor activity in HepG2 cells [387]. In this cell line, *Dunaliella salina* (as *Dunaliella bardawil*) (Chlorophyta) biomass-loaded nanoparticles, whose majority components are β-carotene, LUT, ZX, CX, phytoene, and phytofluene, were effective in inhibiting cell proliferation and inducing apoptosis [388].

The antiproliferative and proapoptotic actions of β-carotene have also been reported in human cervical cancer cells, hepatoma cells, and breast cancer cells, via inhibition of human calcium/calmodulin-dependent protein kinase IV activity [389], as well as in adrenocorticotropic hormone-secreting pituitary adenoma AtT-20 cells [390]. This carotenoid also suppressed cell proliferation in leukemia K562 cells through an increase in PPAR-γ expression [391], as well as increased the growth inhibitory effect of the anticancer drug trichostatin A in the lung carcinoma cell line A549 [392]. β-Carotene has also been shown to have an antiproliferative effect in human breast adenocarcinoma cells via induction of apoptosis and cell cycle arrest [393], as well as suppression of PI3K/Akt and ERK signaling pathways [394]. Similarly, the combination of a low-dose doxorrubicin treatment with several carotenoids, such as β-carotene, LUT, ATX, or FX, was reported to have a cell growth inhibitory effect and a proapoptotic effect in breast cancer cells [395]. Similar results were reported after treatment with β-carotene-loaded solid lipid nanoparticles [396].

5.1.2. In Vivo Studies

In relation to in vivo studies, β-carotene at the doses of 5 and 15 mg/kg twice weekly for 11 weeks was demonstrated to be effective in the reduction of tumor growth in a model of colitis-associated colon cancer in mice via suppression of M2 macrophage polarization [311]. Similarly, this carotenoid administered orally (20, 40, and 60 mg/kg) for 30 days decreased tumor weight and size in a rat model of H22 cell-induced liver cancer [313]. In addition, the chemopreventive role of β-carotene in gastric cancer was demonstrated in a model of tobacco smoke-exposed mice. This carotenoid prevented epithelial–mesenchymal transition, which is involved in the gastric cancer development, through inhibition of Notch pathway activation [315]. Another paper evidenced that β-carotene in combination with 5-fluorouracil suppressed tumor growth and induced apoptosis in a mouse model of Eca109 cells (an esophageal squamous cell carcinoma cell line) [317]. Similarly, this carotenoid administered at the dose of 16 mg/kg twice a week for 7 weeks showed antiproliferative effects in a xenograft model of prostate cancer [319].

As regards extracranial solid tumors, oral pretreatment with β-carotene reduced tumor growth in a neuroblastoma model, as well as induced cell differentiation and inhibited cancer cell stemness via down-regulation of different cancer stem cell markers [320]. In the same model, these authors confirmed the anticarcinogenic effects of this carotenoid on the murine liver microenvironment of a metastatic neuroblastoma through suppression of proliferation and angiogenesis, as well as inhibition of apoptosis by up-regulating of Bcl-2 and down-regulating Bax protein [397]. Finally, β-carotene-loaded lipid polymer hybrid or zein nanoparticles were shown to reduce tumor growth in a model of chemically induced breast cancer in rats and this effect was enhanced when the carotenoid was co-administered with methotrexate [321,322].

5.1.3. Human Studies

Previous human studies have reported that reduced levels of β-carotene can be detected in patients with different cancers, including oral cancer [398], breast cancer [399], prostate cancer [400], pancreatic cancer [338], and malignant pleural mesothelioma [401]. Moreover, numerous epidemiological studies have indicated that dietary intakes of β-carotene, obtained from fruits and vegetables, may reduce cancer mortality [402] and protect against the development of some gastrointestinal cancers, such as esophageal cancer [318], gastric cancer [316], colon cancer [312], pancreatic cancer, and hepatocellular carcinoma [314,324]. Likewise, consumption of this carotenoid exerted a chemopreventive effect against the development of breast cancer [323,403], lung cancer [404], head and neck cancer [333], and non-Hodgkin lymphoma [325]. However, other human studies have reported contradictory results since β-carotene supplementation was associated with higher risk of developing cancer, such as breast cancer [405] and lung cancer in smokers [406]. These effects may be explained due to the antioxidant properties of this carotenoid, which would lead to a reduction in ROS production with the consequent apoptosis inhibition. In conclusion, further studies for β-carotene are needed to assess this potential association.

5.2. Lutein

5.2.1. In Vitro Studies

Several in vitro studies have reported the anticancer properties of LUT in breast cancer. In this regard, LUT inhibited cell growth and induced apoptosis in two breast cancer lines, the non-invasive MCF-7 and invasive MDA-MB-231 cells. The mechanisms underlying these effects were associated with an inhibition of the transcription factor Nrf2 and its target genes SOD-2 and HO-1, as well as a down-regulation of cell survival markers such as pAkt, pERK, and NF-κB [407]. Other mechanisms involved in the anti-breast cancer effects of this carotenoid include inhibition of glycolysis [408], suppression of cell cycle progression, stimulation of p53 signaling, and an increase in cellular heat shock protein 60 expression [409]. Moreover, LUT inhibited cell invasion and migration under hypoxic conditions through down-regulation of the transcription factor hairy and enhancer of split-1 (HES1) in MCF-7 and MDA-MB-231 cells [410]. In the same cell lines, the epoxide form of LUT exhibited higher cytotoxic and proapoptotic activity than LUT [411]. Likewise, LUT-loaded nanoparticles exhibited an antiproliferative effect in MCF-7 cells [412].

The antiproliferative and proapoptotic actions of LUT have also been described in other cancer cell lines, including sarcoma S180 cells [413], colon adenocarcinoma cells [414], prostate cancer (PC-3) cells [415], A549 lung cancer cells [416], and lymphoid leukaemia cell lines [417].

5.2.2. In Vivo Studies

As regards preclinical animal studies, the chemoprotective effect of dietary LUT (0.002%) administered either 8 weeks before or after the induction of neoplasia was reported in dimethylhydrazine-induced colon cancer. This carotenoid reduced tumor incidence and down-regulated some proteins involved in cell proliferation, such as K-ras, Akt/protein kinase B, and β-catenin [326]. Moreover, LUT (50 and 250 mg/kg) effectively inhibited carcinogenesis in a model of N-nitrosodiethylamine-induced hepatocellular carcinoma in rats via suppression of cytochrome P450 phase I enzyme activity and induction of detoxifying phase II enzymes [328]. More recently, it has been reported that daily administration of LUT (50 mg/kg) for 30 days inhibited tumor growth in a murine breast cancer model induced by injection of 4T1 cells [329]. Similar results were found when this carotenoid (40 mg/kg) was administered to mice inoculated with sarcoma S180 cells; interestingly, the growth inhibitory effect was higher when this carotenoid was co-administered with doxorubicin [413].

5.2.3. Human Studies

The protective effects of dietary LUT and ZX in the prevention of cancer have been revealed in human epidemiological studies, which reported that consumption of these carotenoids reduced the risk of different cancers, such as bladder cancer [331], breast cancer [330], renal cell carcinoma [332], head and neck cancer [333], and non-Hodgkin lymphoma [325]. Similarly, it has been reported that intake of LUT and ZX was inversely related with a decreased risk of gastrointestinal cancers, including oral and pharyngeal cancer [334], esophageal cancer [318], colon cancer [327], and pancreatic cancer [335].

5.3. Zeaxanthin

5.3.1. In Vitro and Animal Studies

The in vitro anticancer effects of ZX have been recently reported in HT-29 cells [378,414] as well as in several human gastric cancer cells. This carotenoid exhibited cytotoxic effects and induced G2/M cell cycle and apoptosis in gastric cancer cells by up-regulating several proapoptotic factors, such as Bax, and down-regulating some antiapoptotic proteins, such as Bcl-2, among others. Moreover, these authors suggested that LUT-induced ROS production may induce regulation of the MAPK signaling pathway and, consequently, activate apoptosis [418]. A bioguided study of the microalga *Cyanophora paradoxa* (Glaucophyta) reported a marked antiproliferative activity of different fractions rich in ZX and BCX in A-2058 melanoma cells [419]. Other papers evidenced the potential of ZX as an antimelanoma agent since this carotenoid induced apoptosis of human uveal melanoma cells [420], as well as suppressed platelet-derived growth factor and melanoma cell-induced fibroblast migration [421]. A preclinical study in mice reported that intravitreal injection of ZX markedly supressed the tumor growth and invasion in a model of human uveal melanoma induced by injection of C918 cells [337].

5.3.2. Human Studies

As regards human studies, in the section on LUT the chemopreventive effects of intake of LUT and ZX in the development of many tumors have already been mentioned. In addition, other studies have described an inverse association between low plasma levels of ZX and increased risk of pancreatic cancer [338] and ovarian cancer [339].

5.4. Astaxanthin

5.4.1. In Vitro Studies

Several studies have reported the anticancer activity of this red pigment carotenoid. In this regard, a study evaluated the role of ATX on pontin, a conserved ATPase of the AAA+ (ATPases associated with various cellular activities) superfamily overexpressed in many cancers. This carotenoid modulated the expression of pontin, which led to a reduction in the proliferation and migration of breast cancer cells when compared to normal breast cells [422]. Recently, the role of ATX has been reported as a novel metastasis inhibitor on the human breast cell line T47D through activation of different tumor metastasis suppressors such as maspin, Kai1, breast cancer metastasis suppressor 1, and mitogen-activated protein kinase kinase 4 [423]. In addition, the cytotoxic effect of ATX against ovarian carcinoma cells via promotion of apoptosis and inactivation of the NF-κB signaling pathway has recently been reported [424].

ATX has also shown antiproliferative effects in leukemia K562 cells by PPAR-γ inhibition [425]. In addition, this compound may induce G0/G1 or G2/M cell cycle arrest, modulate epigenetic alterations (e.g., cell cycle regulator genes or growth factors), and inhibit angiogenesis and metastasis in different cancer cell lines including glioblastoma [426–428]. These mechanisms were also observed in murine hepatoma cells H22 [429] and in several human adenocarcinoma gastric cell lines such as AGS, KATO-III, MKN-45, and SNU-1 [430]. Additionally, this carotenoid induced mitochondrial membrane damage, decreasing its transmembrane potential and the function of electron transport, which promoted the expression of proapoptotic proteins in rat hepatocellular carcinoma cells [431]. Furthermore, ATX evidenced protective effects against the gastric disease associated with *H. pylori* infection by promoting autophagy through AMPK pathway activation and reducing the oxidative stress in the gastric adenocarcinoma cell line AGS [432].

Regarding colon cancer, ATX has been reported to inhibit cancer cell growth not only by arresting cell cycle progression but also by promoting apoptosis via an increase in caspase 3 expression in colon cancer cells [433]. Additionally, this carotenoid was able to promote the expression of Bax, p53, p21, and p27 and the phosphorylation of p38, JNK, and ERK1/2. Moreover, cyclin D1 and Bcl-2 expression and Akt phosphorylation were found to be significantly decreased by ATX treatment, suggesting a protective role against colon cancer cells [434], MCF-7 breast cancer cells [435], and glioblastoma [426]. It is worth highlighting that the three stereoisomers of ATX (*S*, *R*, and a mixture of *S:meso:R*) exhibited antiproliferative activity in HCT116 and HT29 colon cancer cells via apoptosis induction and cell cycle arrest; however, terminal ring structures were not involved in these antitumor effects since no significant differences were detected between the three stereoisomers [436]. Concerning skin cancer, ATX has been shown to decrease tyrosinase activity on human dermal fibroblasts, which can lead to a malignant transformation of normal melanocytes and promote skin cancer [437].

5.4.2. In Vivo Studies

Previous in vivo studies have reported the anticancer activity of ATX in gastrointestinal cancers. In this line, the chemoprotective effect of ATX administered orally (15 mg/kg) for 16 weeks was reported in dimethylhydrazine-induced colon cancer in rats through apoptosis induction via down-regulation of ERK-2, NF-κB, and COX-2 [349]. Similar results were demonstrated after ATX treatment (200 ppm in the diet) in the experimental model of colitis-associated colon cancer induced by azoxymethane (AOM)/DSS in mice [254]. Likewise, dietary intake of ATX at the same dose suppressed AOM-induced colonic premalignant lesion development in mice via attenuation of oxidative stress markers and inactivation of NF-κB [255]. Regarding oral cancer, ATX effectively inhibited carcinogenesis in 7,12-dimethylbenz[a]anthracene (DMBA)-induced buccal pouch cancer in hamsters via down-regulation of NF-κB and Wnt/β-catenin signaling pathways. In addition, this carotenoid induced caspase-mediated mitochondrial apoptosis through attenuation of the antiapoptotic Bcl-2, p-Bad, and surviving expression and up-regulation of the proapoptotic proteins Bax and Bad [351]. In the same model, an ATX-enriched diet (15 mg/kg) suppressed tumor progression via inhibition of the JAK/STAT3 signaling pathway and its downstream targets cyclin D1, MMP-2 and -9, and VEGF, preventing cell proliferation and invasion and, consequently, regulating tumor microvascular density [352]. In addition, ATX supplementation at the dose of 25 mg/kg effectively suppressed tumorigenesis in a rat model of N-nitrosomethylbenzylamine-induced esophageal cancer by down-regulating NF-κB and its target gene COX-2 [350]. Likewise, the chemopreventive effects of dietary ATX (200 ppm) were also reported in diethylnitrosamine (DEN)-induced hepatic cancer in obese mice via attenuation of oxidative stress and an increase in serum adiponectin levels [347].

Regarding skin cancer, the chemopreventive role of ATX (200 µg/kg) was demonstrated in a rat model of UV-DMBA-induced skin tumorigenesis through inhibition of tyrosinase activity and modulation of oxidative stress [438]. In the same line, nitroastaxanthin, the main reaction product of ATX with peroxynitrite, reduced the number of papillomas in a two-stage carcinogensis model on mouse skin initiated by DMBA and promoted by TPA [439]. Moreover, an oral nanoemulsion containing 15 mg/kg of ATX has been found to suppress lung metastatic melanoma by apoptosis activation via down-regulation of Bcl-2, ERK, and NF-κB in B16F10 cell-injected mice [354]. Likewise, in a xenograft model induced by human mammary tumor cells, a diet containing 0.005% ATX for 8 weeks reduced tumor growth and regulated immune response when this carotenoid was administered before tumor initiation, increasing NK cell populations and plasma IFN-γ levels. However, mice fed ATX after tumor initiation exhibited a faster tumor growth and increased plasma levels of IL-6 and TNF-α, showing the importance of a good antioxidant status prior to tumor initiation [348]. Additionally, this carotenoid administered orally at the dose of 100 mg/kg suppressed tumor growth and induced apoptosis via caspase-3 activation in a xenograft model of prostate cancer in nude mice [353].

5.4.3. Human Studies

ATX is considered as a phytonutrient with strong anti-inflammatory and antioxidant activity. Moreover, the European Food Safety Authority (EFSA) recently reported that the intake of 8 mg ATX per day is safe [440], although no toxic effect has been shown with an exceeded EFSA dose recommendation [437]. Nevertheless, although further clinical studies are needed to complete the anticancer activity, ATX supplementation in the human diet has been shown to regulate inflammatory activity [441], enhance the immune response [442], reduce the risk of cardiovascular disease [443], promote eye health, and improve cognitive function [444].

A common metabolic alteration in the tumor microenvironment is lipid accumulation, which is associated with immune dysfunction [445]. In this line, the most studied ATX-mediated pathways in humans are the low-density lipoprotein peroxidation and blood lipid profiles, which increase atherosclerosis risk [446]. Moreover, the relation between abnormal lipid metabolism and liver cancer has been demonstrated. In this regard, and in line with animal experimentation, ATX could be a good candidate for hepatocellular carcinoma, although further clinical data are necessary [345].

5.5. Fucoxanthin

5.5.1. In Vitro Studies

Previous in vitro studies have reported the anticancer activity of FX in gastrointestinal cancers. In this line, FX has been shown to have growth-inhibitory effects on gastric adenocarcinoma cells by suppression of cyclin B1 and myeloid cell leukemia 1 protein via the JAK/STAT signaling pathway [447,448]. Additionally, the anticancer actions of this carotenoid were associated with autophagy and apoptosis induction through an increase in beclin-1, microtubule-associated protein 1 light chain 3, and cleaved caspase-3, and a reduction in Bcl-2 in gastric cancer cells [449]. Similarly, the cytotoxic activity of FX via up-regulation of autophagy and apoptosis was reported in B666-1 nasopharyngeal cancer cells [450]. Regarding colon cancer, FX exhibited cytotoxic effects in HCT116 and HT29 cells, demonstrating a higher cytotoxicity when the carotenoid was combined with 5-fluorouracil [451]. In addition, FX demonstrated anticancer properties by reducing beta-glucuronidase activity in DLD-1 colorectal cancer cells [452]. Interestingly, fucoxanthinol evidenced a more potent proapoptotic effect than FX in HCT116 cells via suppression of NF-κB activation [453]. Additionally, other studies using FX nanogels or nanoparticles to increase its bioavailability reported that these formulations exhibited a greater pro-oxidative activity than free FX, stimulating ROS-triggered apoptosis in Caco-2 cells [454,455]. In relation to hepatic cancer, FX in combination with cisplatin evidenced a higher antiproliferative activity than treatment with cisplatin alone in human hepatoma HepG2 cells through down-regulation of NF-κB expression as well as an increase in the Bax/Bcl-2 ratio [456]. In the same cell line, an FX-rich fraction from the microalga *Chaetoceros calcitrans* (Bacillariophyta) demonstrated proapoptotic effects via inhibition of antioxidant gene expression and MAPK signaling [457].

On the other hand, FX and its metabolite fucoxanthinol inhibited viability in two breast cancer lines, the non-invasive MCF-7 and the invasive MDA-MB-231 cells, by inducing apoptosis. These effects were more prominent with fucoxanthinol and correlated with a suppression of NF-κB pathway activation [458]. Moreover, FX reduced migration and invasion of MDA-MB-231 cells as well as inhibited tumor-induced lymphangiogenesis in human lymphatic endothelial cells [459]. In cervical tumors, FX was reported to have cytotoxic activity in the human cervical cancer cell line HeLa through suppression of the Akt/mechanistic target of rapamycin (mTOR) pathway and the subsequent autophagy induction [460]. Additionally, the mechanisms underlying the proapoptotic effects of FX in HeLa cells were associated with a down-regulation of PI3K/Akt, NF-κB, and the oncogene histone cluster 1 H3 family member [365,461,462].

Regarding lung cancer, FX exhibited growth inhibitory effects in several lung carcinoma cell lines by up-regulation of the proapoptotic genes PUMA (p53 up-regulated modulator of apoptosis) and Fas, as well as suppression of Bcl-2 levels [361]. Moreover, this carotenoid induced apoptosis in the human bladder cancer T24 cells via attenuation of mortalin expression, which is considered as an antiapoptotic factor that binds to p53, thus inhibiting its apoptotic activity [463]. Similarly, FX suppressed the mortalin–p53 interaction, leading to p53 nuclear translocation and activation in different cancer cells [464]. This carotenoid and its deacetylated product, fucoxanthinol, also exhibited antiosteosarcoma activity via attenuation of migration and invasion and activation of apoptosis in different osteosarcoma cell lines. The mechanisms underlying these effects may be related to down-regulation of Akt and AP-1 pathways [465]. In relation to skin, the anticancer effects of FX were demonstrated in mouse melanoma B16F10 cells, via cell cycle arrest in the G0/G1 phase and apoptosis induction [366] as well as metastasis inhibition [466]. Furthermore, FX and ATX supressed TPA-induced neoplastic transformation of mouse skin JB6 P+ cells, an in vitro model for tumor promotion, via activation of the Nrf2 pathway [467].

As regards central nervous system tumors, FX has been reported to inhibit cell proliferation, invasion, and angiogenesis as well as induced ROS-triggered apoptosis in several glioblastoma cells [468,469]. The molecular antitumorigenic mechanisms of FX involved suppression of PI3K/Akt/mTOR and p38 signaling pathways as well as modulation of the MAPK pathway [364,470]. In relation to B cell malignancies, FX and fucoxanthinol exhibited antiproliferative and proapoptotic effects in Burkitt's and Hodgkin's lymphoma cell lines through NF-κB activation with the consequent down-regulation of antiapoptotic proteins (Bcl-2 and X-linked inhibitor of apoptosis protein), and cell cycle regulatory proteins (cyclins D1 and D2) [471]. Similar results were described after treatment of primary effusion lymphoma cells with FX and its metabolite; in addition, their antineoplastic actions were associated with suppression of PI3K/Akt and AP-1 activation [472]. Additionally, the proapoptotic activity of FX was demonstrated in HL-60 leukemia cells due to its pro-oxidative effects and the subsequent down-regulation of the Bcl-xL signalling pathway [473]. Moreover, the antileukemia activity of FX was confirmed in two cancer cell lines representative of advanced stages of chronic myelogenous leukemia [474].

5.5.2. In Vivo Studies

Previous in vivo studies have demonstrated the protective effect of FX in colorectal carcinogenesis. In this respect, FX at the dose of 30 mg/kg for 8 weeks was effective in supressing adenocarcinoma incidence and development of the tumor microenvironment in a model of inflammation-associated colorectal cancer by AOM/DSS [355]. In the same model, these authors demonstrated that FX treatment reduced salivary glycine content over time, suggesting that it may be a good predictor for cancer chemopreventive actions of FX [356]. Additionally, the mechanisms involved in the anti-colon cancer effects of this carotenoid were related to modulation of gut microbiota [357], as well as an induction of anoikis (detachment-induced cell death) though down-regulation of integrin signaling-related proteins [358]. In addition, dietary FX for 5 weeks inhibited colon carcinogenesis in DSS-treated Apc$^{Min/+}$ mice, a model of human familial adenomatous polyposis, by down-regulating cyclin D1 levels [359].

Regarding lung cancer, the chemopreventive role of FX was demonstrated in a mouse model of benzo(A)pyrene-induced lung cancer through apoptosis induction by enhanced caspase 9 and 3 levels and reduced expression of Bcl2 protein [360]. Additionally, FX administration at the dose of 50 mg/kg for 5 weeks attenuated A549 tumor xenograft growth in nude mice via apoptosis induction [361]. Furthermore, a recent study demonstrated the antimetastatic activity of FX in a lung metastatic tumor model in A549-bearing mice [362].

On the other hand, FX administered orally for 15 weeks (50 mg/kg) effectively inhibited carcinogenesis in a model of DEN-induced hepatocellular carcinoma in rats via an increase in the endogenous antioxidant defence system [363]. In xenograft models, this carotenoid administered at the dose of 200 mg/kg for 28 days showed antiproliferative and proapoptotic effects as well as reduced invasion and migration in a xenograft of glioblastoma through suppression of PI3K/Akt/mTOR and p38 pathways [364]. In addition, oral administration of FX (10 and 20 mg/kg) for 5 weeks effectively inhibited tumor growth in a cervical cancer xenograft model in nude mice [365]. Similarly, intraperitoneal administration of this carotenoid suppressed melanoma tumor mass in B16F10 cell-injected mice [366]. Additionally, FX exhibited antitumor growth and proapoptotic effects in mice bearing sarcoma 180 xenografts through suppression of STAT3/epidermal growth factor receptor signaling [367].

5.6. β-Cryptoxanthin

5.6.1. In Vitro Studies

Several in vitro studies evidenced the antiproliferative, antimigratory, and antiapoptotic effects of BCX in different gastric cancer cells [368,369]. Likewise, this carotenoid inhibited cell viability and induced apoptosis in HCT116 colon cancer cells [475], as well as supressed the migration and invasion of lung cancer cells [372].

5.6.2. In Vivo Studies

Animal studies have demonstrated the chemopreventive effects of BCX in different gastrointestinal cancers. In this regard, oral administration of BCX (5 and 10 mg/kg) for 20 days in a gastric cancer xenograft model in nude mice effectively inhibited tumor growth and angiogenesis and induced apoptosis [369]. Similarly, this carotenoid in combination with the chemotherapeutic drug oxaliplatin exhibited antitumor growth effects on nude mice bearing HCT116 xenografts [475]. Another paper demonstrated that dietary BCX for 24 weeks suppressed the progression of chemically and highly refined carbohydrate diet-induced hepatocellular carcinoma in mice. The mechanisms underlying this effect involved an increase in p53 acetylation, with the subsequent induction of apoptosis and the reduction in HIF-1α and its down-stream targets, MMP-2 and MMP-9 [370].

As regards lung cancer, it has been demonstrated that dietary BCX (10 and 20 mg/kg diet) reduced tumor size and multiplicity in a chemically induced lung cancer model via up-regulation of the tumor suppressors SIRT-1, p53, and retinoic acid receptor-β [371]. Later, these authors reported that pre-treatment with BCX supplementation (1 and 10 mg/kg diet) supressed tumor promotion in a model of a nicotine-derived carcinogen-induced lung tumorigenesis through down-regulation of nicotinic acetylcholine receptor α7, highly involved in lung cancer development [372].

5.6.3. Human Studies

Finally, several human studies have described that high serum BCX levels were associated with reduced risk of non-Hodgkin lymphoma [374], colon cancer [375], head and neck cancer [333], breast cancer [376], renal cell carcinoma [377], and lung cancer death in current smokers [373].

6. Conclusions

Microalgae have widely drawn scientists' attention since they are a rich source of bioactive compounds. Their basic and cheap growth requirements make them attractive to be used on a large scale by pharmaceutical, food, and cosmetic industries for health promotion. Carotenoids are one of the most abundant components in microalgae and have been shown to have significant beneficial effects for health. There are two types of carotenoids: carotenes (hydrocabon carotenoids) and xanthophylls (oxygenate derivatives, including ZX, ATX, FX, LUT, α- and BCX, and CX). A multitude of in vitro and in vivo studies and some human studies have evidenced the anti-inflammatory, antioxidant, and antitumor activities of microalgal carotenoids. In this regard, they have been reported to have beneficial effects on many inflammatory diseases, including colitis, non-alcoholic fatty liver, type 2 diabetes mellitus, asthma, arthritis, AMD, AD, and psoriasis, among others. Furthermore, they have been demonstrated to exhibit chemopreventive effects in numerous types of cancer, such as gastric, colon, liver, pancreas, skin, lung, glioblastoma, breast, and prostate. However, further studies, including clinical trials, are required to better evaluate the efficacy and safety of carotenoids and establish recommendations for optimal doses to be used in the prevention and treatment of different inflammatory disorders and cancer.

Author Contributions: Conceptualization, J.Á.-R. and E.T.; writing—original draft preparation, J.Á.-R., S.G.-G., A.R.-L., V.M., and E.T.; writing—review and editing, J.Á.-R. and E.T. All authors have read and agreed to the published version of the manuscript.

Funding: VI Plan Propio Universidad de Sevilla; Proyecto: 2021/00000196—Grupo De Investigación En Farmacología Molecular Y Aplicada.

Institutional Review Board Statement: Not applicable.

Informed Consent Statement: Not applicable.

Data Availability Statement: Not applicable.

Acknowledgments: We would like to thank Mario A. Gómez-Hurtado for the technical support with chemical structures.

Conflicts of Interest: The authors declare no conflict of interest.

References

1. Irigoien, X.; Hulsman, J.; Harris, R.P. Global biodiversity patterns of marine phytoplankton and zooplankton. *Nature* **2004**, *429*, 863–867. [CrossRef]
2. Norsker, N.H.; Barbosa, M.J.; Vermuë, M.H.; Wijffels, R.H. Microalgal production—A close look at the economics. *Biotechnol. Adv.* **2011**, *29*, 24–27. [CrossRef] [PubMed]
3. Acién, F.G.; Fernández, J.M.; Magán, J.J.; Molina, E. Production cost of a real microalgae production plant and strategies to reduce it. *Biotechnol. Adv.* **2012**, *30*, 1344–1353. [CrossRef] [PubMed]
4. Posten, C.; Schaub, G. Microalgae and terrestrial biomass as source for fuels—A process view. *J. Biotechnol.* **2009**, *142*, 64–69. [CrossRef]
5. Zhu, L.D.; Li, Z.H.; Hiltunen, E. Strategies for lipid production improvement in microalgae as a biodiesel feedstock. *Biomed Res. Int.* **2016**, *2016*, 8792548. [CrossRef]
6. Smith, V.H.; Sturm, B.S.M.; deNoyelles, F.J.; Billings, S.A. The ecology of algal biodiesel production. *Trends Ecol. Evol.* **2010**, *25*, 301–309. [CrossRef]
7. Popp, J.; Harangi-Rákos, M.; Gabnai, Z.; Balogh, P.; Antal, G.; Bai, A. Biofuels and their co-products as livestock feed: Global economic and environmental implications. *Molecules* **2016**, *21*, 285. [CrossRef]
8. Rumin, J.; Nicolau, E.; de Oliveira, R.G.; Fuentes-Grünewald, C.; Picot, L. Analysis of scientific research driving microalgae market opportunities in Europe. *Mar. Drugs* **2020**, *18*, 264. [CrossRef] [PubMed]
9. Raff, J.D.; Njegic, B.; Chang, W.L.; Gordon, M.S.; Dabdub, D.; Gerber, R.B.; Finlayson-Pitts, B.J. Chlorine activation indoors and outdoors via surface-mediated reactions of nitrogen oxides with hydrogen chloride. *Proc. Natl. Acad. Sci. USA* **2009**, *106*, 13647–13654. [CrossRef] [PubMed]

10. González, Y.; Torres-Mendoza, D.; Jones, G.E.; Fernandez, P.L. Marine diterpenoids as potential anti-inflammatory agents. *Mediat. Inflamm.* **2015**, *2015*, 263543. [CrossRef]
11. Eseberri, I.; Gómez-Zorita, S.; Trepiana, J.; González-Arceo, M.; Aguirre, L.; Milton-Laskibar, I.; González, M.; Fernández-Quintela, A.; Portillo, M.P. Anti-obesity effects of microalgae. *Int. J. Mol. Sci.* **2020**, *21*, 41. [CrossRef]
12. Lauritano, C.; Helland, K.; Riccio, G.; Andersen, J.H.; Ianora, A.; Hansen, E.H. Lysophosphatidylcholines and chlorophyll-derived molecules from the diatom *Cylindrotheca closterium* with anti-inflammatory activity. *Mar. Drugs* **2020**, *18*, 166. [CrossRef]
13. Markou, G.; Iconomou, D.; Sotiroudis, T.; Israilides, C.; Muylaert, K. Exploration of using stripped ammonia and ash from poultry litter for the cultivation of the cyanobacterium *Arthrospira platensis* and the green microalga *Chlorella vulgaris*. *Bioresour. Technol.* **2015**, *196*, 459–468. [CrossRef]
14. Yu, X.; Chen, L.; Zhang, W. Chemicals to enhance microalgal growth and accumulation of high-value bioproducts. *Front. Microbiol.* **2015**, *6*, 56. [CrossRef] [PubMed]
15. Singh, N.; Roy, K.; Goyal, A.; Moholkar, V.S. Investigations in ultrasonic enhancement of β-carotene production by isolated microalgal strain *Tetradesmus obliquus* SGM19. *Ultrason. Sonochem.* **2019**, *58*, 104697. [CrossRef] [PubMed]
16. Ahmad, I.; Sharma, A.K.; Daniell, H.; Kumar, S. Altered lipid composition and enhanced lipid production in green microalga by introduction of brassica diacylglycerol acyltransferase 2. *Plant Biotechnol. J.* **2015**, *13*, 540–550. [CrossRef]
17. Venkata Mohan, S.; Hemalatha, M.; Chakraborty, D.; Chatterjee, S.; Ranadheer, P.; Kona, R. Algal biorefinery models with self-sustainable closed loop approach: Trends and prospective for blue-bioeconomy. *Bioresour. Technol.* **2020**, *295*, 122128. [CrossRef] [PubMed]
18. PatentScope Database. World Intelectual Propiety Organization. Available online: https://patentscope.wipo.int/search/es/search.jsf (accessed on 6 February 2021).
19. Magri, M. Una Nueva Microalga Chlorella Para la Producción de Aceite Vegetal Para Biodiésel y Unidades de Energía de Cogeneración. Spanish Patent No. ES2755158, 21 April 2020.
20. Fernández Acién, G.F.; Fernández Sevilla, J.M.; Molina Grima, E.; Gómez Serrano, C. Sistema de Eliminación de Metales Pesados en Aguas Mediante Microalgas. Spanish Patent No. ES2642462, 16 November 2017.
21. Frazao de Andrade, A.; Figueiredo Porto, A.L.; De Araujo Viana Marques, D.; De Lima Filho, J.L.; Madruga Lima Ribeiro, M.H.; Nunes Herculano, P.; Pedrosa Bezerra, R.; Goncalves De Melo, R.; Pedrosa Brandão Costa, R.M.; Da Silva, V.A. Formulação Tópica em Gel Com Atividade Cicatrizante Contendo Extrato de Microalga. British Patent No. BR102018077212, 7 July 2020.
22. Leclere-Bienfait, S.; Bredif, S. Extract of Chlamydomonas Acidophila, Method for Preparing Same and Cosmetic Compositions and Dermatological Compositions Comprising Same. French Patent No. WO2020136283, 2 July 2020.
23. Herrera Valencia, V.A.; Peraza Echeverría, S.; Beltrán Aguilar, A.G. Inducible Crgpdh3 Promoter of Chlamydomonas Reinhardtii and the Ese Thereof for the Expression of Recombinant Proteins. Mexican Patent No. WO2020130772, 25 June 2020.
24. Riquelme Salamanca, C.E.; Silva Aciares, F.R.; Gonzalez Cortes, L.A.; Marticorena de la Rosa, P.A. Método de Cultivo al Exterior u "Outdoor" de la Microalga Muriellopsis sp. para Producir Biomasa Con Alto Contenido en Luteína y Bajo Contenido en Metales Que Tiene Buenas Propiedades Antioxidantes y Util para Preparar Alimento Animal o de Consumo Humano. Chile Patent No. WO2019071364, 18 April 2019.
25. Yueming, L.; Jianchun, X.; Lina, X.; Xiuluan, X.; Bingzheng, X. Method for Comprehensively Extracting EPA and Fucoxanthin from Phaeodactylum Tricornutum. Chinese Patent No. CN111205179, 9 January 2020.
26. Nakashima, A.; Suzuki, K.; Sugawara, T.; Manabe, Y. Agent for Suppressing Increment of Blood Glucose Level, Diabetes Preventing Agent, and Food Composition. Japanese Patent No. WO2020045647, 5 March 2020.
27. Napolitano, G.; Fasciolo, G.; Salbitani, G.; Venditti, P. *Chlorella sorokiniana* dietary supplementation increases antioxidant capacities and reduces ros release in mitochondria of hyperthyroid rat liver. *Antioxidants* **2020**, *9*, 883. [CrossRef] [PubMed]
28. Talero, E.; García-Mauriño, S.; Ávila-Román, J.; Rodríguez-Luna, A.; Alcaide, A.; Motilva, V. Bioactive compounds isolated from microalgae in chronic inflammation and cancer. *Mar. Drugs* **2015**, *13*, 6152–6209. [CrossRef]
29. Meléndez-Martínez, A.J.; Stinco, C.M.; Mapelli-Brahm, P. Skin carotenoids in public health and nutricosmetics: The emerging roles and applications of the UV radiation-absorbing colourless carotenoids phytoene and phytofluene. *Nutrients* **2019**, *11*, 1093. [CrossRef]
30. Foong, L.C.; Loh, C.W.L.; Ng, H.S.; Lan, J.C.W. Recent development in the production strategies of microbial carotenoids. *World J. Microbiol. Biotechnol.* **2021**, *37*, 12. [CrossRef] [PubMed]
31. Silva, S.C.; Ferreira, I.C.; Dias, M.; Barreiro, M.F. Microalgae-derived pigments: A 10-year bibliometric review and industry and market trend analysis. *Molecules* **2020**, *25*, 3406. [CrossRef] [PubMed]
32. Han, S.-I.; Kim, S.; Lee, C.; Choi, Y.E. Blue-red LED wavelength shifting strategy for enhancing beta-carotene production from halotolerant microalga, *Dunaliella salina*. *J. Microbiol.* **2019**, *57*, 101–106. [CrossRef]
33. Hassaan, M.S.; Mohammady, E.Y.; Soaudy, M.R.; Sabae, S.A.; Mahmoud, A.M.A.; El-Haroun, E.R. Comparative study on the effect of dietary β-carotene and phycocyanin extracted from *Spirulina platensis* on immune-oxidative stress biomarkers, genes expression and intestinal enzymes, serum biochemical in Nile tilapia, *Oreochromis niloticus*. *Fish Shellfish Immunol.* **2021**, *108*, 63–72. [CrossRef] [PubMed]
34. Rathod, J.P.; Vira, C.; Lali, A.M.; Prakash, G. Metabolic engineering of *Chlamydomonas reinhardtii* for enhanced β-carotene and lutein production. *Appl. Biochem. Biotechnol.* **2020**, *190*, 1457–1469. [CrossRef]

35. Di Lena, G.; Casini, I.; Lucarini, M.; Lombardi-Boccia, G. Carotenoid profiling of five microalgae species from large-scale production. *Food Res. Int.* **2019**, *120*, 810–818. [CrossRef]
36. Low, K.L.; Idris, A.; Mohd Yusof, N. Novel protocol optimized for microalgae lutein used as food additives. *Food Chem.* **2020**, *307*, 125631. [CrossRef]
37. Jalali Jivan, M.; Abbasi, S. Nano based lutein extraction from marigold petals: Optimization using different surfactants and co-surfactants. *Heliyon* **2019**, *5*, e01572. [CrossRef]
38. Wang, X.; Zhang, M.M.; Sun, Z.; Liu, S.F.; Qin, Z.H.; Mou, J.H.; Zhou, Z.G.; Lin, C.S.K. Sustainable lipid and lutein production from Chlorella mixotrophic fermentation by food waste hydrolysate. *J. Hazard. Mater.* **2020**, *400*, 123258. [CrossRef]
39. Saha, S.K.; Kazipet, N.; Murray, P. The carotenogenic Dunaliella salina CCAP 19/20 produces enhanced levels of carotenoid under specific nutrients limitation. *Biomed. Res. Int.* **2018**, *2018*, 7532897. [CrossRef]
40. Xie, Y.; Lu, K.; Zhao, X.; Ma, R.; Chen, J.; Ho, S.H. Manipulating nutritional conditions and salinity-gradient stress for enhanced lutein production in marine microalga *Chlamydomonas* sp. *Biotechnol. J.* **2019**, *14*, e1800380. [CrossRef]
41. Ahmed, F.; Fanning, K.; Netzel, M.; Schenk, P.M. Induced carotenoid accumulation in *Dunaliella salina* and *Tetraselmis suecica* by plant hormones and UV-C radiation. *Appl. Microbiol. Biotechnol.* **2015**, *99*, 9407–9416. [CrossRef] [PubMed]
42. Wojtasiewicz, B.; Stoń-Egiert, J. Bio-optical characterization of selected cyanobacteria strains present in marine and freshwater ecosystems. *J. Appl. Phycol.* **2016**, *28*, 2299–2314. [CrossRef] [PubMed]
43. Lee, M.-Y.; Min, B.-S.; Chang, C.-S.; Jin, E. Isolation and characterization of a xanthophyll aberrant mutant of the green alga *Nannochloropsis oculata*. *Mar. Biotechnol.* **2006**, *8*, 238–245. [CrossRef]
44. Singh, D.; Puri, M.; Wilkens, S.; Mathur, A.S.; Tuli, D.K.; Barrow, C.J. Characterization of a new zeaxanthin producing strain of *Chlorella saccharophila* isolated from New Zealand marine waters. *Bioresour. Technol.* **2013**, *143*, 308–314. [CrossRef] [PubMed]
45. El-Baz, F.K.; Hussein, R.A.; Saleh, D.O.; Jaleel, G.A.R.A. Zeaxanthin isolated from *Dunaliella salina* microalgae ameliorates age associated cardiac dysfunction in rats through stimulation of retinoid receptors. *Mar. Drugs* **2019**, *17*, 290. [CrossRef] [PubMed]
46. Manfellotto, F.; Stella, G.R.; Ferrante, M.I.; Falciatore, A.; Brunet, C. Engineering the unicellular alga *Phaeodactylum tricornutum* for enhancing carotenoid production. *Antioxidants* **2020**, *9*, 757. [CrossRef]
47. Sun, K.M.; Gao, C.; Zhang, J.; Tang, X.; Wang, Z.; Zhang, X.; Li, Y. Rapid formation of antheraxanthin and zeaxanthin in seconds in microalgae and its relation to non-photochemical quenching. *Photosynth. Res.* **2020**, *144*, 317–326. [CrossRef]
48. Johnson, E.A.; An, G.H. Astaxanthin from microbial sources. *Crit. Rev. Biotechnol.* **1991**, *11*, 297–326. [CrossRef]
49. Mularczyk, M.; Michalak, I.; Marycz, K. Astaxanthin and other nutrients from *Haematococcus pluvialis*—Multifunctional applications. *Mar. Drugs* **2020**, *18*, 459. [CrossRef]
50. Mao, X.; Lao, Y.; Sun, H.; Li, X.; Yu, J.; Chen, F. Time-resolved transcriptome analysis during transitions of sulfur nutritional status provides insight into triacylglycerol (TAG) and astaxanthin accumulation in the green alga *Chromochloris zofingiensis*. *Biotechnol. Biofuels* **2020**, *13*, 128. [CrossRef] [PubMed]
51. Janchot, K.; Rauytanapanit, M.; Honda, M.; Hibino, T.; Sirisattha, S.; Praneenararat, T.; Kageyama, H.; Waditee-Sirisattha, R. Effects of potassium chloride-induced stress on the carotenoids canthaxanthin, astaxanthin, and lipid accumulations in the green Chlorococcal microalga strain TISTR 9500. *J. Eukaryot. Microbiol.* **2019**, *66*, 778–787. [CrossRef] [PubMed]
52. Rajput, A.; Singh, D.P.; Khattar, J.S.; Swatch, G.K.; Singh, Y. Evaluation of growth and carotenoid production by a green microalga *Scenedesmus quadricauda* PUMCC 4.1.40. under optimized culture conditions. *J. Basic Microbiol.* **2021**. [CrossRef] [PubMed]
53. Singh, D.P.; Khattar, J.S.; Rajput, A.; Chaudhary, R.; Singh, R. High production of carotenoids by the green microalga *Asterarcys quadricellulare* PUMCC 5.1.1 under optimized culture conditions. *PLoS ONE* **2019**, *14*, e0221930. [CrossRef] [PubMed]
54. Méresse, S.; Fodil, M.; Fleury, F.; Chénais, B. Fucoxanthin, a marine-derived carotenoid from brown seaweeds and microalgae: A promising bioactive compound for cancer therapy. *Int. J. Mol. Sci.* **2020**, *21*, 9273. [CrossRef]
55. Bustamam, M.S.A.; Pantami, H.A.; Azizan, A.; Shaari, K.; Min, C.C.; Abas, F.; Nagao, N.; Maulidiani, M.; Banerjee, S.; Sulaiman, F.; et al. Complementary analytical platforms of NMR spectroscopy and LCMS analysis in the metabolite profiling of *Isochrysis galbana*. *Mar. Drugs* **2021**, *19*, 139. [CrossRef]
56. Lu, X.; Sun, H.; Zhao, W.; Cheng, K.W.; Chen, F.; Liu, B. A hetero-photoautotrophic two-stage cultivation process for production of fucoxanthin by the marine diatom *Nitzschia laevis*. *Mar. Drugs* **2018**, *16*, 219. [CrossRef]
57. Dogdu Okcu, G.; Eustance, E.; Lai, Y.J.S.; Rittmann, B.E. Evaluation of co-culturing a diatom and a coccolithophore using different silicate concentrations. *Sci. Total Environ.* **2021**, *769*. [CrossRef]
58. Kanamoto, A.; Kato, Y.; Yoshida, E.; Hasunuma, T.; Kondo, A. Development of a method for fucoxanthin production using the Haptophyte marine microalga *Pavlova* sp. OPMS 30543. *Mar. Biotechnol.* **2021**, *23*, 331–341. [CrossRef]
59. Havaux, M.; Niyogi, K.K. The violaxanthin cycle protects plants from photooxidative damage by more than one mechanism. *Proc. Natl. Acad. Sci. USA* **1999**, *96*, 8762–8767. [CrossRef]
60. Park, S.B.; Yun, J.H.; Ryu, A.J.; Yun, J.; Kim, J.W.; Lee, S.; Choi, S.; Cho, D.H.; Choi, D.Y.; Lee, Y.J.; et al. Development of a novel *Nannochloropsis* strain with enhanced violaxanthin yield for large-scale production. *Microb. Cell Fact.* **2021**, *20*, 43. [CrossRef] [PubMed]
61. Ahmad, N.; Mounsef, J.R.; Lteif, R. A simple and fast experimental protocol for the extraction of xanthophylls from microalga *Chlorella luteoviridis*. *Prep. Biochem. Biotechnol.* **2021**, 1–5. [CrossRef] [PubMed]

62. Schüler, L.M.; Bombo, G.; Duarte, P.; Santos, T.F.; Maia, I.B.; Pinheiro, F.; Marques, J.; Jacinto, R.; Schulze, P.S.C.; Pereira, H.; et al. Carotenoid biosynthetic gene expression, pigment and n-3 fatty acid contents in carotenoid-rich *Tetraselmis striata* CTP4 strains under heat stress combined with high light. *Bioresour. Technol.* **2021**, *337*, 125385. [CrossRef] [PubMed]
63. Martins, C.B.; Ferreira, O.; Rosado, T.; Gallardo, E.; Silvestre, S.; Santos, L.M.A. Eustigmatophyte strains with potential interest in cancer prevention and treatment: Partial chemical characterization and evaluation of cytotoxic and antioxidant activity. *Biotechnol. Lett.* **2021**, *43*, 1487–1502. [CrossRef]
64. Lohr, M.; Wilhelm, C. Xanthophyll synthesis in diatoms: Quantification of putative intermediates and comparison of pigment conversion kinetics with rate constants derived from a model. *Planta* **2001**, *212*, 382–391. [CrossRef]
65. Inbaraj, B.S.; Chien, J.T.; Chen, B.H. Improved high performance liquid chromatographic method for determination of carotenoids in the microalga *Chlorella pyrenoidosa*. *J. Chromatogr. A* **2006**, *1102*, 193–199. [CrossRef]
66. Markina, Z.V.; Orlova, T.Y.; Vasyanovich, Y.A.; Vardavas, A.I.; Stivaktakis, P.D.; Vardavas, C.I.; Kokkinakis, M.N.; Rezaee, R.; Ozcagli, E.; Golokhvast, K.S. *Porphyridium purpureum* microalga physiological and ultrastructural changes under copper intoxication. *Toxicol. Rep.* **2021**, *8*, 988–993. [CrossRef] [PubMed]
67. Juin, C.; Bonnet, A.; Nicolau, E.; Bérard, J.B.; Devillers, R.; Thiéry, V.; Cadoret, J.P.; Picot, L. UPLC-MSE profiling of phytoplankton metabolites: Application to the identification of pigments and structural analysis of metabolites in *Porphyridium purpureum*. *Mar. Drugs* **2015**, *13*, 2541–2558. [CrossRef]
68. Rebelo, B.A.; Farrona, S.; Ventura, M.R.; Abranches, R. Canthaxanthin, a red-hot carotenoid: Applications, synthesis, and biosynthetic evolution. *Plants* **2020**, *9*, 1039. [CrossRef]
69. Lotan, T.; Hirschberg, J. Cloning and expression in *Escherichia coli* of the gene encoding beta-C-4-oxygenase, that converts beta-carotene to the ketocarotenoid canthaxanthin in *Haematococcus pluvialis*. *FEBS Lett.* **1995**, *364*, 125–128. [CrossRef] [PubMed]
70. Hua-Bin, L.; Fan, K.W.; Chen, F. Isolation and purification of canthaxanthin from the microalga *Chlorella zofingiensis* by high-speed counter-current chromatography. *J. Sep. Sci.* **2006**, *29*, 699–703. [CrossRef]
71. Anila, N.; Simon, D.P.; Chandrashekar, A.; Ravishankar, G.A.; Sarada, R. Metabolic engineering of *Dunaliella salina* for production of ketocarotenoids. *Photosynth. Res.* **2016**, *127*, 321–333. [CrossRef]
72. Kumar, T.S.; Josephine, A.; Sreelatha, T.; Azger Dusthackeer, V.N.; Mahizhaveni, B.; Dharani, G.; Kirubagaran, R.; Raja Kumar, S. Fatty acids-carotenoid complex: An effective anti-TB agent from the chlorella growth factor-extracted spent biomass of *Chlorella vulgaris*. *J. Ethnopharmacol.* **2020**, *249*, 112392. [CrossRef] [PubMed]
73. Pereira, H.; Custódio, L.; Rodrigues, M.J.; De Sousa, C.B.; Oliveira, M.; Barreira, L.; Neng, N.D.R.; Nogueira, J.M.F.; Alrokayan, S.A.; Mouffouk, F.; et al. Biological activities and chemical composition of methanolic extracts of selected autochthonous microalgae strains from the Red Sea. *Mar. Drugs* **2015**, *13*, 3531–3549. [CrossRef] [PubMed]
74. Grama, B.S.; Chader, S.; Khelifi, D.; Agathos, S.N.; Jeffryes, C. Induction of canthaxanthin production in a *Dactylococcus* microalga isolated from the Algerian Sahara. *Bioresour. Technol.* **2014**, *151*, 297–305. [CrossRef]
75. Germolec, D.R.; Shipkowski, K.A.; Frawley, R.P.; Evans, E. Markers of Inflammation. *Methods Mol. Biol.* **2018**, *1803*, 57–79. [CrossRef] [PubMed]
76. Panigrahy, D.; Gilligan, M.M.; Serhan, C.N.; Kashfi, K. Resolution of inflammation: An organizing principle in biology and medicine. *Pharmacol. Ther.* **2021**, *227*, 107879. [CrossRef]
77. Chiurchiù, V.; Leuti, A.; Maccarrone, M. Bioactive lipids and chronic inflammation: Managing the fire within. *Front. Immunol.* **2018**, *9*, 38. [CrossRef]
78. Doyle, R.; Sadlier, D.M.; Godson, C. Pro-resolving lipid mediators: Agents of anti-ageing? *Semin. Immunol.* **2018**, *40*, 36–48. [CrossRef]
79. Fullerton, J.N.; Gilroy, D.W. Resolution of inflammation: A new therapeutic frontier. *Nat. Rev. Drug Discov.* **2016**, *15*, 551–567. [CrossRef]
80. Sun, L.; Wang, X.; Saredy, J.; Yuan, Z.; Yang, X.; Wang, H.L. Innate-adaptive immunity interplay and redox regulation in immune response. *Redox Biol.* **2020**, *37*, 101759. [CrossRef]
81. Mu, X.; Li, Y.; Fan, G.-C. Tissue-resident macrophages in the control of infection and resolution of inflammation. *Shock* **2021**, *55*, 14–23. [CrossRef] [PubMed]
82. Mills, C.D.; Kincaid, K.; Alt, J.M.; Heilman, M.J.; Hill, A.M. M-1/M-2 macrophages and the Th1/Th2 paradigm. *J. Immunol.* **2000**, *164*, 6166–6173. [CrossRef] [PubMed]
83. Sica, A.; Mantovani, A. Macrophage plasticity and polarization: In vivo veritas. *J. Clin. Invest.* **2012**, *122*, 787–795. [CrossRef] [PubMed]
84. Italiani, P.; Boraschi, D. From monocytes to M1/M2 macrophages: Phenotypical vs. functional differentiation. *Front. Immunol.* **2014**, *5*, 514. [CrossRef]
85. Adams, N.M.; Grassmann, S.; Sun, J.C. Clonal expansion of innate and adaptive lymphocytes. *Nat. Rev. Immunol.* **2020**, *20*, 694–707. [CrossRef]
86. Golstein, P.; Griffiths, G.M. An early history of T cell-mediated cytotoxicity. *Nat. Rev. Immunol.* **2018**, *18*, 527–535. [CrossRef]
87. Kourtzelis, I.; Hajishengallis, G.; Chavakis, T. Phagocytosis of apoptotic cells in resolution of inflammation. *Front. Immunol.* **2020**, *11*, 553. [CrossRef]
88. Obata-Ninomiya, K.; Domeier, P.P.; Ziegler, S.F. Basophils and eosinophils in nematode infections. *Front. Immunol.* **2020**, *11*, 583824. [CrossRef]

89. Xia, M.; Wang, B.; Wang, Z.; Zhang, X.; Wang, X. Epigenetic regulation of NK cell-mediated antitumor immunity. *Front. Immunol.* **2021**, *12*, 672328. [CrossRef]
90. Gilroy, D.W.; Edin, M.L.; Maeyer, R.P.H.D.; Bystrom, J.; Newson, J.; Lih, F.B.; Stables, M.; Zeldin, D.C.; Bishop-Bailey, D. CYP450-derived oxylipins mediate inflammatory resolution. *Proc. Natl. Acad. Sci. USA* **2016**, *113*, E3240–E3249. [CrossRef]
91. Jaén, R.I.; Sánchez-García, S.; Fernández-Velasco, M.; Boscá, L.; Prieto, P. Resolution-based therapies: The potential of lipoxins to treat human diseases. *Front. Immunol.* **2021**, *12*, 658840. [CrossRef] [PubMed]
92. Kwon, Y. Immuno-resolving ability of resolvins, protectins, and maresins derived from omega-3 fatty acids in metabolic syndrome. *Mol. Nutr. Food Res.* **2020**, *64*, e1900824. [CrossRef]
93. Serhan, C.N.; Levy, B.D. Resolvins in inflammation: Emergence of the pro-resolving superfamily of mediators. *J. Clin. Invest.* **2018**, *128*, 2657–2669. [CrossRef] [PubMed]
94. Gupta, J.; Gupta, R. Nutraceutical status and scientific strategies for enhancing production of omega-3 fatty acids from microalgae and their role in healthcare. *Curr. Pharm. Biotechnol.* **2020**, *21*, 1616–1631. [CrossRef]
95. Balkwill, F.R.; Mantovani, A. Cancer-related inflammation: Common themes and therapeutic opportunities. *Semin. Cancer Biol.* **2012**, *22*, 33–40. [CrossRef] [PubMed]
96. Coussens, L.M.; Werb, Z. Inflammation and cancer. *Nature* **2002**, *420*, 860–867. [CrossRef] [PubMed]
97. Gómez-Valenzuela, F.; Escobar, E.; Pérez-Tomás, R.; Montecinos, V.P. The inflammatory profile of the tumor microenvironment, orchestrated by cyclooxygenase-2, promotes epithelial-mesenchymal transition. *Front. Oncol.* **2021**, *11*, 686792. [CrossRef]
98. Cortese, N.; Carriero, R.; Laghi, L.; Mantovani, A.; Marchesi, F. Prognostic significance of tumor-associated macrophages: Past, present and future. *Semin. Immunol.* **2020**, *48*, 101408. [CrossRef]
99. Nywening, T.M.; Wang-Gillam, A.; Sanford, D.E.; Belt, B.A.; Panni, R.Z.; Cusworth, B.M.; Toriola, A.T.; Nieman, R.K.; Worley, L.A.; Yano, M.; et al. Targeting tumour-associated macrophages with CCR2 inhibition in combination with FOLFIRINOX in patients with borderline resectable and locally advanced pancreatic cancer: A single-centre, open-label, dose-finding, non-randomised, phase 1b trial. *Lancet. Oncol.* **2016**, *17*, 651–662. [CrossRef]
100. Cannarile, M.A.; Weisser, M.; Jacob, W.; Jegg, A.M.; Ries, C.H.; Rüttinger, D. Colony-stimulating factor 1 receptor (CSF1R) inhibitors in cancer therapy. *J. Immunother. Cancer* **2017**, *5*, 53. [CrossRef]
101. Cortese, N.; Donadon, M.; Rigamonti, A.; Marchesi, F. Macrophages at the crossroads of anticancer strategies. *Front. Biosci. Landmark* **2019**, *24*, 1271–1283. [CrossRef]
102. Vonderheide, R.H. CD40 agonist antibodies in cancer immunotherapy. *Annu. Rev. Med.* **2020**, *71*, 47–58. [CrossRef] [PubMed]
103. Advani, R.; Flinn, I.; Popplewell, L.; Forero, A.; Bartlett, N.L.; Ghosh, N.; Kline, J.; Roschewski, M.; LaCasce, A.; Collins, G.P.; et al. CD47 blockade by Hu5F9-G4 and rituximab in Non-Hodgkin's lymphoma. *N. Engl. J. Med.* **2018**, *379*, 1711–1721. [CrossRef]
104. Pan, X.; Zhang, K.; Shen, C.; Wang, X.; Wang, L.; Huang, Y.Y. Astaxanthin promotes M2 macrophages and attenuates cardiac remodeling after myocardial infarction by suppression inflammation in rats. *Chin. Med. J.* **2020**, *133*, 1786–1797. [CrossRef]
105. Zbakh, H.; Zubía, E.; de Los Reyes, C.; Calderón-Montaño, J.M.; Motilva, V. Anticancer activities of meroterpenoids isolated from the brown alga *Cystoseira usneoides* against the human colon cancer cells HT-29. *Foods* **2020**, *9*, 300. [CrossRef] [PubMed]
106. Ávila-Román, J.; Talero, E.; de los Reyes, C.; García-Mauriño, S.; Motilva, V. Microalgae-derived oxylipins decrease inflammatory mediators by regulating the subcellular location of NFκB and PPAR-γ. *Pharmacol. Res.* **2018**, *128*, 220–230. [CrossRef] [PubMed]
107. Wang, L.; Hauenstein, A.V. The NLRP3 inflammasome: Mechanism of action, role in disease and therapies. *Mol. Asp. Med.* **2020**, *76*, 100889. [CrossRef] [PubMed]
108. Ramos-Tovar, E.; Muriel, P. Molecular mechanisms that link oxidative stress, inflammation, and fibrosis in the liver. *Antioxidants* **2020**, *9*, 1279. [CrossRef] [PubMed]
109. Holley, C.L.; Schroder, K. The rOX-stars of inflammation: Links between the inflammasome and mitochondrial meltdown. *Clin. Transl. Immunol.* **2020**, *9*, e01109. [CrossRef]
110. Farkhondeh, T.; Pourbagher-Shahri, A.M.; Azimi-Nezhad, M.; Forouzanfar, F.; Brockmueller, A.; Ashrafizadeh, M.; Talebi, M.; Shakibaei, M.; Samargandian, S. Roles of Nrf2 in gastric cancer: Targeting for therapeutic strategies. *Molecules* **2021**, *26*, 3157. [CrossRef] [PubMed]
111. Loboda, A.; Damulewicz, M.; Pyza, E.; Jozkowicz, A.; Dulak, J. Role of Nrf2/HO-1 system in development, oxidative stress response and diseases: An evolutionarily conserved mechanism. *Cell. Mol. Life Sci.* **2016**, *73*, 3221–3247. [CrossRef]
112. Mirzaei, S.; Mohammadi, A.T.; Gholami, M.H.; Hashemi, F.; Zarrabi, A.; Zabolian, A.; Hushmandi, K.; Makvandi, P.; Samec, M.; Liskova, A.; et al. Nrf2 signaling pathway in cisplatin chemotherapy: Potential involvement in organ protection and chemoresistance. *Pharmacol. Res.* **2021**, *167*, 105575. [CrossRef]
113. Zimta, A.A.; Cenariu, D.; Irimie, A.; Magdo, L.; Nabavi, S.M.; Atanasov, A.G.; Berindan-Neagoe, I. The role of Nrf2 activity in cancer development and progression. *Cancers* **2019**, *11*, 1755. [CrossRef]
114. Carambia, A.; Schuran, F.A. The aryl hydrocarbon receptor in liver inflammation. *Semin. Immunopathol.* **2021**, *43*, 563–575. [CrossRef]
115. Bock, K.W. Aryl hydrocarbon receptor (AHR) functions: Balancing opposing processes including inflammatory reactions. *Biochem. Pharmacol.* **2020**, *178*, 114093. [CrossRef]
116. Liu, L.; Tang, Z.; Zeng, Y.; Liu, Y.; Zhou, L.; Yang, S.; Wang, D. Role of necroptosis in infection-related, immune-mediated, and autoimmune skin diseases. *J. Dermatol.* **2021**, *48*, 1129–1138. [CrossRef] [PubMed]

117. Song, S.; Ding, Y.; Dai, G.L.; Zhang, Y.; Xu, M.T.; Shen, J.R.; Chen, T.T.; Chen, Y.; Meng, G.L. Sirtuin 3 deficiency exacerbates diabetic cardiomyopathy via necroptosis enhancement and NLRP3 activation. *Acta Pharmacol. Sin.* **2020**, *42*, 230–241. [CrossRef]
118. Aggarwal, V.; Tuli, H.S.; Varol, A.; Thakral, F.; Yerer, M.B.; Sak, K.; Varol, M.; Jain, A.; Khan, M.A.; Sethi, G. Role of reactive oxygen species in cancer progression: Molecular mechanisms and recent advancements. *Biomolecules* **2019**, *9*, 735. [CrossRef] [PubMed]
119. Lee, D.Y.; Song, M.Y.; Kim, E.H. Role of oxidative stress and Nrf2/keap1 signaling in colorectal cancer: Mechanisms and therapeutic perspectives with phytochemicals. *Antioxidants* **2021**, *10*, 743. [CrossRef]
120. Tarafdar, A.; Pula, G. The role of NADPH oxidases and oxidative stress in neurodegenerative disorders. *Int. J. Mol. Sci.* **2018**, *19*, 3824. [CrossRef] [PubMed]
121. Shin, J.; Song, M.H.; Oh, J.W.; Keum, Y.S.; Saini, R.K. Pro-oxidant actions of carotenoids in triggering apoptosis of cancer cells: A review of emerging evidence. *Antioxidants* **2020**, *9*, 532. [CrossRef] [PubMed]
122. Black, H.S.; Boehm, F.; Edge, R.; Truscott, T.G. The benefits and risks of certain dietary carotenoids that exhibit both anti-and pro-oxidative mechanisms—A comprehensive review. *Antioxidants* **2020**, *9*, 264. [CrossRef]
123. Ucci, M.; Di Tomo, P.; Tritschler, F.; Cordone, V.G.P.; Lanuti, P.; Bologna, G.; Di Silvestre, S.; Di Pietro, N.; Pipino, C.; Mandatori, D.; et al. Anti-inflammatory role of carotenoids in endothelial cells derived from umbilical cord of women affected by gestational diabetes mellitus. *Oxid. Med. Cell. Longev.* **2019**, *2019*, 8184656. [CrossRef]
124. Di Tomo, P.; Canali, R.; Ciavardelli, D.; Di Silvestre, S.; De Marco, A.; Giardinelli, A.; Pipino, C.; Di Pietro, N.; Virgili, F.; Pandolfi, A. β-Carotene and lycopene affect endothelial response to TNF-α reducing nitro-oxidative stress and interaction with monocytes. *Mol. Nutr. Food Res.* **2012**, *56*, 217–227. [CrossRef]
125. Cho, S.O.; Kim, M.-H.; Kim, H. β-Carotene inhibits activation of NF-κB, activator protein-1, and STAT3 and regulates abnormal expression of some adipokines in 3T3-L1 adipocytes. *J. Cancer Prev.* **2018**, *23*, 37–43. [CrossRef]
126. Lesmana, R.; Felia Yusuf, I.; Goenawan, H.; Achadiyani, A.; Khairani, A.F.; Nur Fatimah, S.; Supratman, U. Low dose of β-carotene regulates inflammation, reduces caspase signaling, and correlates with autophagy activation in cardiomyoblast cell lines. *Med. Sci. Monit. Basic Res.* **2020**, *26*, e928648. [CrossRef]
127. Yang, G.; Lee, H.E.; Moon, S.; Ko, K.M.; Koh, J.H.; Seok, J.K.; Min, J.; Heo, T.; Kang, H.C.; Cho, Y.; et al. Direct binding to NLRP3 pyrin domain is a novel strategy to prevent NLRP3-driven inflammation and gouty arthritis. *Arthritis Rheumatol.* **2020**, *72*, 1192–1202. [CrossRef]
128. Li, R.; Hong, P.; Zheng, X. β-carotene attenuates lipopolysaccharide-induced inflammation via inhibition of the NF-κB, JAK2/STAT3 and JNK/p38 MAPK signaling pathways in macrophages. *Anim. Sci. J.* **2019**, *90*, 140–148. [CrossRef]
129. Lin, H.W.; Chang, T.J.; Yang, D.J.; Chen, Y.C.; Wang, M.; Chang, Y.Y. Regulation of virus-induced inflammatory response by β-carotene in RAW264.7 cells. *Food Chem.* **2012**, *134*, 2169–2175. [CrossRef]
130. Trivedi, P.P.; Jena, G.B. Mechanistic insight into beta-carotene-mediated protection against ulcerative colitis-associated local and systemic damage in mice. *Eur. J. Nutr.* **2015**, *54*, 639–652. [CrossRef] [PubMed]
131. Yang, Y.; Li, R.; Hui, J.; Li, L.; Zheng, X. β-Carotene attenuates LPS-induced rat intestinal inflammation via modulating autophagy and regulating the JAK2/STAT3 and JNK/p38 MAPK signaling pathways. *J. Food Biochem.* **2021**, *45*, e13544. [CrossRef]
132. Li, R.; Li, L.; Hong, P.; Lang, W.; Hui, J.; Yang, Y.; Zheng, X. β-Carotene prevents weaning-induced intestinal inflammation by modulating gut microbiota in piglets. *Anim. Biosci.* **2021**, *34*, 1221–1234. [CrossRef]
133. Latief, U.; Ahmad, R. β-Carotene inhibits NF-κB and restrains diethylnitrosamine-induced hepatic inflammation in Wistar rats. *Int. J. Vitam. Nutr. Res.* **2020**, 1–10. [CrossRef] [PubMed]
134. El-Din, S.H.S.; El-Lakkany, N.M.; El-Naggar, A.A.; Hammam, O.A.; El-Latif, H.A.A.; Ain-Shoka, A.A.; Ebeid, F.A. Effects of rosuvastatin and/or β-carotene on non-alcoholic fatty liver in rats. *Res. Pharm. Sci.* **2015**, *10*, 275–287.
135. Relevy, N.Z.; Harats, D.; Harari, A.; Ben-Amotz, A.; Bitzur, R.; Rühl, R.; Shaish, A. Vitamin A-deficient diet accelerated atherogenesis in apolipoprotein E(−/−) mice and dietary β -carotene prevents this consequence. *Biomed Res. Int.* **2015**, *2015*, 758723. [CrossRef]
136. Kaliappan, G.; Nagarajan, P.; Moorthy, R.; Kalai Gana Selvi, S.; Avinash Raj, T.; Mahesh Kumar, J. Ang II induce kidney damage by recruiting inflammatory cells and up regulates PPAR gamma and Renin 1 gene: Effect of β carotene on chronic renal damage. *J. Thromb. Thrombolysis* **2013**, *36*, 277–285. [CrossRef]
137. Takahashi, N.; Kake, T.; Hasegawa, S.; Imai, M. Effects of post-administration of β-carotene on diet-induced atopic dermatitis in hairless mice. *J. Oleo Sci.* **2019**, *68*, 793–802. [CrossRef]
138. Kake, T.; Imai, M.; Takahashi, N. Effects of β-carotene on oxazolone-induced atopic dermatitis in hairless mice. *Exp. Dermatol.* **2019**, *28*, 1044–1050. [CrossRef]
139. Horváth, G.; Kemény, Á.; Barthó, L.; Molnár, P.; Deli, J.; Szente, L.; Bozó, T.; Pál, S.; Sándor, K.; Szőke, É.; et al. Effects of some natural carotenoids on TRPA1- and TRPV1-induced neurogenic inflammatory processes *in vivo* in the mouse skin. *J. Mol. Neurosci.* **2015**, *56*, 113–121. [CrossRef]
140. Zhou, L.; Ouyang, L.; Lin, S.; Chen, S.; Liu, Y.J.; Zhou, W.; Wang, X. Protective role of β-carotene against oxidative stress and neuroinflammation in a rat model of spinal cord injury. *Int. Immunopharmacol.* **2018**, *61*, 92–99. [CrossRef]
141. Zainal, Z.; Rahim, A.A.; Khaza'ai, H.; Chang, S.K. Effects of palm oil tocotrienol-rich fraction (TRF) and carotenes in ovalbumin (OVA)-challenged asthmatic brown Norway rats. *Int. J. Mol. Sci.* **2019**, *20*, 1764. [CrossRef]

142. Fuke, N.; Aizawa, K.; Suganuma, H.; Takagi, T.; Naito, Y. Effect of combined consumption of *Lactobacillus brevis* KB290 and β-carotene on minor diarrhoea-predominant irritable bowel syndrome-like symptoms in healthy subjects: A randomised, double-blind, placebo-controlled, parallel-group trial. *Int. J. Food Sci. Nutr.* **2017**, *68*, 973–986. [CrossRef]
143. Asemi, Z.; Alizadeh, S.A.; Ahmad, K.; Goli, M.; Esmaillzadeh, A. Effects of beta-carotene fortified synbiotic food on metabolic control of patients with type 2 diabetes mellitus: A double-blind randomized cross-over controlled clinical trial. *Clin. Nutr.* **2016**, *35*, 819–825. [CrossRef] [PubMed]
144. Cho, S.; Lee, D.H.; Won, C.H.; Kim, S.M.; Lee, S.; Lee, M.J.; Chung, J.H. Differential effects of low-dose and high-dose beta-carotene supplementation on the signs of photoaging and type I procollagen gene expression in human skin in vivo. *Dermatology* **2010**, *221*, 160–171. [CrossRef]
145. Ribeiro, D.; Sousa, A.; Nicola, P.; Ferreira de Oliveira, J.M.P.; Rufino, A.T.; Silva, M.; Freitas, M.; Carvalho, F.; Fernandes, E. β-Carotene and its physiological metabolites: Effects on oxidative status regulation and genotoxicity in in vitro models. *Food Chem. Toxicol.* **2020**, *141*, 111392. [CrossRef] [PubMed]
146. Wang, L.; Ding, C.; Zeng, F.; Zhu, H. Low levels of serum β-carotene and β-carotene/retinol ratio are associated with histological severity in nonalcoholic fatty liver disease patients. *Ann. Nutr. Metab.* **2019**, *74*, 156–164. [CrossRef]
147. Chambaneau, A.; Filaire, M.; Jubert, L.; Bremond, M.; Filaire, E. Nutritional Intake, Physical Activity and Quality of Life in COPD Patients. *Int. J. Sports Med.* **2016**, *37*, 730–737. [CrossRef] [PubMed]
148. Freitas, F.; Brucker, N.; Durgante, J.; Bubols, G.; Bulcão, R.; Moro, A.; Charão, M.; Baierle, M.; Nascimento, S.; Gauer, B.; et al. Urinary 1-hydroxypyrene is associated with oxidative stress and inflammatory biomarkers in acute myocardial infarction. *Int. J. Environ. Res. Public Health* **2014**, *11*, 9024–9037. [CrossRef] [PubMed]
149. Epplein, M.; Signorello, L.B.; Zheng, W.; Cai, Q.; Hargreaves, M.K.; Michel, A.; Pawlita, M.; Fowke, J.H.; Correa, P.; Blot, W.J. *Helicobacter pylori* prevalence and circulating micronutrient levels in a low-income United States population. *Cancer Prev. Res.* **2011**, *4*, 871–878. [CrossRef]
150. Muzáková, V.; Kand'ár, R.; Meloun, M.; Skalický, J.; Královec, K.; Záková, P.; Vojtíšek, P. Inverse correlation between plasma Beta-carotene and interleukin-6 in patients with advanced coronary artery disease. *Int. J. Vitam. Nutr. Res.* **2010**, *80*, 369–377. [CrossRef]
151. Munia, I.; Gafray, L.; Bringer, M.A.; Goldschmidt, P.; Proukhnitzky, L.; Jacquemot, N.; Cercy, C.; Otman, K.R.B.; Errera, M.H.; Ranchon-Cole, I. Cytoprotective effects of natural highly bio-available vegetable derivatives on human-derived retinal cells. *Nutrients* **2020**, *12*, 879. [CrossRef]
152. Ge, Y.; Zhang, A.; Sun, R.; Xu, J.; Yin, T.; He, H.; Gou, J.; Kong, J.; Zhang, Y.; Tang, X. Penetratin-modified lutein nanoemulsion in-situ gel for the treatment of age-related macular degeneration. *Expert Opin. Drug Deliv.* **2020**, *17*, 603–619. [CrossRef]
153. Bian, Q.; Gao, S.; Zhou, J.; Qin, J.; Taylor, A.; Johnson, E.J.; Tang, G.; Sparrow, J.R.; Gierhart, D.; Shang, F. Lutein and zeaxanthin supplementation reduces photooxidative damage and modulates the expression of inflammation-related genes in retinal pigment epithelial cells. *Free Radic. Biol. Med.* **2012**, *53*, 1298–1307. [CrossRef] [PubMed]
154. Li, S.Y.; Fung, F.K.C.; Fu, Z.J.; Wong, D.; Chan, H.H.L.; Lo, A.C.Y. Anti-inflammatory effects of lutein in retinal ischemic/hypoxic injury: In vivo and in vitro studies. *Investig. Ophthalmol. Vis. Sci.* **2012**, *53*, 5976–5984. [CrossRef]
155. Fung, F.K.C.; Law, B.Y.K.; Lo, A.C.Y. Lutein attenuates both apoptosis and autophagy upon cobalt (II) chloride-induced hypoxia in rat Muller cells. *PLoS ONE* **2016**, *11*, e0167828. [CrossRef]
156. Chao, S.C.; Nien, C.W.; Iacob, C.; Hu, D.N.; Huang, S.C.; Lin, H.Y. Effects of lutein on hyperosmoticity-induced upregulation of IL-6 in cultured corneal epithelial cells and its relevant signal pathways. *J. Ophthalmol.* **2016**, *2016*, 8341439. [CrossRef] [PubMed]
157. Pongcharoen, S.; Warnnissorn, P.; Lertkajornsin, O.; Limpeanchob, N.; Sutheerawattananonda, M. Protective effect of silk lutein on ultraviolet B-irradiated human keratinocytes. *Biol. Res.* **2013**, *46*, 39–45. [CrossRef]
158. Chen, C.Y.O.; Smith, A.; Liu, Y.; Du, P.; Blumberg, J.B.; Garlick, J. Photoprotection by pistachio bioactives in a 3-dimensional human skin equivalent tissue model. *Int. J. Food Sci. Nutr.* **2017**, *68*, 712–718. [CrossRef] [PubMed]
159. Oh, J.; Kim, J.H.; Park, J.G.; Yi, Y.; Park, K.W.; Rho, H.S.; Lee, M.; Yoo, J.W.; Kang, S.; Hong, Y.D.; et al. Radical scavenging activity-based and AP-1-targeted anti-inflammatory effects of lutein in macrophage-like and skin keratinocytic cells. *Mediat. Inflamm.* **2013**, *2013*, 787042. [CrossRef]
160. Qiao, Y.Q.; Jiang, P.F.; Gao, Y.Z. Lutein prevents osteoarthritis through Nrf2 activation and downregulation of inflammation. *Arch. Med. Sci.* **2018**, *14*, 617–624. [CrossRef] [PubMed]
161. Wu, W.; Li, Y.; Wu, Y.; Zhang, Y.; Wang, Z.; Liu, X. Lutein suppresses inflammatory responses through Nrf2 activation and NF-κB inactivation in lipopolysaccharide-stimulated BV-2 microglia. *Mol. Nutr. Food Res.* **2015**, *59*, 1663–1673. [CrossRef]
162. Chung, R.W.S.; Leanderson, P.; Lundberg, A.K.; Jonasson, L. Lutein exerts anti-inflammatory effects in patients with coronary artery disease. *Atherosclerosis* **2017**, *262*, 87–93. [CrossRef]
163. Phan, M.A.T.; Bucknall, M.; Arcot, J. Effect of different anthocyanidin glucosides on lutein uptake by Caco-2 cells, and their combined activities on anti-oxidation and anti-inflammation in vitro and ex vivo. *Molecules* **2018**, *23*, 2035. [CrossRef]
164. Tuzcu, M.; Orhan, C.; Muz, O.E.; Sahin, N.; Juturu, V.; Sahin, K. Lutein and zeaxanthin isomers modulates lipid metabolism and the inflammatory state of retina in obesity-induced high-fat diet rodent model. *BMC Ophthalmol.* **2017**, *17*, 129. [CrossRef]
165. Kamoshita, M.; Toda, E.; Osada, H.; Narimatsu, T.; Kobayashi, S.; Tsubota, K.; Ozawa, Y. Lutein acts via multiple antioxidant pathways in the photo-stressed retina. *Sci. Rep.* **2016**, *6*, 30226. [CrossRef]

166. Wang, W.; Tam, K.C.; Ng, T.C.; Goit, R.K.; Chan, K.L.S.; Lo, A.C.Y. Long-term lutein administration attenuates retinal inflammation and functional deficits in early diabetic retinopathy using the Ins2 Akita/+ mice. *BMJ Open Diabetes Res. Care* **2020**, *8*, e001519. [CrossRef]
167. Sasaki, M.; Ozawa, Y.; Kurihara, T.; Kubota, S.; Yuki, K.; Noda, K.; Kobayashi, S.; Ishida, S.; Tsubota, K. Neurodegenerative influence of oxidative stress in the retina of a murine model of diabetes. *Diabetologia* **2010**, *53*, 971–979. [CrossRef] [PubMed]
168. Yeh, P.T.; Huang, H.W.; Yang, C.M.; Yang, W.S.; Yang, C.H. Astaxanthin inhibits expression of retinal oxidative stress and inflammatory mediators in streptozotocin-induced diabetic rats. *PLoS ONE* **2016**, *11*, e0146438. [CrossRef]
169. Padmanabha, S.; Vallikannan, B. Fatty acids modulate the efficacy of lutein in cataract prevention: Assessment of oxidative and inflammatory parameters in rats. *Biochem. Biophys. Res. Commun.* **2018**, *500*, 435–442. [CrossRef] [PubMed]
170. Padmanabha, S.; Vallikannan, B. Fatty acids influence the efficacy of lutein in the modulation of α-crystallin chaperone function: Evidence from selenite induced cataract rat model. *Biochem. Biophys. Res. Commun.* **2020**, *529*, 425–431. [CrossRef]
171. He, R.R.; Tsoi, B.; Lan, F.; Yao, N.; Yao, X.S.; Kurihara, H. Antioxidant properties of lutein contribute to the protection against lipopolysaccharide-induced uveitis in mice. *Chin. Med.* **2011**, *6*, 38. [CrossRef] [PubMed]
172. Chao, S.C.; Vagaggini, T.; Nien, C.W.; Huang, S.C.; Lin, H.Y. Effects of lutein and zeaxanthin on LPS-induced secretion of IL-8 by uveal melanocytes and relevant signal pathways. *J. Ophthalmol.* **2015**, *2015*, 152854. [CrossRef] [PubMed]
173. Muz, O.E.; Orhan, C.; Erten, F.; Tuzcu, M.; Ozercan, I.H.; Singh, P.; Morde, A.; Padigaru, M.; Rai, D.; Sahin, K. A novel integrated active herbal formulation ameliorates dry eye syndrome by inhibiting inflammation and oxidative stress and enhancing glycosylated phosphoproteins in rats. *Pharmaceuticals* **2020**, *13*, 295. [CrossRef] [PubMed]
174. Han, H.; Cui, W.; Wang, L.; Xiong, Y.; Liu, L.; Sun, X.; Hao, L. Lutein prevents high fat diet-induced atherosclerosis in ApoE-deficient mice by inhibiting NADPH oxidase and increasing PPAR expression. *Lipids* **2015**, *50*, 261–273. [CrossRef]
175. Kim, J.E.; Leite, J.O.; deOgburn, R.; Smyth, J.A.; Clark, R.M.; Fernandez, M.L. A Lutein-enriched diet prevents cholesterol accumulation and decreases oxidized LDL and inflammatory cytokines in the aorta of guinea pigs. *J. Nutr.* **2011**, *141*, 1458–1463. [CrossRef]
176. Kim, J.E.; Clark, R.M.; Park, Y.; Lee, J.; Fernandez, M.L. Lutein decreases oxidative stress and inflammation in liver and eyes of guinea pigs fed a hypercholesterolemic diet. *Nutr. Res. Pract.* **2012**, *6*, 113–119. [CrossRef]
177. Shimazu, Y.; Kobayashi, A.; Endo, S.; Takemura, J.; Takeda, M. Effect of lutein on the acute inflammation-induced c-Fos expression of rat trigeminal spinal nucleus caudalis and C1 dorsal horn neurons. *Eur. J. Oral Sci.* **2019**, *127*, 379–385. [CrossRef]
178. Syoji, Y.; Kobayashi, R.; Miyamura, N.; Hirohara, T.; Kubota, Y.; Uotsu, N.; Yui, K.; Shimazu, Y.; Takeda, M. Suppression of hyperexcitability of trigeminal nociceptive neurons associated with inflammatory hyperalgesia following systemic administration of lutein via inhibition of cyclooxygenase-2 cascade signaling. *J. Inflamm.* **2018**, *15*, 4–13. [CrossRef]
179. AbuBakr, H.O.; Aljuaydi, S.H.; Abou-Zeid, S.M.; El-Bahrawy, A. Burn-induced multiple organ injury and protective effect of lutein in rats. *Inflammation* **2018**, *41*, 760–772. [CrossRef]
180. Tan, D.; Yu, X.; Chen, M.; Chen, J.; Xu, J. Lutein protects against severe traumatic brain injury through anti-inflammation and antioxidative effects via ICAM-1/Nrf-2. *Mol. Med. Rep.* **2017**, *16*, 4235–4240. [CrossRef]
181. Li, H.; Huang, C.; Zhu, J.; Gao, K.; Fang, J.; Li, H. Lutein suppresses oxidative stress and inflammation by Nrf2 activation in an osteoporosis rat model. *Med. Sci. Monit.* **2018**, *24*, 5071–5075. [CrossRef]
182. Du, S.Y.; Zhang, Y.L.; Bai, R.X.; Ai, Z.L.; Xie, B.S.; Yang, H.Y. Lutein prevents alcohol-induced liver disease in rats by modulating oxidative stress and inflammation. *Int. J. Clin. Exp. Med.* **2015**, *8*, 8785–8793. [PubMed]
183. Cheng, F.; Zhang, Q.; Yan, F.F.; Wan, J.F.; Lin, C.S. Lutein protects against ischemia/reperfusion injury in rat skeletal muscle by modulating oxidative stress and inflammation. *Immunopharmacol. Immunotoxicol.* **2015**, *37*, 329–334. [CrossRef]
184. Clemons, T.E.; Sangiovanni, J.P.; Danis, R.P.; Frederick, L.; Iii, F.; Elman, M.J.; Antoszyk, A.; Ruby, A.; Orth, D.; Bressler, S.B.; et al. Secondary analyses of the effects of lutein/zeaxanthin on age-related macular degeneration progression AREDS2 report No. 3. *JAMA Ophthalmol.* **2014**, *132*, 142–149. [CrossRef]
185. Agrón, E.; Mares, J.; Clemons, T.E.; Swaroop, A.; Chew, E.Y.; Keenan, T.D.L. Dietary nutrient intake and progression to late age-related macular degeneration in the Age-Related Eye Disease Studies 1 and 2. *Ophthalmology* **2020**, *128*, 425–442. [CrossRef]
186. Korobelnik, J.F.; Rougier, M.B.; Delyfer, M.N.; Bron, A.; Merle, B.M.J.; Savel, H.; Chêne, G.; Delcourt, C.; Creuzot-Garcher, C. Effect of dietary supplementation with lutein, zeaxanthin, and ω-3 on macular pigment: A randomized clinical trial. *JAMA Ophthalmol.* **2017**, *135*, 1259–1266. [CrossRef]
187. Huang, Y.M.; Dou, H.L.; Huang, F.F.; Xu, X.R.; Zou, Z.Y.; Lin, X.M. Effect of supplemental lutein and zeaxanthin on serum, macular pigmentation, and visual performance in patients with early age-related macular degeneration. *Biomed. Res. Int.* **2015**, *2015*, 564738. [CrossRef]
188. Huang, Y.M.; Dou, H.L.; Huang, F.F.; Xu, X.R.; Zou, Z.Y.; Lu, X.R.; Lin, X.M. Changes following supplementation with lutein and zeaxanthin in retinal function in eyes with early age-related macular degeneration: A randomised, double-blind, placebo-controlled trial. *Br. J. Ophthalmol.* **2015**, *99*, 371–375. [CrossRef] [PubMed]
189. García-Layana, A.; Recalde, S.; Alamán, A.S.; Robredo, P.F. Effects of lutein and docosahexaenoic acid supplementation on macular pigment optical density in a randomized controlled trial. *Nutrients* **2013**, *5*, 543–551. [CrossRef]
190. Wolf-Schnurrbusch, U.E.K.; Zinkernagel, M.S.; Munk, M.R.; Ebneter, A.; Wolf, S. Oral lutein supplementation enhances macular pigment density and contrast sensitivity but not in combination with polyunsaturated fatty acids. *Investig. Ophthalmol. Vis. Sci.* **2015**, *56*, 8069–8074. [CrossRef]

191. Grether-Beck, S.; Marini, A.; Jaenicke, T.; Stahl, W.; Krutmann, J. Molecular evidence that oral supplementation with lycopene or lutein protects human skin against ultraviolet radiation: Results from a double-blinded, placebo-controlled, crossover study. *Br. J. Dermatol.* **2017**, *176*, 1231–1240. [CrossRef]
192. Morse, N.L.; Reid, A.J.; St-Onge, M. An open-label clinical trial assessing the efficacy and safety of Bend Skincare Anti-Aging Formula on minimal erythema dose in skin. *Photodermatol. Photoimmunol. Photomed.* **2018**, *34*, 152–161. [CrossRef]
193. Granger, C.; Aladren, S.; Delgado, J.; Garre, A.; Trullas, C.; Gilaberte, Y. Prospective evaluation of the efficacy of a food supplement in increasing photoprotection and improving selective markers related to skin photo-ageing. *Dermatol. Ther.* **2020**, *10*, 163–178. [CrossRef]
194. Liu, Y.; Xiong, Y.; Xing, F.; Gao, H.; Wang, X.; He, L.; Ren, C.; Liu, L.; So, K.F.; Xiao, J. Precise regulation of mir-210 is critical for the cellular homeostasis maintenance and transplantation efficacy enhancement of mesenchymal stem cells in acute liver failure therapy. *Cell Transpl.* **2017**, *26*, 805–820. [CrossRef] [PubMed]
195. Zou, X.; Gao, J.; Zheng, Y.; Wang, X.; Chen, C.; Cao, K.; Xu, J.; Li, Y.; Lu, W.; Liu, J.; et al. Zeaxanthin induces Nrf2-mediated phase II enzymes in protection of cell death. *Cell Death Dis.* **2014**, *5*, e1218. [CrossRef]
196. Biswal, M.R.; Justis, B.D.; Han, P.; Li, H.; Gierhart, D.; Dorey, C.K.; Lewin, A.S. Daily zeaxanthin supplementation prevents atrophy of the retinal pigment epithelium (RPE) in a mouse model of mitochondrial oxidative stress. *PLoS ONE* **2018**, *13*, e0203816. [CrossRef]
197. Sahin, K.; Akdemir, F.; Orhan, C.; Tuzcu, M.; Gencoglu, H.; Sahin, N.; Ozercan, I.H.; Ali, S.; Yilmaz, I.; Juturu, V. (3R, 3′R)-zeaxanthin protects the retina from photo-oxidative damage via modulating the inflammation and visual health molecular markers. *Cutan. Ocul. Toxicol.* **2019**, *38*, 161–168. [CrossRef] [PubMed]
198. Gunal, M.Y.; Sakul, A.A.; Caglayan, A.B.; Erten, F.; Kursun, O.E.D.; Kilic, E.; Sahin, K. Protective effect of lutein/zeaxanthin isomers in traumatic brain injury in mice. *Neurotox. Res.* **2021**, *39*, 1543–1550. [CrossRef] [PubMed]
199. El-Akabawy, G.; El-Sherif, N.M. Zeaxanthin exerts protective effects on acetic acid-induced colitis in rats via modulation of pro-inflammatory cytokines and oxidative stress. *Biomed. Pharmacother.* **2019**, *111*, 841–851. [CrossRef]
200. Firdous, A.P.; Kuttan, G.; Kuttan, R. Anti-inflammatory potential of carotenoid meso-zeaxanthin and its mode of action. *Pharm. Biol.* **2015**, *53*, 961–967. [CrossRef]
201. Gao, H.; Lv, Y.; Liu, Y.; Li, J.; Wang, X.; Zhou, Z.; Tipoe, G.L.; Ouyang, S.; Guo, Y.; Zhang, J.; et al. Wolfberry-derived zeaxanthin dipalmitate attenuates ethanol-induced hepatic damage. *Mol. Nutr. Food Res.* **2019**, *63*, e1801339. [CrossRef] [PubMed]
202. Zhou, X.; Gan, T.; Fang, G.; Wang, S.; Mao, Y.; Ying, C. Zeaxanthin improved diabetes-induced anxiety and depression through inhibiting inflammation in hippocampus. *Metab. Brain Dis.* **2018**, *33*, 705–711. [CrossRef] [PubMed]
203. Majeed, M.; Majeed, S.; Nagabhushanam, K. An open-label pilot study on Macumax supplementation for dry-type age-related macular degeneration. *J. Med. Food.* **2021**, *24*, 551–557. [CrossRef] [PubMed]
204. Azar, G.; Quaranta-El Maftouhi, M.; Masella, J.-J.; Mauget-Faysse, M. Macular pigment density variation after supplementation of lutein and zeaxanthin using the Visucam® 200 pigment module: Impact of age-related macular degeneration and lens status. *J. Fr. Ophtalmol.* **2017**, *40*, 303–313. [CrossRef] [PubMed]
205. Radkar, P.; Lakshmanan, P.S.; Mary, J.J.; Chaudhary, S.; Durairaj, S.K. A Novel multi-ingredient supplement reduces inflammation of the eye and improves production and quality of tears in humans. *Ophthalmol. Ther.* **2021**, *10*, 581–599. [CrossRef]
206. Kishimoto, Y.; Tani, M.; Uto-Kondo, H.; Iizuka, M.; Saita, E.; Sone, H.; Kurata, H.; Kondo, K. Astaxanthin suppresses scavenger receptor expression and matrix metalloproteinase activity in macrophages. *Eur. J. Nutr.* **2010**, *49*, 119–126. [CrossRef]
207. Farruggia, C.; Kim, M.; Bae, M.; Lee, Y.; Pham, T.X.; Yang, Y.; Joo, M.; Park, Y.; Lee, J. Astaxanthin exerts anti-inflammatory and antioxidant effects in macrophages in NRF2-dependent and independent manners. *J. Nutr. Biochem.* **2018**, *62*, 202–209. [CrossRef]
208. Cai, X.; Chen, Y.; Xie, X.; Yao, D.; Ding, C.; Chen, M. Astaxanthin prevents against lipopolysaccharide-induced acute lung injury and sepsis via inhibiting activation of MAPK/NF-κB. *Am. J. Transl. Res.* **2019**, *11*, 1884–1894.
209. Kang, H.; Lee, Y.; Bae, M.; Park, Y.-K.; Lee, J.-Y. Astaxanthin inhibits alcohol-induced inflammation and oxidative stress in macrophages in a Sirtuin 1-dependent manner. *J. Nutr. Biochem.* **2020**, *85*, 108477. [CrossRef]
210. Binatti, E.; Zoccatelli, G.; Zanoni, F.; Donà, G.; Mainente, F.; Chignola, R. Phagocytosis of astaxanthin-loaded microparticles modulates TGFβ production and intracellular ROS levels in J774A.1 macrophages. *Mar. Drugs* **2021**, *19*, 163. [CrossRef] [PubMed]
211. Hyang, Y.; Koh, H.; Kim, D. Down-regulation of IL-6 production by astaxanthin via ERK-, MSK-, and NF-κB-mediated signals in activated microglia. *Int. Immunopharmacol.* **2010**, *10*, 1560–1572. [CrossRef]
212. Wen, X.; Xiao, L.; Zhong, Z.; Wang, L.; Li, Z.; Pan, X. Astaxanthin acts via LRP-1 to inhibit inflammation and reverse lipopolysaccharide-induced M1/M2 polarization of microglial cells. *Oncotarget* **2017**, *8*, 69370–69385. [CrossRef] [PubMed]
213. Kim, R.E.; Shin, C.Y.; Han, S.H.; Kwon, K.J. Astaxanthin suppresses PM2.5-induced neuroinflammation by regulating Akt phosphorylation in BV-2 microglial cells. *Int. J. Mol. Sci.* **2020**, *21*, 7227. [CrossRef] [PubMed]
214. Han, J.H.; Lee, Y.S.; Im, J.H.; Ham, Y.W.; Lee, H.P.; Han, S.B. Astaxanthin ameliorates lipopolysaccharide-induced neuroinflammation, oxidative stress and memory dysfunction through inactivation of the signal transducer and activator of transcription 3 pathway. *Mar. Drugs* **2019**, *17*, 123. [CrossRef] [PubMed]
215. Peng, Y.J.; Lu, J.W.; Liu, F.C.; Lee, C.H.; Lee, H.S.; Ho, Y.J.; Hsieh, T.H.; Wu, C.C.; Wang, C.C. Astaxanthin attenuates joint inflammation induced by monosodium urate crystals. *FASEB J.* **2020**, *34*, 11215–11226. [CrossRef] [PubMed]

216. Terazawa, S.; Nakajima, H.; Shingo, M.; Niwano, T.; Imokawa, G. Astaxanthin attenuates the UVB-induced secretion of prostaglandin E 2 and interleukin-8 in human keratinocytes by interrupting MSK1 phosphorylation in a ROS depletion—Independent manner. *Exp. Dermatol.* 2012, 21, 11–17. [CrossRef] [PubMed]
217. Li, H.; Li, J.; Hou, C.; Li, J.; Peng, H.; Wang, Q. The effect of astaxanthin on inflammation in hyperosmolarity of experimental dry eye model *in vitro* and *in vivo*. *Exp. Eye Res.* 2020, 197, 108113. [CrossRef]
218. Wan, F.C.; Zhang, C.; Jin, Q.; Wei, C.; Zhao, H.B.; Zhang, X.L.; You, W.; Liu, X.M.; Liu, G.F.; Liu, Y.F.; et al. Protective effects of astaxanthin on lipopolysaccharide-induced inflammation in bovine endometrial epithelial cells. *Biol. Reprod.* 2020, 102, 339–347. [CrossRef]
219. Kim, S.H.; Lim, J.W.; Kim, H. Astaxanthin inhibits mitochondrial dysfunction and and interleukin-8 expression in *Helicobacter pylori*-infected gastric epithelial cells. *Nutrients* 2018, 10, 1320. [CrossRef] [PubMed]
220. Hwang, Y.; Kim, K.; Kim, S.; Mun, S.; Hong, S. Suppression Effect of Astaxanthin on Osteoclast Formation *In Vitro* and Bone Loss *In Vivo*. *Int. J. Mol. Sci.* 2018, 19, 912. [CrossRef] [PubMed]
221. Bhuvaneswari, S.; Baskaran, Y. Astaxanthin reduces hepatic endoplasmic reticulum stress and nuclear factor-κB-mediated inflammation in high fructose and high fat diet-fed mice. *Cell Stress Chaperones* 2014, 19, 183–191. [CrossRef] [PubMed]
222. Ni, Y.; Nagashimada, M.; Zhuge, F.; Zhan, L.; Nagata, N.; Tsutsui, A.; Nakanuma, Y.; Kaneko, S.; Ota, T. Astaxanthin prevents and reverses diet-induced insulin resistance and steatohepatitis in mice: A comparison with vitamin E. *Sci. Rep.* 2015, 5, 17192. [CrossRef]
223. Jia, Y.; Wu, C.; Kim, J.; Kim, B.; Lee, S. Astaxanthin reduces hepatic lipid accumulations in high-fat-fed C57BL/6J mice via activation of peroxisome proliferator-activated receptor (PPAR) alpha and inhibition of PPAR gamma and Akt. *J. Nutr. Biochem.* 2016, 28, 9–18. [CrossRef]
224. Han, J.H.; Ju, J.H.; Lee, Y.S.; Park, J.H.; Yeo, I.J.; Park, M.H.; Roh, Y.S. Astaxanthin alleviated ethanol-induced liver injury by inhibition of oxidative stress and inflammatory responses via blocking of STAT3 activity. *Sci. Rep.* 2018, 8, 14090. [CrossRef]
225. Liu, H.; Liu, M.; Fu, X.; Zhang, Z.; Zhu, L.; Zheng, X.; Liu, J. Astaxanthin prevents alcoholic fatty liver disease by modulating mouse gut microbiota. *Nutrients* 2018, 10, 1298. [CrossRef]
226. Zhang, J.; Zhang, S.; Bi, J.; Gu, J.; Deng, Y.; Liu, C. Astaxanthin pretreatment attenuates acetaminophen-induced liver injury in mice. *Int. Immunopharmacol.* 2017, 45, 26–33. [CrossRef]
227. Shen, M.; Chen, K.; Lu, J.; Cheng, P.; Xu, L.; Dai, W.; Wang, F.; He, L.; Zhang, Y.; Chengfen, W.; et al. Protective effect of astaxanthin on liver fibrosis through modulation of TGF- β 1 expression and autophagy. *Mediat. Inflamm.* 2014, 2014, 954502. [CrossRef]
228. Zhang, Z.; Guo, C.; Jiang, H.; Han, B.; Wang, X.; Li, S.; Lv, Y.; Lv, Z.; Zhu, Y. Inflammation response after the cessation of chronic arsenic exposure and post-treatment of natural astaxanthin in liver: Potential role of cytokine-mediated cell-cell interactions. *Food Funct.* 2020, 11, 9252–9262. [CrossRef]
229. Iskender, H.; Yenice, G.; Terim Kapakin, K.A.; Dokumacioglu, E.; Sevim, C.; Hayirli, A.; Altun, S. Effects of high fructose diet on lipid metabolism and the hepatic NF-κB/SIRT-1 pathway. *Biotech. Histochem.* 2021, 1–9. [CrossRef]
230. Chiu, C.; Chang, C.; Lin, S.; Chyau, C.; Peng, R. improved hepatoprotective effect of liposome-encapsulated astaxanthin in lipopolysaccharide-induced acute hepatotoxicity. *Int. J. Mol. Sci.* 2016, 17, 1128. [CrossRef] [PubMed]
231. Guo, S.; Guo, L.; Fang, Q.; Yu, M.; Zhang, L.; You, C.; Wang, X.; Liu, Y.; Han, C. Astaxanthin protects against early acute kidney injury in severely burned rats by inactivating the TLR4/MyD88/NF-κB axis and upregulating heme oxygenase-1. *Sci. Rep.* 2021, 11, 6679. [CrossRef] [PubMed]
232. Xie, W.J.; Hou, G.; Wang, L.; Wang, S.S.; Xiong, X.X. Astaxanthin suppresses lipopolysaccharide-induced myocardial injury by regulating MAPK and PI3K/AKT/mTOR/GSK3β signaling. *Mol. Med. Rep.* 2020, 22, 3338–3346. [CrossRef]
233. Zhuge, F.; Ni, Y.; Wan, C.; Liu, F.; Fu, Z. Anti-diabetic effects of astaxanthin on an STZ-induced diabetic model in rats. *Endocr. J.* 2021, 68, 451–459. [CrossRef]
234. Feng, W.; Wang, Y.; Guo, N.; Huang, P.; Mi, Y. Effects of astaxanthin on inflammation and insulin resistance in a mouse model of gestational diabetes mellitus. *Dose Response* 2020, 18, 1559325820926765. [CrossRef]
235. Liu, Y.; Yang, L.; Guo, Y.; Zhang, T.; Qiao, X.; Wang, J.; Xu, J.; Xue, C. Hydrophilic astaxanthin: PEGylated astaxanthin fights diabetes by enhancing the solubility and oral absorbability. *J. Agric. Food Chem.* 2020, 68, 3649–3655. [CrossRef] [PubMed]
236. Janani, R.; Anitha, R.E.; Perumal, M.K.; Divya, P.; Baskaran, V. Astaxanthin mediated regulation of VEGF through HIF1α and XBP1 signaling pathway: An insight from ARPE-19 cell and streptozotocin mediated diabetic rat model. *Exp. Eye Res.* 2021, 206, 108555. [CrossRef]
237. Xu, L.; Zhu, J.; Yin, W.; Ding, X. Astaxanthin improves cognitive deficits from oxidative stress, nitric oxide synthase and inflammation through upregulation of PI3K/Akt in diabetes rat. *Int. J. Clin. Exp. Pathol.* 2015, 8, 6083–6094.
238. Feng, Y.; Chu, A.; Luo, Q.; Wu, M.; Shi, X.; Chen, Y. The protective effect of astaxanthin on cognitive function via inhibition of oxidative stress and inflammation in the brains of chronic T2DM rats. *Front. Pharmacol.* 2018, 9, 748. [CrossRef]
239. Jiang, X.; Chen, L.; Shen, L.; Chen, Z.; Xu, L.; Zhang, J.; Yu, X. Trans-astaxanthin attenuates lipopolysaccharide-induced neuroin fl ammation and depressive-like behavior in mice. *Brain Res.* 2016, 1649, 30–37. [CrossRef]
240. Zhao, T.; Ma, D.; Mulati, A.; Zhao, B.; Liu, F.; Liu, X. Development of astaxanthin-loaded layer-by-layer emulsions: Physicochemical properties and improvement of LPS-induced neuroinflammation in mice. *Food Funct.* 2021, 12, 5333–5350. [CrossRef]
241. Wang, M.; Deng, X.; Xie, Y.; Chen, Y. Astaxanthin attenuates neuroinflammation in status epilepticus rats by regulating the ATP-P2X7R signal. *Drug Des. Devel. Ther.* 2020, 14, 1651–1662. [CrossRef] [PubMed]

242. Zhang, X.; Zhang, X.; Zhang, Q.; Wu, Q.; Li, W.; Jiang, T.; Hang, C. Astaxanthin reduces matrix metalloproteinase-9 expression and activity in the brain after experimental subarachnoid hemorrhage in rats. *Brain Res.* **2015**, *1624*, 113–124. [CrossRef]
243. Zhang, X.; Lu, Y.; Wu, Q.; Dai, H.; Li, W.; Lv, S.; Zhou, X.; Zhang, X.; Hang, C.; Wang, J. Astaxanthin mitigates subarachnoid hemorrhage injury primarily by increasing sirtuin 1 and inhibiting the Toll-like receptor 4 signaling pathway. *FASEB J.* **2019**, *33*, 722–737. [CrossRef]
244. Jiang, X.; Yan, Q.; Liu, F.; Jing, C.; Ding, L.; Zhang, L. Chronic trans-astaxanthin treatment exerts antihyperalgesic effect and corrects co-morbid depressive like behaviors in mice with chronic pain. *Neurosci. Lett.* **2018**, *662*, 36–43. [CrossRef] [PubMed]
245. Fakhri, S.; Dargahi, L.; Abbaszadeh, F.; Jorjani, M. Astaxanthin attenuates neuroinflammation contributed to the neuropathic pain and motor dysfunction following compression spinal cord injury. *Brain Res. Bull.* **2018**, *143*, 217–224. [CrossRef]
246. Fu, J.; Sun, H.; Wei, H.; Dong, M.; Zhang, Y.; Xu, W.; Fang, Y.; Zhao, J. Astaxanthin alleviates spinal cord ischemia- reperfusion injury via activation of PI3K/Akt/GSK-3β pathway in rats. *J. Orthop. Surg. Res.* **2020**, *15*, 275. [CrossRef]
247. Chen, M.H.; Wang, T.J.; Chen, L.J.; Jiang, M.Y.; Wang, Y.J.; Tseng, G.F.; Chen, J.R. The effects of astaxanthin treatment on a rat model of Alzheimer's disease. *Brain Res. Bull.* **2021**, *172*, 151–163. [CrossRef] [PubMed]
248. Yang, B.-B.; Zou, M.; Zhao, L.; Zhang, Y.-K. Astaxanthin attenuates acute cerebral infarction via Nrf-2/HO-1 pathway in rats. *Curr. Res. Transl. Med.* **2021**, *69*, 103271. [CrossRef]
249. Sun, K.; Luo, J.; Jing, X.; Guo, J.; Yao, X.; Hao, X.; Ye, Y.; Lin, J.; Wang, G.; Guo, F. Astaxanthin protects against osteoarthritis via Nrf2: A guardian of cartilage homeostasis. *Aging* **2019**, *11*, 10513–10531. [CrossRef] [PubMed]
250. Kumar, A.; Dhaliwal, N.; Dhaliwal, J.; Dharavath, R.N.; Chopra, K. Astaxanthin attenuates oxidative stress and inflammatory responses in complete Freund-adjuvant-induced arthritis in rats. *Pharmacol. Rep.* **2020**, *72*, 104–114. [CrossRef]
251. Park, M.H.; Jung, J.C.; Hill, S.; Cartwright, E.; Dohnalek, M.H.; Yu, M.; Jun, H.J.; Han, S.B.; Hong, J.T.; Son, D.J. FlexPro MD®, a combination of krill oil, astaxanthin and hyaluronic acid, reduces pain behavior and inhibits inflammatory response in monosodium iodoacetate-induced osteoarthritis in rats. *Nutrients* **2020**, *12*, 956. [CrossRef]
252. Han, H.; Lim, J.W.; Kim, H. Astaxanthin inhibits *Helicobacter pylori*-induced inflammatory and oncogenic responses in gastric mucosal tissues of mice. *J. Cancer Prev.* **2020**, *25*, 244–251. [CrossRef] [PubMed]
253. Chen, Y.; Zhao, S.; Jiao, D.; Yao, B.; Yang, S.; Li, P.; Long, M. Astaxanthin alleviates ochratoxin a-induced cecum injury and inflammation in mice by regulating the diversity of cecal microbiota and TLR4/MyD88/NF-κB signaling pathway. *Oxid. Med. Cell. Longev.* **2021**, *2021*, 8894491. [CrossRef] [PubMed]
254. Yasui, Y.; Hosokawa, M.; Mikami, N.; Miyashita, K.; Tanaka, T. Dietary astaxanthin inhibits colitis and colitis-associated colon carcinogenesis in mice via modulation of the inflammatory cytokines. *Chem. Biol. Interact.* **2011**, *193*, 79–87. [CrossRef] [PubMed]
255. Kochi, T.; Shimizu, M.; Sumi, T.; Kubota, M.; Shirakami, Y.; Tanaka, T. Inhibitory effects of astaxanthin on azoxymethane- induced colonic preneoplastic lesions in C57/BL/KsJ- db/db mice. *BMC Gastroenterol.* **2014**, *14*, 212. [CrossRef] [PubMed]
256. Zhang, H.; Yang, W.; Li, Y.; Hu, L.; Dai, Y.; Chen, J.; Xu, S. Astaxanthin ameliorates cerulein-induced acute pancreatitis in mice. *Int. Immunopharmacol.* **2018**, *56*, 18–28. [CrossRef] [PubMed]
257. Hwang, Y.; Hong, S.; Mun, S.; Kim, S.-J.; Lee, S.; Kim, J.; Kang, K.; Yee, S. The protective effects of astaxanthin on the OVA-induced asthma mice model. *Molecules* **2017**, *22*, 2019. [CrossRef]
258. Bi, J.; Cui, R.; Li, Z.; Liu, C.; Zhang, J. Astaxanthin alleviated acute lung injury by inhibiting oxidative/nitrative stress and the inflammatory response in mice. *Biomed. Pharmacother.* **2017**, *95*, 974–982. [CrossRef]
259. Xu, W.; Wang, M.; Cui, G.; Li, L.; Jiao, D.; Yao, B.; Xu, K.; Chen, Y.; Long, M.; Yang, S.; et al. Astaxanthin protects OTA-induced lung injury in mice through the Nrf2/NF-κB pathway. *Toxins* **2019**, *11*, 540. [CrossRef]
260. Park, J.H.; Yeo, I.J.; Han, J.H.; Suh, J.W.; Lee, H.P.; Hong, J.T. Anti-inflammatory effect of astaxanthin in phthalic anhydride-induced atopic dermatitis animal model. *Exp. Dermatol.* **2018**, *27*, 378–385. [CrossRef]
261. Park, J.H.; Yeo, I.J.; Jang, J.S.; Kim, K.C.; Park, M.H.; Lee, H.P.; Han, S.; Hong, J.T. Combination effect of titrated extract of *Centella asiatica* and astaxanthin in a mouse model of phthalic anhydride-induced atopic dermatitis. *Allergy Asthma Immunol. Res.* **2019**, *11*, 548–559. [CrossRef]
262. Lee, Y.S.; Jeon, S.H.; Ham, H.J.; Lee, H.P.; Song, M.J.; Hong, J.T. Improved anti-inflammatory effects of liposomal astaxanthin on a phthalic anhydride-induced atopic dermatitis model. *Front. Immunol.* **2020**, *11*, 565285. [CrossRef]
263. Yoshihisa, Y.; Andoh, T.; Matsunaga, K.; Ur Rehman, M.; Maoka, T.; Shimizu, T. Efficacy of astaxanthin for the treatment of atopic dermatitis in a murine model. *PLoS ONE* **2016**, *11*, e0152288. [CrossRef]
264. Harada, F.; Morikawa, T.; Lennikov, A.; Mukwaya, A.; Schaupper, M.; Uehara, O.; Takai, R.; Yoshida, K.; Sato, J.; Horie, Y.; et al. Protective effects of oral astaxanthin nanopowder against ultraviolet-induced photokeratitis in mice. *Oxid. Med. Cell. Longev.* **2017**, *2017*, 1956104. [CrossRef] [PubMed]
265. Fang, Q.; Guo, S.; Zhou, H.; Han, R.; Wu, P.; Han, C. Astaxanthin protects against early burn-wound progression in rats by attenuating oxidative stress-induced inflammation and mitochondria-related apoptosis. *Sci. Rep.* **2017**, *7*, 41440. [CrossRef] [PubMed]
266. Tominaga, K.; Hongo, N.; Fujishita, M.; Takahashi, Y.; Adachi, Y. Protective effects of astaxanthin on skin deterioration. *J. Clin. Biochem. Nutr.* **2017**, *61*, 33–39. [CrossRef]
267. Ito, N.; Seki, S.; Ueda, F. The protective role of astaxanthin for UV-induced skin deterioration in healthy people—A randomized, double-blind, placebo-controlled trial. *Nutrients* **2018**, *10*, 817. [CrossRef]

268. Ito, N.; Saito, H.; Seki, S.; Ueda, F.; Asada, T. Effects of composite supplement containing astaxanthin and sesamin on cognitive functions in people with mild cognitive impairment: A randomized, double-blind, placebo-controlled trial. *J. Alzheimer's Dis.* **2018**, *62*, 1767–1775. [CrossRef] [PubMed]
269. Imai, A.; Oda, Y.; Ito, N.; Seki, S.; Nakagawa, K.; Miyazawa, T.; Ueda, F. Effects of dietary supplementation of astaxanthin and sesamin on daily fatigue: A randomized, double-blind, placebo-controlled, two-way crossover study. *Nutrients* **2018**, *10*, 281. [CrossRef] [PubMed]
270. Mashhadi, N.S.; Zakerkish, M.; Mohammadiasl, J.; Zarei, M.; Mohammadshahi, M.; Haghighizadeh, M.H. Astaxanthin improves glucose metabolism and reduces blood pressure in patients with type 2 diabetes mellitus. *Asia Pac. J. Clin. Nutr.* **2018**, *27*, 341–346. [CrossRef] [PubMed]
271. Shokri-mashhadi, N.; Tahmasebi, M.; Mohammadiasl, J.; Zakerkish, M.; Mohammadshahi, M. The antioxidant and anti-inflammatory effects of astaxanthin supplementation on the expression of miR-146a and miR-126 in patients with type 2 diabetes mellitus: A randomised, double-blind, placebo-controlled clinical trial. *Int. J. Clin. Pract.* **2021**, *75*, e14022. [CrossRef]
272. Heo, S.; Yoon, W.; Kim, K.; Oh, C.; Choi, Y.; Yoon, K.; Kang, D.; Qian, Z.; Choi, I.; Jung, W. Anti-inflammatory effect of fucoxanthin derivatives isolated from *Sargassum siliquastrum* in lipopolysaccharide-stimulated RAW 264.7 macrophage. *Food Chem. Toxicol.* **2012**, *50*, 3336–3342. [CrossRef]
273. Kim, K.; Heo, S.; Yoon, W.; Kang, S.; Ahn, G.; Yi, T.; Jeon, Y. Fucoxanthin inhibits the inflammatory response by suppressing the activation of NF-κB and MAPKs in lipopolysaccharide-induced RAW 264.7 macrophages. *Eur. J. Pharmacol.* **2010**, *649*, 369–375. [CrossRef] [PubMed]
274. Li, S.; Ren, X.; Wang, Y.; Hu, J.; Wu, H. Fucoxanthin alleviates palmitate-induced inflammation in RAW 264.7 cells through improving lipid metabolism and attenuating mitochondrial dysfunction. *Food Funct.* **2020**, *11*, 3361–3370. [CrossRef] [PubMed]
275. Rodríguez-Luna, A.; Ávila-Román, J.; Oliveira, H.; Motilva, V.; Talero, E. Fucoxanthin-containing cream prevents epidermal hyperplasia and UVB-induced skin erythema in mice. *Mar. Drugs* **2018**, *16*, 378. [CrossRef]
276. Pangestuti, R.; Vo, T.; Ngo, D.; Kim, S. Fucoxanthin ameliorates inflammation and oxidative reponses in microglia. *J. Agric. Food Chem.* **2013**, *61*, 3876–3883. [CrossRef]
277. Zhao, D.; Hwan, S.; Yoon, K.; Chun, S.; Yao, M. Anti-neuroinflammatory effects of fucoxanthin via inhibition of Akt/NF-κB and MAPKs/AP-1 pathways and activation of PKA/CREB pathway in lipopolysaccharide-activated BV-2 microglial cells. *Neurochem. Res.* **2017**, *42*, 667–677. [CrossRef]
278. Young, S.; Sun, W.; Lee, D.; Choi, G.; Yim, M.; Min, J.; Jung, W.; Gwang, S.; Seo, S.; Jae, S.; et al. Fucoxanthin inhibits pro fibrotic protein expression *in vitro* and attenuates bleomycin-induced lung fibrosis in vivo. *Eur. J. Pharmacol.* **2017**, *811*, 199–207. [CrossRef]
279. Rodríguez-Luna, A.; Ávila-Román, J.; Oliveira, H.; Motilva, V.; Talero, E. Fucoxanthin and rosmarinic acid combination has anti-inflammatory effects through regulation of NLRP3 inflammasome in UVB-exposed HaCaT keratinocytes. *Mar. Drugs* **2019**, *17*, 451. [CrossRef]
280. Tavares, R.S.N.; Kawakami, C.M.; de Castro Pereira, K.; do Amaral, G.T.; Benevenuto, C.G.; Maria-Engler, S.S.; Colepicolo, P.; Debonsi, H.M.; Gaspar, L.R. Fucoxanthin for topical administration, a phototoxic vs. photoprotective potential in a tiered strategy assessed by in vitro methods. *Antioxidants* **2020**, *9*, 328. [CrossRef] [PubMed]
281. Tavares, R.S.N.; Maria-Engler, S.S.; Colepicolo, P.; Debonsi, H.M.; Schäfer-Korting, M.; Marx, U.; Gaspar, L.R.; Zoschke, C. Skin irritation testing beyond tissue viability: Fucoxanthin effects on inflammation, homeostasis, and metabolism. *Pharmaceutics* **2020**, *12*, 136. [CrossRef]
282. Chiang, Y.F.; Chen, H.Y.; Chang, Y.J.; Shih, Y.H.; Shieh, T.M.; Wang, K.L.; Hsia, S.M. Protective effects of fucoxanthin on high glucose and 4-hydroxynonenal (4-HNE)-induced injury in human retinal pigment epithelial cells. *Antioxidants* **2020**, *9*, 1176. [CrossRef]
283. Hwang, P.A.; Phan, N.N.; Lu, W.J.; Ngoc Hieu, B.T.; Lin, Y.C. Low-molecular-weight fucoidan and high-stability fucoxanthin from brown seaweed exert prebiotics and anti-inflammatory activities in Caco-2 cells. *Food Nutr. Res.* **2016**, *60*, 32033. [CrossRef]
284. Maeda, H.; Kanno, S.; Kodate, M.; Hosokawa, M.; Miyashita, K. Fucoxanthinol, metabolite of fucoxanthin, improves obesity-induced inflammation in adipocyte cells. *Mar. Drugs* **2015**, *13*, 4799–4813. [CrossRef] [PubMed]
285. Seo, M.; Seo, Y.; Pan, C.; Lee, O.; Kim, K.; Lee, B. Fucoxanthin suppresses lipid accumulation and ROS production during differentiation in 3T3-L1 adipocytes. *Phytother. Res.* **2016**, *30*, 1802–1808. [CrossRef] [PubMed]
286. Hosokawa, M.; Miyashita, T.; Nishikawa, S.; Emi, S.; Tsukui, T.; Beppu, F.; Okada, T.; Miyashita, K. Fucoxanthin regulates adipocytokine mRNA expression in white adipose tissue of diabetic/obese KK-Ay mice. *Arch. Biochem. Biophys.* **2010**, *504*, 17–25. [CrossRef]
287. Chang, Y.; Chen, Y.; Huang, W.; Liou, C. Fucoxanthin attenuates fatty acid-induced lipid accumulation in FL83B hepatocytes through regulated Sirt1/AMPK signaling pathway. *Biochem. Biophys. Res. Commun* **2018**, *495*, 197–203. [CrossRef]
288. Natsume, C.; Aoki, N.; Aoyama, T.; Senda, K.; Matsui, M.; Ikegami, A.; Tanaka, K.; Azuma, Y.T.; Fujita, T. Fucoxanthin ameliorates atopic dermatitis symptoms by regulating keratinocytes and regulatory innate lymphoid cells. *Int. J. Mol. Sci.* **2020**, *21*, 2180. [CrossRef] [PubMed]
289. Choi, J.; Kim, N.; Kim, S.; Lee, N.; Kim, S. Fucoxanthin inhibits the inflammation response in paw edema model through suppressing MAPKs, Akt, and NF-κB. *J. Biochem. Mol. Toxicol.* **2016**, *30*, 111–119. [CrossRef]

290. Yang, Y.; Tong, Q.; Zheng, S.; Zhou, M.; Zeng, Y.-M.; Zhou, T.-T. Anti-inflammatory effect of fucoxanthin on dextran sulfate sodium-induced colitis in mice. *Nat. Prod. Res.* **2020**, *34*, 1791–1795. [CrossRef] [PubMed]
291. Gong, D.; Chu, W.; Jiang, L.; Geng, C.; Li, J.; Ishikawa, N. Effect of fucoxanthin alone and in combination with d-glucosamine hydrochloride on carrageenan/kaolin-induced experimental arthritis in rats. *Phytother. Res.* **2014**, *28*, 1054–1063. [CrossRef]
292. Jiang, X.; Wang, G.; Lin, Q.; Tang, Z.; Yan, Q.; Yu, X. Fucoxanthin prevents lipopolysaccharide-induced depressive-like behavior in mice via AMPK-NF-κB pathway. *Metab. Brain Dis.* **2019**, *34*, 431–442. [CrossRef]
293. Li, X.; Huang, R.; Liu, K.; Li, M.; Luo, H.; Cui, L.; Huang, L.; Luo, L. Fucoxanthin attenuates LPS-induced acute lung injury via inhibition of the TLR4/MyD88 signaling axis. *Aging (Albany NY)*. **2020**, *13*, 2655–2667. [CrossRef]
294. Yang, X.; Guo, G.; Dang, M.; Yan, L.; Kang, X.; Jia, K.; Ren, H. Assessment of the therapeutic effects of fucoxanthin by attenuating inflammation in ovalbumin-induced asthma in an experimental animal model. *J. Environ. Pathol. Toxicol. Oncol.* **2019**, *38*, 229–238. [CrossRef]
295. Wu, S.-J.; Liou, C.-J.; Chen, Y.-L.; Cheng, S.-C.; Huang, W.-C. Fucoxanthin ameliorates oxidative stress and airway inflammation in tracheal epithelial cells and asthmatic mice. *Cells* **2021**, *10*, 1311. [CrossRef] [PubMed]
296. Tan, C.; Hou, Y. First evidence for the anti-inflammatory activity of fucoxanthin in high-fat-diet-induced obesity in mice and the antioxidant functions in PC12 cells. *Inflammation* **2014**, *37*, 443–450. [CrossRef] [PubMed]
297. Sun, X.; Zhao, H.; Liu, Z.; Sun, X.; Zhang, D.; Wang, S.; Xu, Y.; Zhang, G.; Wang, D. Modulation of gut microbiota by fucoxanthin during alleviation of obesity in high-fat diet-fed mice. *J. Agric. Food Chem.* **2020**, *68*, 5118–5128. [CrossRef] [PubMed]
298. Grasa-López, A.; Miliar-García, Á.; Quevedo-Corona, L.; Paniagua-Castro, N.; Escalona-Cardoso, G.; Reyes-Maldonado, E. *Undaria pinnatifida* and fucoxanthin ameliorate lipogenesis and markers of both inflammation and cardiovascular dysfunction in an animal model of diet-induced obesity. *Mar. Drugs* **2016**, *14*, 148. [CrossRef] [PubMed]
299. Ha, A.W.; Na, S.J.; Kim, W.K. Antioxidant effects of fucoxanthin rich powder in rats fed with high fat diet. *Nutr. Res. Pr.* **2013**, *7*, 475. [CrossRef] [PubMed]
300. Kong, Z.; Sudirman, S.; Hsu, Y.; Su, C.; Kuo, H. Fucoxanthin-rich brown algae extract improves male reproductive function on streptozotocin-nicotinamide-induced diabetic rat model. *Int. J. Mol. Sci.* **2019**, *20*, 4485. [CrossRef] [PubMed]
301. Takatani, N.; Kono, Y.; Beppu, F.; Okamatsu-ogura, Y. Fucoxanthin inhibits hepatic oxidative stress, inflammation, and fibrosis in diet-induced nonalcoholic steatohepatitis model mice. *Biochem. Biophys. Res. Commun.* **2020**, *528*, 305–310. [CrossRef]
302. Zheng, J.; Tian, X.; Zhang, W.; Zheng, P.; Huang, F. Protective effects of fucoxanthin against alcoholic liver injury by activation of Nrf2-mediated antioxidant defense and inhibition of TLR4-mediated inflammation. *Mar. Drugs* **2019**, *17*, 552. [CrossRef]
303. Shih, P.H.; Shiue, S.J.; Chen, C.N.; Cheng, S.W.; Lin, H.Y.; Wu, L.W.; Wu, M.S. Fucoidan and fucoxanthin attenuate hepatic steatosis and inflammation of NAFLD through modulation of leptin/adiponectin axis. *Mar. Drugs* **2021**, *19*, 148. [CrossRef]
304. Orhan, C.; Tuzcu, M.; Gencoglu, H.; Sahin, E.; Sahin, N.; Ozercan, I.H.; Namjoshi, T.; Srivastava, V.; Morde, A.; Rai, D.; et al. Different doses of β-cryptoxanthin may secure the retina from photooxidative injury resulted from common LED sources. *Oxid. Med. Cell. Longev.* **2021**, *2021*, 6672525. [CrossRef]
305. Sahin, K.; Orhan, C.; Akdemir, F.; Tuzcu, M.; Sahin, N.; Yılmaz, I.; Juturu, V. β-Cryptoxanthin ameliorates metabolic risk factors by regulating NF-κB and Nrf2 pathways in insulin resistance induced by high-fat diet in rodents. *Food Chem. Toxicol.* **2017**, *107*, 270–279. [CrossRef]
306. Ni, Y.; Nagashimada, M.; Zhan, L.; Nagata, N.; Kobori, M.; Sugiura, M.; Ogawa, K.; Kaneko, S.; Ota, T. Prevention and reversal of lipotoxicity-induced hepatic insulin resistance and steatohepatitis in mice by an antioxidant carotenoid, β-cryptoxanthin. *Endocrinology* **2015**, *156*, 987–999. [CrossRef] [PubMed]
307. Zhang, F.; Shi, D.; Wang, X.; Zhang, Y.; Duan, W.; Li, Y. β-cryptoxanthin alleviates myocardial ischaemia/reperfusion injury by inhibiting NF-κB-mediated inflammatory signalling in rats. *Arch. Physiol. Biochem.* **2020**, 1–8. [CrossRef]
308. Park, G.; Horie, T.; Fukasawa, K.; Ozaki, K.; Onishi, Y.; Kanayama, T.; Iezaki, T.; Kaneda, K.; Sugiura, M.; Hinoi, E. Amelioration of the development of osteoarthritis by daily intake of β-cryptoxanthin. *Biol. Pharm. Bull.* **2017**, *40*, 1116–1120. [CrossRef]
309. Liu, C.; Bronson, R.T.; Russell, R.M.; Wang, X.D. β-Cryptoxanthin supplementation prevents cigarette smoke-induced lung inflammation, oxidative damage, and squamous metaplasia in ferrets. *Cancer Prev. Res.* **2011**, *4*, 1255–1266. [CrossRef]
310. Haidari, F.; Hojhabrimanesh, A.; Helli, B.; Seyedian, S.S.; Ahmadi-Angali, K. An energy-restricted high-protein diet supplemented with β-cryptoxanthin alleviated oxidative stress and inflammation in nonalcoholic fatty liver disease: A randomized controlled trial. *Nutr. Res.* **2020**, *73*, 15–26. [CrossRef]
311. Lee, N.Y.; Kim, Y.; Kim, Y.S.; Shin, J.H.; Rubin, L.P.; Kim, Y. β-Carotene exerts anti-colon cancer effects by regulating M2 macrophages and activated fibroblasts. *J. Nutr. Biochem.* **2020**, *82*, 108402. [CrossRef]
312. Lu, M.S.; Fang, Y.J.; Chen, Y.M.; Luo, W.P.; Pan, Z.Z.; Zhong, X.; Zhang, C.X. Higher intake of carotenoid is associated with a lower risk of colorectal cancer in Chinese adults: A case–control study. *Eur. J. Nutr.* **2015**, *54*, 619–628. [CrossRef] [PubMed]
313. Cui, B.; Liu, S.; Wang, Q.; Lin, X. Effect of β-carotene on immunity function and tumour growth in hepatocellular carcinoma rats. *Molecules* **2012**, *17*, 8595–8603. [CrossRef] [PubMed]
314. Zhang, D.M.; Luo, Y.; Yishake, D.; Liu, Z.Y.; He, T.T.; Luo, Y.; Zhang, Y.J.; Fang, A.P.; Zhu, H.L. Prediagnostic dietary intakes of vitamin A and β-carotene are associated with hepatocellular-carcinoma survival. *Food Funct.* **2020**, *11*, 759–767. [CrossRef] [PubMed]
315. Lu, L.; Chen, J.; Li, M.; Tang, L.; Wu, R.; Jin, L.; Liang, Z. β-carotene reverses tobacco smoke-induced gastric EMT via Notch pathway *in vivo*. *Oncol. Rep.* **2018**, *39*, 1867–1873. [CrossRef] [PubMed]

316. Kim, J.H.; Lee, J.; Choi, I.J.; Kim, Y.-I.; Kwon, O.; Kim, H.; Kim, J. Dietary carotenoids intake and the risk of gastric cancer: A case—control study in Korea. *Nutrients* **2018**, *10*, 1031. [CrossRef]
317. Zhang, Y.; Zhu, X.; Huang, T.; Chen, L.; Liu, Y.; Li, Q.; Song, J.; Ma, S.; Zhang, K.; Yang, B.; et al. β-Carotene synergistically enhances the anti-tumor effect of 5-fluorouracil on esophageal squamous cell carcinoma *in vivo* and *in vitro*. *Toxicol. Lett.* **2016**, *261*, 49–58. [CrossRef]
318. Ge, X.X.; Xing, M.Y.; Yu, L.F.; Shen, P. Carotenoid intake and esophageal cancer risk: A meta-analysis. *Asian Pac. J. Cancer Prev.* **2013**, *14*, 1911–1918. [CrossRef]
319. Yang, C.M.; Yen, Y.T.; Huang, C.S.; Hu, M.L. Growth inhibitory efficacy of lycopene and β-carotene against androgen-independent prostate tumor cells xenografted in nude mice. *Mol. Nutr. Food Res.* **2011**, *55*, 606–612. [CrossRef]
320. Lim, J.Y.; Kim, Y.S.; Kim, K.M.; Min, S.J.; Kim, Y. β-Carotene inhibits neuroblastoma tumorigenesis by regulating cell differentiation and cancer cell stemness. *Biochem. Biophys. Res. Commun.* **2014**, *450*, 1475–1480. [CrossRef] [PubMed]
321. Jain, A.; Sharma, G.; Kushwah, V.; Garg, N.K.; Kesharwani, P.; Ghoshal, G.; Singh, B.; Shivhare, U.S.; Jain, S.; Katare, O.P. Methotrexate and beta-carotene loaded-lipid polymer hybrid nanoparticles: A preclinical study for breast cancer. *Nanomedicine* **2017**, *12*, 1851–1872. [CrossRef] [PubMed]
322. Jain, A.; Sharma, G.; Kushwah, V.; Ghoshal, G.; Jain, A.; Singh, B.; Shivhare, U.S.; Jain, S.; Katare, O.P. Beta carotene-loaded zein nanoparticles to improve the biopharmaceutical attributes and to abolish the toxicity of methotrexate: A preclinical study for breast cancer. *Artif. Cells Nanomed. Biotechnol.* **2018**, *46*, 402–412. [CrossRef] [PubMed]
323. He, J.; Gu, Y.; Zhang, S. Vitamin A and breast cancer survival: A systematic review and meta-analysis. *Clin. Breast Cancer* **2018**, *18*, e1389–e1400. [CrossRef] [PubMed]
324. Lai, G.Y.; Weinstein, S.J.; Albanes, D.; Taylor, P.R.; Virtamo, J.; McGlynn, K.A.; Freedman, N.D. Association of serum α-tocopherol, β-carotene, and retinol with liver cancer incidence and chronic liver disease mortality. *Br. J. Cancer* **2014**, *111*, 2163–2171. [CrossRef] [PubMed]
325. Chen, F.; Hu, J.; Liu, P.; Li, J.; Wei, Z.; Liu, P. Carotenoid intake and risk of non-Hodgkin lymphoma: A systematic review and dose-response meta-analysis of observational studies. *Ann. Hematol.* **2017**, *96*, 957–965. [CrossRef]
326. Reynoso-Camacho, R.; González-Jasso, E.; Ferriz-Martínez, R.; Villalón-Corona, B.; Loarca-Pina, G.F.; Salgado, L.M.; Ramos-Gomez, M. Dietary supplementation of lutein reduces colon carcinogenesis in DMH-treated rats by modulating K-ras, PKB, and β-catenin proteins. *Nutr. Cancer* **2011**, *63*, 39–45. [CrossRef]
327. Kim, J.; Lee, J.; Oh, J.H.; Chang, H.J.; Sohn, D.K.; Kwon, O.; Shin, A.; Kim, J. Dietary lutein plus zeaxanthin intake and DICER1 rs3742330 A > G polymorphism relative to colorectal cancer risk. *Sci. Rep.* **2019**, *9*, 3406. [CrossRef]
328. Sindhu, E.R.; Firdous, A.P.; Ramnath, V.; Kuttan, R. Effect of carotenoid lutein on N-nitrosodiethylamine-induced hepatocellular carcinoma and its mechanism of action. *Eur. J. Cancer Prev.* **2013**, *22*, 320–327. [CrossRef]
329. Baraya, Y.S.A.; Yankuzo, H.M.; Wong, K.K.; Yaacob, N.S. Strobilanthes crispus bioactive subfraction inhibits tumor progression and improves hematological and morphological parameters in mouse mammary carcinoma model. *J. Ethnopharmacol.* **2021**, *267*, 113522. [CrossRef]
330. Yan, B.; Lu, M.S.; Wang, L.; Mo, X.F.; Luo, W.P.; Du, Y.F.; Zhang, C.X. Specific serum carotenoids are inversely associated with breast cancer risk among Chinese women: A case-control study. *Br. J. Nutr.* **2016**, *115*, 129–137. [CrossRef]
331. Wu, S.; Liu, Y.; Michalek, J.E.; Mesa, R.A.; Parma, D.L.; Rodriguez, R.; Mansour, A.M.; Svatek, R.; Tucker, T.C.; Ramirez, A.G. Carotenoid intake and circulating carotenoids are inversely associated with the risk of bladder cancer: A dose-response meta-analysis. *Adv. Nutr.* **2020**, *11*, 630–643. [CrossRef]
332. Bock, C.H.; Ruterbusch, J.J.; Holowatyj, A.N.; Steck, S.E.; Van Dyke, A.L.; Ho, W.J.; Cote, M.L.; Hofmann, J.N.; Davis, F.; Graubard, B.I.; et al. Renal cell carcinoma risk associated with lower intake of micronutrients. *Cancer Med.* **2018**, *7*, 4087–4097. [CrossRef]
333. Leoncini, E.; Edefonti, V.; Hashibe, M.; Parpinel, M.; Cadoni, G.; Ferraroni, M.; Serraino, D.; Matsuo, K.; Olshan, A.F.; Zevallos, J.P.; et al. Carotenoid intake and head and neck cancer: A pooled analysis in the International Head and Neck Cancer Epidemiology Consortium. *Eur. J. Epidemiol.* **2016**, *31*, 369–383. [CrossRef] [PubMed]
334. Bravi, F.; Bosetti, C.; Filomeno, M.; Levi, F.; Garavello, W.; Galimberti, S.; Negri, E.; La Vecchia, C. Foods, nutrients and the risk of oral and pharyngeal cancer. *Br. J. Cancer* **2013**, *109*, 2904–2910. [CrossRef] [PubMed]
335. Jansen, R.J.; Robinson, D.P.; Stolzenberg-Solomon, R.Z.; William, R.; De Andrade, M.; Oberg, A.L.; Rabe, K.G.; Anderson, K.E.; Janet, E.; Sinha, R.; et al. Nutrients from fruit and vegetable consumption reduce the risk of pancreatic cancer. *J. Gastrointest. Cancer* **2013**, *44*, 152–161. [CrossRef] [PubMed]
336. Arunkumar, R.; Gorusupudi, A.; Li, B.; Blount, J.D.; Nwagbo, U.; Kim, H.J.; Sparrow, J.R.; Bernstein, P.S. Lutein and zeaxanthin reduce A2E and iso-A2E levels and improve visual performance in Abca4-/-/Bco2-/- double knockout mice. *Exp. Eye Res.* **2021**, *209*, 108680. [CrossRef]
337. Xu, X.L.; Hu, D.N.; Iacob, C.; Jordan, A.; Gandhi, S.; Gierhart, D.L.; Rosen, R. Effects of zeaxanthin on growth and invasion of human uveal melanoma in nude mouse model. *J. Ophthalmol.* **2015**, *2015*, 392305. [CrossRef]
338. Jeurnink, S.M.; Ros, M.M.; Leenders, M.; Van Duijnhoven, F.J.B.; Siersema, P.D.; Jansen, E.H.J.M.; Van Gils, C.H.; Bakker, M.F.; Overvad, K.; Roswall, N.; et al. Plasma carotenoids, vitamin C, retinol and tocopherols levels and pancreatic cancer risk within the European Prospective Investigation into Cancer and Nutrition: A nested case-control study: Plasma micronutrients and pancreatic cancer risk. *Int. J. Cancer* **2015**, *136*, E665–E676. [CrossRef]

339. Terlikowska, K.M.; Dobrzycka, B.; Kinalski, M.; Terlikowski, S.J. Serum concentrations of carotenoids and fat-soluble vitamins in relation to nutritional status of patients with ovarian cancer. *Nutr. Cancer* **2021**, *73*, 1480–1488. [CrossRef]
340. Kim, D.; Kim, Y.; Kim, Y. Effects of β-carotene on expression of selected MicroRNAs, histone acetylation, and DNA methylation in colon cancer stem cells. *J. Cancer Prev.* **2019**, *24*, 224–232. [CrossRef] [PubMed]
341. Ke, Y.; Bu, S.; Ma, H.; Gao, L.; Cai, Y.; Zhang, Y.; Zhou, W. Preventive and therapeutic effects of astaxanthin on depressive-like behaviors in high-fat diet and streptozotocin-treated rats. *Front. Pharmacol.* **2020**, *10*, 1621. [CrossRef] [PubMed]
342. Huang, L.J.; Chen, W.P. Astaxanthin ameliorates cartilage damage in experimental osteoarthritis. *Mod. Rheumatol.* **2015**, *25*, 768–771. [CrossRef] [PubMed]
343. Akduman, H.; Tayman, C.; Çakir, U.; Çakir, E.; Dilli, D.; Türkmenoğlu, T.T.; Gönel, A. Astaxanthin prevents lung injury due to hyperoxia and inflammation. *Comb. Chem. High Throughput Screen.* **2020**. [CrossRef]
344. Kim, H.; Ahn, Y.T.; Lee, G.S.; Cho, S.I.; Kim, J.M.; Lee, C.; Lim, B.K.; Ju, S.A.; An, W.G. Effects of astaxanthin on dinitrofluorobenzene-induced contact dermatitis in mice. *Mol. Med. Rep.* **2015**, *12*, 3632–3638. [CrossRef]
345. Li, J.; Guo, C.; Wu, J. Astaxanthin in liver health and disease: A potential therapeutic agent. *Drug Des. Devel. Ther.* **2020**, *14*, 2275–2285. [CrossRef]
346. Prabhu, P.N.; Ashokkumar, P.; Sudhandiran, G. Antioxidative and antiproliferative effects of astaxanthin during the initiation stages of 1,2-dimethyl hydrazine-induced experimental colon carcinogenesis. *Fundam. Clin. Pharmacol.* **2009**, *23*, 225–234. [CrossRef]
347. Ohno, T.; Shimizu, M.; Shirakami, Y.; Miyazaki, T.; Ideta, T.; Kochi, T.; Kubota, M.; Sakai, H.; Tanaka, T.; Moriwaki, H. Preventive effects of astaxanthin on diethylnitrosamine-induced liver tumorigenesis in C57/BL/KsJ-db/db obese mice. *Hepatol. Res.* **2016**, *46*, E201–E209. [CrossRef]
348. Nakao, R.; Nelson, O.L.; Park, J.S.; Mathison, B.D.; Thompson, P.A.; Chew, B.P. Effect of dietary astaxanthin at different stages of mammary tumor initiation in BALB/c mice. *Anticancer Res.* **2010**, *30*, 2171–2175. [PubMed]
349. Nagendraprabhu, P.; Sudhandiran, G. Astaxanthin inhibits tumor invasion by decreasing extracellular matrix production and induces apoptosis in experimental rat colon carcinogenesis by modulating the expressions of ERK-2, NF-kB and COX-2. *Invest. New Drugs* **2011**, *29*, 207–224. [CrossRef]
350. Cui, L.; Xu, F.; Wang, M.; Li, L.; Qiao, T.; Cui, H.; Li, Z.; Sun, C. Dietary natural astaxanthin at an early stage inhibits N-nitrosomethylbenzylamine–induced esophageal cancer oxidative stress and inflammation via downregulation of NFκB and COX2 in F344 rats. *Onco Targets Ther.* **2019**, *12*, 5087–5096. [CrossRef] [PubMed]
351. Kavitha, K.; Thiyagarajan, P.; Rathna, J.; Mishra, R.; Nagini, S. Chemopreventive effects of diverse dietary phytochemicals against DMBA-induced hamster buccal pouch carcinogenesis via the induction of Nrf2-mediated cytoprotective antioxidant, detoxification, and DNA repair enzymes. *Biochimie* **2013**, *95*, 1629–1639. [CrossRef] [PubMed]
352. Kowshik, J.; Baba, A.B.; Giri, H.; Reddy, G.D.; Dixit, M.; Nagini, S. Astaxanthin inhibits JAK/STAT-3 signaling to abrogate cell proliferation, invasion and angiogenesis in a hamster model of oral cancer. *PLoS ONE* **2014**, *9*, e109114. [CrossRef] [PubMed]
353. Ni, X.; Yu, H.; Wang, S.; Zhang, C.; Shen, S. Astaxanthin inhibits PC-3 xenograft prostate tumor growth in nude mice. *Mar. Drugs* **2017**, *15*, 66. [CrossRef]
354. Haung, H.Y.; Wang, Y.C.; Cheng, Y.C.; Kang, W.; Hu, S.H.; Liu, D.; Xiao, C.; Wang, H.M.D.; Ali, D. A novel oral astaxanthin nanoemulsion from *Haematococcus pluvialis* induces apoptosis in lung metastatic melanoma. *Oxid. Med. Cell. Longev.* **2020**, *2020*, 2647670. [CrossRef]
355. Terasaki, M.; Masaka, S.; Fukada, C.; Houzaki, M.; Endo, T.; Tanaka, T.; Maeda, H.; Miyashita, K.; Mutoh, M. Salivary glycine is a significant predictor for the attenuation of polyp and tumor microenvironment formation by fucoxanthin in AOM/DSS mice. *In Vivo* **2019**, *33*, 365–374. [CrossRef] [PubMed]
356. Terasaki, M.; Kimura, R.; Kubota, A.; Kojima, H.; Tanaka, T.; Maeda, H.; Miyashita, K.; Mutoh, M. Continuity of tumor microenvironmental suppression in AOM/DSS mice by fucoxanthin may be able to track with salivary glycine. *In Vivo* **2020**, *34*, 3205–3215. [CrossRef]
357. Terasaki, M.; Uehara, O.; Ogasa, S.; Sano, T.; Kubota, A.; Kojima, H.; Tanaka, T.; Maeda, H.; Miyashita, K.; Mutoh, M. Alteration of fecal microbiota by fucoxanthin results in prevention of colorectal cancer in AOM/DSS mice. *Carcinogenesis* **2021**, *42*, 210–219. [CrossRef]
358. Terasaki, M.; Ikuta, M.; Kojima, H.; Tanaka, T.; Maeda, H.; Miyashita, K.; Mutoh, M. Dietary fucoxanthin induces anoikis in colorectal adenocarcinoma by suppressing integrin signaling in a murine colorectal cancer model. *J. Clin. Med.* **2019**, *9*, 90. [CrossRef] [PubMed]
359. Terasaki, M.; Hamoya, T.; Kubota, A.; Kojima, H.; Tanaka, T.; Maeda, H.; Miyashita, K.; Mutoh, M. Fucoxanthin prevents colorectal cancer development in dextran sodium sulfate-treated ApcMin/+ mice. *Anticancer Res.* **2021**, *41*, 1299–1305. [CrossRef]
360. Chen, W.; Zhang, H.; Liu, Y. Anti-inflammatory and apoptotic signaling effect of fucoxanthin on benzo(A)pyrene-induced lung cancer in mice. *J. Environ. Pathol. Toxicol. Oncol.* **2019**, *38*, 239–251. [CrossRef]
361. Mei, C.H.; Zhou, S.C.; Zhu, L.; Ming, J.X.; Zeng, F.D.; Xu, R. Antitumor effects of Laminaria extract fucoxanthin on lung cancer. *Mar. Drugs* **2017**, *15*, 39. [CrossRef] [PubMed]
362. Ming, J.X.; Wang, Z.C.; Huang, Y.; Ohishi, H.; Wu, R.J.; Shao, Y.; Wang, H.; Qin, M.Y.; Wu, Z.L.; Li, Y.Y.; et al. Fucoxanthin extracted from *Laminaria japonica* inhibits metastasis and enhances the sensitivity of lung cancer to gefitinib. *J. Ethnopharmacol.* **2021**, *265*, 113302. [CrossRef]

363. Jin, X.; Zhao, T.; Shi, D.; Ye, M.B.; Yi, Q. Protective role of fucoxanthin in diethylnitrosamine-induced hepatocarcinogenesis in experimental adult rats. *Drug Dev. Res.* **2019**, *80*, 209–217. [CrossRef] [PubMed]
364. Liu, Y.; Zheng, J.; Zhang, Y.; Wang, Z.; Yang, Y.; Bai, M.; Dai, Y. Fucoxanthin activates apoptosis via inhibition of PI3K/Akt/mTOR pathway and suppresses invasion and migration by restriction of p38-MMP-2/9 pathway in human glioblastoma cells. *Neurochem. Res.* **2016**, *41*, 2728–2751. [CrossRef]
365. Ye, G.; Lu, Q.; Zhao, W.; Du, D.; Jin, L.; Liu, Y. Fucoxanthin induces apoptosis in human cervical cancer cell line HeLa via PI3K/Akt pathway. *Tumor Biol.* **2014**, *35*, 11261–11267. [CrossRef]
366. Kim, K.N.; Ahn, G.; Heo, S.J.; Kang, S.M.; Kang, M.C.; Yang, H.M.; Kim, D.; Roh, S.W.; Kim, S.K.; Jeon, B.T.; et al. Inhibition of tumor growth *in vitro* and *in vivo* by fucoxanthin against melanoma B16F10 cells. *Environ. Toxicol. Pharmacol.* **2013**, *35*, 39–46. [CrossRef]
367. Wang, J.; Chen, S.; Xu, S.; Yu, X.; Ma, D.; Hu, X.; Cao, X. *In vivo* induction of apoptosis by fucoxanthin, a marine carotenoid, associated with down-regulating STAT3/EGFR signaling in sarcoma 180 (S180) xenografts-bearing mice. *Mar. Drugs* **2012**, *10*, 2055–2068. [CrossRef] [PubMed]
368. Wu, C.; Han, L.; Riaz, H.; Wang, S.; Cai, K.; Yang, L. The chemopreventive effect of β-cryptoxanthin from mandarin on human stomach cells (BGC-823). *Food Chem.* **2013**, *136*, 1122–1129. [CrossRef]
369. Gao, M.; Dang, F.; Deng, C. β-Cryptoxanthin induced anti-proliferation and apoptosis by G0/G1 arrest and AMPK signal inactivation in gastric cancer. *Eur. J. Pharmacol.* **2019**, *859*, 172528. [CrossRef]
370. Lim, J.Y.; Liu, C.; Hu, K.Q.; Smith, D.E.; Wu, D.; Lamon-Fava, S.; Ausman, L.M.; Wang, X.D. Xanthophyll β-cryptoxanthin inhibits highly refined carbohydrate diet–promoted hepatocellular carcinoma progression in mice. *Mol. Nutr. Food Res.* **2020**, *64*, e1900949. [CrossRef] [PubMed]
371. Iskandar, A.R.; Liu, C.; Smith, D.E.; Hu, K.Q.; Choi, S.W.; Ausman, L.M.; Wang, X.D. β-cryptoxanthin restores nicotine-reduced lung SIRT1 to normal levels and inhibits nicotine-promoted lung tumorigenesis and emphysema in A/J mice. *Cancer Prev. Res.* **2013**, *6*, 309–320. [CrossRef] [PubMed]
372. Iskandar, A.R.; Miao, B.; Li, X.; Hu, K.Q.; Liu, C.; Wang, X.D. β-Cryptoxanthin reduced lung tumor multiplicity and inhibited lung cancer cell motility by downregulating nicotinic acetylcholine receptor A7 signaling. *Cancer Prev. Res.* **2016**, *9*, 875–886. [CrossRef] [PubMed]
373. Min, K.B.; Min, J.Y. Serum carotenoid levels and risk of lung cancer death in US adults. *Cancer Sci.* **2014**, *105*, 736–743. [CrossRef] [PubMed]
374. Li, S.; Zhu, X.; Zhu, L.; Hu, X.; Wen, S. Associations between serum carotenoid levels and the risk of non-Hodgkin lymphoma: A case-control study. *Br. J. Nutr.* **2020**, *124*, 1311–1319. [CrossRef]
375. Huang, J.; Lu, M.S.; Fang, Y.J.; Xu, M.; Huang, W.Q.; Pan, Z.Z.; Chen, Y.M.; Zhang, C.X. Serum carotenoids and colorectal cancer risk: A case-control study in Guangdong, China. *Mol. Nutr. Food Res.* **2017**, *61*, 1700267. [CrossRef]
376. Wang, L.; Li, B.; Pan, M.X.; Mo, X.F.; Chen, Y.M.; Zhang, C.X. Specific carotenoid intake is inversely associated with the risk of breast cancer among Chinese women. *Br. J. Nutr.* **2014**, *111*, 1686–1695. [CrossRef] [PubMed]
377. Brock, K.E.; Ke, L.; Gridley, G.; Chiu, B.C.H.; Ershow, A.G.; Lynch, C.F.; Graubard, B.I.; Cantor, K.P. Fruit, vegetables, fibre and micronutrients and risk of US renal cell carcinoma. *Br. J. Nutr.* **2012**, *108*, 1077–1085. [CrossRef]
378. Jinendiran, S.; Dahms, H.U.; Dileep Kumar, B.S.; Kumar Ponnusamy, V.; Sivakumar, N. Diapolycopenedioic-acid-diglucosyl ester and keto-myxocoxanthin glucoside ester: Novel carotenoids derived from Exiguobacterium acetylicum S01 and evaluation of their anticancer and anti-inflammatory activities. *Bioorg. Chem.* **2020**, *103*, 104149. [CrossRef]
379. Storniolo, C.E.; Sacanella, I.; Lamuela-Raventos, R.M.; Moreno, J.J. Bioactive compounds of Mediterranean cooked tomato sauce (sofrito) modulate intestinal epithelial cancer cell growth through oxidative stress/arachidonic acid cascade regulation. *ACS Omega* **2020**, *5*, 17071–17077. [CrossRef]
380. Park, Y.; Choi, J.; Lim, J.W.; Kim, H. β-Carotene-induced apoptosis is mediated with loss of Ku proteins in gastric cancer AGS cells. *Genes Nutr.* **2015**, *10*, 467. [CrossRef]
381. Park, Y.; Lee, H.; Lim, J.W.; Kim, H. Inhibitory effect of β-carotene on *Helicobacter pylori*-induced TRAF expression and hyper-proliferation in gastric epithelial cells. *Antioxidants* **2019**, *8*, 637. [CrossRef] [PubMed]
382. Kim, D.; Lim, J.W.; Kim, H. β-carotene Inhibits Expression of c-Myc and Cyclin E in *Helicobacter pylori*-infected Gastric Epithelial Cells. *J. Cancer Prev.* **2019**, *24*, 192–196. [CrossRef]
383. Zhu, X.; Zhang, Y.; Li, Q.; Yang, L.; Zhang, N.; Ma, S.; Zhang, K.; Song, J.; Guan, F. β-Carotene induces apoptosis in human esophageal squamous cell carcinoma cell lines via the Cav-1/AKT/NF-κB signaling pathway. *J. Biochem. Mol. Toxicol.* **2016**, *30*, 148–157. [CrossRef]
384. Ngoc, N.B.; Lv, P.; Zhao, W.E. Suppressive effects of lycopene and β-carotene on the viability of the human esophageal squamous carcinoma cell line EC109. *Oncol. Lett.* **2018**, *15*, 6727–6732. [CrossRef] [PubMed]
385. Dutta, S.; Surapaneni, B.K.; Bansal, A. Marked inhibition of cellular proliferation in the normal human esophageal epithelial cells and human esophageal squamous cancer cells in culture by carotenoids: Role for prevention and early treatment of esophageal cancer. *Asian Pac. J. Cancer Prev.* **2018**, *19*, 3251–3256. [CrossRef] [PubMed]
386. Huei-Yan, C.; Chih-Min, Y.; Jen-Yin, C.; Te-Cheng, Y.; Miao-Lin, H. Multicarotenoids at physiological levels inhibit metastasis in human hepatocarcinoma SK-Hep-1 cells. *Nutr. Cancer* **2015**, *67*, 676–686. [CrossRef]

387. Yurtcu, E.; Iseri, O.D.; Sahin, F.I. Effects of ascorbic acid and β-carotene on HepG2 human hepatocellular carcinoma cell line. *Mol. Biol. Rep.* **2011**, *38*, 4265–4272. [CrossRef]
388. Kunjiappan, S.; Panneerselvam, T.; Somasundaram, B.; Sankaranarayanan, M.; Parasuraman, P.; Joshi, S.D.; Arunachalam, S.; Murugan, I. Design graph theoretical analysis and *in silico* modeling of *Dunaliella bardawil* biomass encapsulated N-succinyl chitosan nanoparticles for enhanced anticancer activity. *Anticancer. Agents Med. Chem.* **2018**, *18*, 1900–1918. [CrossRef] [PubMed]
389. Naz, H.; Khan, P.; Tarique, M.; Rahman, S.; Meena, A.; Ahamad, S.; Luqman, S.; Islam, A.; Ahmad, F.; Hassan, M.I. Binding studies and biological evaluation of β-carotene as a potential inhibitor of human calcium/calmodulin-dependent protein kinase IV. *Int. J. Biol. Macromol.* **2017**, *96*, 161–170. [CrossRef]
390. Haddad, N.F.; Teodoro, A.J.; Leite de Oliveira, F.; Soares, N.; de Mattos, R.M.; Hecht, F.; Dezonne, R.S.; Vairo, L.; dos Santos Goldenberg, R.C.; Gomes, F.C.A.; et al. Lycopene and Beta-carotene induce growth inhibition and proapoptotic effects on ACTH-secreting pituitary adenoma cells. *PLoS ONE* **2013**, *8*, e62773. [CrossRef]
391. Zhang, X.; Zhao, W.E.; Hu, L.; Zhao, L.; Huang, J. Carotenoids inhibit proliferation and regulate expression of peroxisome proliferators-activated receptor gamma (PPARγ) in K562 cancer cells. *Arch. Biochem. Biophys.* **2011**, *512*, 96–106. [CrossRef] [PubMed]
392. Shiau, R.J.; Chen, K.Y.; Der Wen, Y.; Chuang, C.H.; Yeh, S.L. Genistein and β-carotene enhance the growth-inhibitory effect of trichostatin A in A549 cells. *Eur. J. Nutr.* **2010**, *49*, 19–25. [CrossRef] [PubMed]
393. Sowmya Shree, G.; Yogendra Prasad, K.; Arpitha, H.S.; Deepika, U.R.; Nawneet Kumar, K.; Mondal, P.; Ganesan, P. β-carotene at physiologically attainable concentration induces apoptosis and down-regulates cell survival and antioxidant markers in human breast cancer (MCF-7) cells. *Mol. Cell. Biochem.* **2017**, *436*, 1–12. [CrossRef]
394. Gloria, N.F.; Soares, N.; Brand, C.; Oliveira, F.L.; Borojevic, R.; Teodoro, A.J. Lycopene and Beta-carotene induce cell-cycle arrest and apoptosis in human breast cancer cell lines. *Anticancer Res.* **2014**, *34*, 1377–1386.
395. Vijay, K.; Sowmya, P.R.R.; Arathi, B.P.; Shilpa, S.; Shwetha, H.J.; Raju, M.; Baskaran, V.; Lakshminarayana, R. Low-dose doxorubicin with carotenoids selectively alters redox status and upregulates oxidative stress-mediated apoptosis in breast cancer cells. *Food Chem. Toxicol.* **2018**, *118*, 675–690. [CrossRef] [PubMed]
396. Jain, A.; Sharma, G.; Thakur, K.; Raza, K.; Shivhare, U.S.; Ghoshal, G.; Katare, O.P. Beta-carotene-encapsulated solid lipid nanoparticles (BC-SLNs) as promising vehicle for cancer: An investigative assessment. *AAPS PharmSciTech.* **2019**, *20*, 100. [CrossRef]
397. Lim, J.Y.; Kim, Y.-S.; Kim, Y. β-carotene regulates the murine liver microenvironment of a metastatic neuroblastoma. *J. Cancer Prev.* **2013**, *18*, 337–345. [CrossRef]
398. Chan, M.Y.; Lee, B.J.; Chang, P.S.; Hsiao, H.Y.; Hsu, L.P.; Chang, C.H.; Lin, P.T. The risks of ubiquinone and β-carotene deficiency and metabolic disorders in patients with oral cancer. *BMC Cancer* **2020**, *20*, 310. [CrossRef]
399. Rosa, C.; Franca, C.; Vieira, S.L.; Carvalho, A.; Penna, A.; Nogueira, C.; Lessa, S.; Ramalho, A. Reduction of serum concentrations and synergy between retinol, β-carotene, and zinc according to cancer staging and different treatment modalities prior to radiation therapy in women with breast cancer. *Nutrients* **2019**, *11*, 2953. [CrossRef]
400. Nordström, T.; Van Blarigan, E.L.; Ngo, V.; Roy, R.; Weinberg, V.; Song, X.; Simko, J.; Carroll, P.R.; Chan, J.M.; Paris, P.L. Associations between circulating carotenoids, genomic instability and the risk of high-grade prostate cancer. *Prostate* **2016**, *76*, 339–348. [CrossRef]
401. Emri, S.; Kilickap, S.; Kadilar, C.; Halil, M.G.; Akay, H.; Besler, T. Serum levels of alpha-tocopherol, vitamin C, beta-carotene, and retinol in malignant pleural mesothelioma. *Asian Pac. J. Cancer Prev.* **2012**, *13*, 3025–3029. [CrossRef] [PubMed]
402. Huang, J.; Weinstein, S.J.; Yu, K.; Männistö, S.; Albanes, D. Serum Beta-carotene and overall and cause-specific mortality: A prospective cohort study. *Circ. Res.* **2018**, *123*, 1339–1349. [CrossRef] [PubMed]
403. Pantavos, A.; Ruiter, R.; Feskens, E.F.; De Keyser, C.E.; Hofman, A.; Stricker, B.H.; Franco, O.H.; Kiefte-De Jong, J.C. Total dietary antioxidant capacity, individual antioxidant intake and breast cancer risk: The Rotterdam study. *Int. J. Cancer* **2015**, *136*, 2178–2186. [CrossRef]
404. Yu, N.; Su, X.; Wang, Z.; Dai, B.; Kang, J. Association of dietary vitamin A and β-carotene intake with the risk of lung cancer: A meta-analysis of 19 publications. *Nutrients* **2015**, *7*, 9309–9324. [CrossRef]
405. Tayyem, R.F.; Mahmoud, R.I.; Shareef, M.H.; Marei, L.S. Nutrient intake patterns and breast cancer risk among Jordanian women: A case-control study. *Epidemiol. Health* **2019**, *41*, e2019010. [CrossRef]
406. Middha, P.; Weinstein, S.J.; Männistö, S.; Albanes, D.; Mondul, A.M. β-Carotene supplementation and lung cancer incidence in the Alpha-tocopherol, Beta-carotene cancer prevention study: The role of tar and nicotine. *Nicotine Tob. Res.* **2019**, *21*, 1045–1050. [CrossRef] [PubMed]
407. Kavalappa, Y.P.; Gopal, S.S.; Ponesakki, G. Lutein inhibits breast cancer cell growth by suppressing antioxidant and cell survival signals and induces apoptosis. *J. Cell. Physiol.* **2021**, *236*, 1798–1809. [CrossRef]
408. Muhammad, S.N.H.; Yaacob, N.S.; Safuwan, N.A.M.; Fauzi, A.N. Antiglycolytic activities of *Strobilanthes crispus* active fraction and its bioactive components on triple-negative breast cancer cells *in vitro*. *Anticancer Agents Med. Chem.* **2021**. [CrossRef]
409. Gong, X.; Smith, J.R.; Swanson, H.M.; Rubin, L.P. Carotenoid lutein selectively inhibits breast cancer cell growth and potentiates the effect of chemotherapeutic agents through ROS-mediated mechanisms. *Molecules* **2018**, *23*, 905. [CrossRef]
410. Li, Y.; Zhang, Y.; Liu, X.; Wang, M.; Wang, P.; Yang, J.; Zhang, S. Lutein inhibits proliferation, invasion and migration of hypoxic breast cancer cells via downregulation of HES1. *Int. J. Oncol.* **2018**, *52*, 2119–2129. [CrossRef] [PubMed]

411. Behbahani, M. Evaluation of *in vitro* anticancer activity of *Ocimum basilicum*, *Alhagi maurorum*, *Calendula officinalis* and their parasite *Cuscuta campestris*. *PLoS ONE* **2014**, *9*, e116049. [CrossRef]
412. Xu, Y.; Ma, X.Y.; Gong, W.; Li, X.; Huang, H.B.; Zhu, X.M. Nanoparticles based on carboxymethylcellulose-modified rice protein for efficient delivery of lutein. *Food Funct.* **2020**, *11*, 2380–2394. [CrossRef] [PubMed]
413. Luan, R.L.; Wang, P.C.; Yan, M.X.; Chen, J. Effect of lutein and doxorubicin combinatorial therapy on S180 cell proliferation and tumor growth. *Eur. Rev. Med. Pharmacol. Sci.* **2021**, *22*, 1514–1520. [CrossRef]
414. Grudzinski, W.; Piet, M.; Luchowski, R.; Reszczynska, E.; Welc, R.; Paduch, R.; Gruszecki, W.I. Different molecular organization of two carotenoids, lutein and zeaxanthin, in human colon epithelial cells and colon adenocarcinoma cells. *Spectrochim. Acta Part A Mol. Biomol. Spectrosc.* **2018**, *188*, 57–63. [CrossRef] [PubMed]
415. Rafi, M.M.; Kanakasabai, S.; Gokarn, S.V.; Krueger, E.G.; Bright, J.J. Dietary lutein modulates growth and survival genes in prostate cancer cells. *J. Med. Food* **2015**, *18*, 173–181. [CrossRef] [PubMed]
416. Zhang, W.L.; Zhao, Y.N.; Shi, Z.Z.; Cong, D.; Bai, Y.S. Lutein inhibits cell growth and activates apoptosis via the PI3K/AKT/mTOR signaling pathway in A549 human non-small-cell lung cancer cells. *J. Environ. Pathol. Toxicol. Oncol.* **2018**, *37*, 341–350. [CrossRef]
417. Zaini, R.G.; Brandt, K.; Clench, M.R.; Le Maitre, C.L. Effects of bioactive compounds from carrots (*Daucus carota* L.), polyacetylenes, Beta-carotene and lutein on human lymphoid leukaemia cells. *Anticancer Agents Med. Chem.* **2012**, *12*, 640–652. [CrossRef]
418. Sheng, Y.N.; Luo, Y.H.; Liu, S.B.; Xu, W.T.; Zhang, Y.; Zhang, T.; Xue, H.; Zuo, W.B.; Li, Y.N.; Wang, C.Y.; et al. Zeaxanthin induces apoptosis via ROS-regulated MAPK and Akt signaling pathway in human gastric cancer cells. *Onco Targets. Ther.* **2020**, *13*, 10995–11006. [CrossRef]
419. Baudelet, P.H.; Gagez, A.L.; Bérard, J.B.; Juin, C.; Bridiau, N.; Kaas, R.; Thiéry, V.; Cadoret, J.P.; Picot, L. Antiproliferative activity of *Cyanophora paradoxa* pigments in melanoma, breast and lung cancer cells. *Mar. Drugs* **2013**, *11*, 4390–4406. [CrossRef]
420. Bi, M.C.; Rosen, R.; Zha, R.Y.; McCormick, S.A.; Song, E.; Hu, D.N. Zeaxanthin induces apoptosis in human uveal melanoma cells through Bcl-2 family proteins and intrinsic apoptosis pathway. *Evid. Based Complement. Altern. Med.* **2013**, *2013*, 205082. [CrossRef]
421. Wu, N.L.; Chiang, Y.C.; Huang, C.C.; Fang, J.Y.; Chen, D.F.; Hung, C.F. Zeaxanthin inhibits PDGF-BB-induced migration in human dermal fibroblasts. *Exp. Dermatol.* **2010**, *19*, 173–181. [CrossRef]
422. Ahn, Y.T.; Kim, M.S.; Kim, Y.S.; An, W.G. Astaxanthin reduces stemness markers in BT20 and T47D breast cancer stem cells by inhibiting expression of pontin and mutant p53. *Mar. Drugs* **2020**, *18*, 577. [CrossRef]
423. Badak, B.; Aykanat, N.E.B.; Kacar, S.; Sahinturk, V.; Arik, D.; Canaz, F. Effects of astaxanthin on metastasis suppressors in ductal carcinoma. A preliminary study. *Ann. Ital. Chir.* **2021**, *10*, S0003469X21035648.
424. Su, X.-Z.; Chen, R.; Wang, C.-B.; Ouyang, X.-L.; Jiang, Y.; Zhu, M.-Y. Astaxanthin combine with human serum albumin to abrogate cell proliferation, migration, and drug-resistant in human ovarian carcinoma SKOV3 cells. *Anticancer Agents Med. Chem.* **2019**, *19*, 792–801. [CrossRef] [PubMed]
425. Zhao, H.; Gu, H.; Zhang, H.; Li, J.H.; Zhao, W.E. PPARγ-dependent pathway in the growth-inhibitory effects of K562 cells by carotenoids in combination with rosiglitazone. *Biochim. Biophys. Acta Gen. Subj.* **2014**, *1840*, 545–555. [CrossRef] [PubMed]
426. Tsuji, S.; Nakamura, S.; Maoka, T.; Yamada, T.; Imai, T.; Ohba, T.; Yako, T.; Hayashi, M.; Endo, K.; Saio, M.; et al. Antitumour effects of astaxanthin and adonixanthin on glioblastoma. *Mar. Drugs* **2020**, *18*, 474. [CrossRef]
427. Faraone, I.; Sinisgalli, C.; Ostuni, A.; Armentano, M.F.; Carmosino, M.; Milella, L.; Russo, D.; Labanca, F.; Khan, H. Astaxanthin anticancer effects are mediated through multiple molecular mechanisms: A systematic review. *Pharmacol. Res.* **2020**, *155*, 104689. [CrossRef] [PubMed]
428. Ferdous, U.T.; Yusof, Z.N.B. Medicinal prospects of antioxidants from algal sources in cancer therapy. *Front. Pharmacol.* **2021**, *12*, 593116. [CrossRef] [PubMed]
429. Shao, Y.; Ni, Y.; Yang, J.; Lin, X.; Li, J.; Zhang, L. Astaxanthin inhibits proliferation and induces apoptosis and cell cycle arrest of mice H22 hepatoma cells. *Med. Sci. Monit.* **2016**, *22*, 2152. [CrossRef]
430. Kim, J.H.; Park, J.J.; Lee, B.J.; Joo, M.K.; Chun, H.J.; Lee, S.W.; Bak, Y.T. Astaxanthin inhibits proliferation of human gastric cancer cell lines by interrupting cell cycle progression. *Gut Liver* **2016**, *10*, 369. [CrossRef]
431. Song, X.; Zhang, J.; Wang, M.; Liu, W.; Gu, X.; Lv, C.-J. Astaxanthin induces mitochondria-mediated apoptosis in rat hepatocellular carcinoma CBRH-7919 cells. *Biol. Pharm. Bull.* **2011**, *34*, 839–844. [CrossRef] [PubMed]
432. Lee, H.; Lim, J.W.; Kim, H. Effect of astaxanthin on activation of autophagy and inhibition of apoptosis in *Helicobacter pylori*-infected gastric epithelial cell line AGS. *Nutrients* **2020**, *12*, 1750. [CrossRef]
433. Hormozi, M.; Ghoreishi, S.; Baharvand, P. Astaxanthin induces and increases activity of antioxidant enzymes in LS-180 cells. *Artif. Cells Nanomed. Biotechnol.* **2019**, *47*, 891–895. [CrossRef] [PubMed]
434. Palozza, P.; Torelli, C.; Boninsegna, A.; Simone, R.; Catalano, A.; Mele, M.C.; Picci, N. Growth-inhibitory effects of the astaxanthin-rich alga *Haematococcus pluvialis* in human colon cancer cells. *Cancer Lett.* **2009**, *283*, 108–117. [CrossRef]
435. Sowmya, P.R.R.; Arathi, B.P.; Vijay, K.; Baskaran, V.; Lakshminarayana, R. Astaxanthin from shrimp efficiently modulates oxidative stress and allied cell death progression in MCF-7 cells treated synergistically with β-carotene and lutein from greens. *Food Chem. Toxicol.* **2017**, *106*, 58–69. [CrossRef]
436. Liu, X.; Song, M.; Gao, Z.; Cai, X.; Dixon, W.; Chen, X.; Cao, Y.; Xiao, H. Stereoisomers of astaxanthin inhibit human colon cancer cell growth by inducing G2/M cell cycle arrest and apoptosis. *J. Agric. Food Chem.* **2016**, *64*, 7750–7759. [CrossRef] [PubMed]

437. Catanzaro, E.; Bishayee, A.; Fimognari, C. On a beam of light: Photoprotective activities of the marine carotenoids astaxanthin and fucoxanthin in suppression of inflammation and cancer. *Mar. Drugs* **2020**, *18*, 544. [CrossRef] [PubMed]
438. Rao, A.R.; Sindhuja, H.N.; Dharmesh, S.M.; Sankar, K.U.; Sarada, R.; Ravishankar, G.A. Effective inhibition of skin cancer, tyrosinase, and antioxidative properties by astaxanthin and astaxanthin esters from the green alga *Haematococcus pluvialis*. *J. Agric. Food Chem.* **2013**, *61*, 3842–3851. [CrossRef]
439. Maoka, T.; Tokuda, H.; Suzuki, N.; Kato, H.; Etoh, H. Anti-oxidative, anti-tumor-promoting, and anti-carcinogensis activities of nitroastaxanthin and nitrolutein, the reaction products of astaxanthin and lutein with peroxynitrite. *Mar. Drugs* **2012**, *10*, 1391–1399. [CrossRef]
440. Turck, D.; Castenmiller, J.; de Henauw, S.; Hirsch-Ernst, K.I.; Kearney, J.; Maciuk, A.; Mangelsdorf, I.; McArdle, H.J.; Naska, A.; Pelaez, C.; et al. Safety of astaxanthin for its use as a novel food in food supplements. *EFSA J.* **2020**, *18*, 5993. [CrossRef]
441. Desai, S.J.; Prickril, B.; Rasooly, A. Mechanisms of phytonutrient modulation of cyclooxygenase-2 (COX-2) and inflammation related to cancer. *Nutr. Cancer* **2018**, *70*, 350. [CrossRef] [PubMed]
442. Park, J.S.; Chyun, J.H.; Kim, Y.K.; Line, L.L.; Chew, B.P. Astaxanthin decreased oxidative stress and inflammation and enhanced immune response in humans. *Nutr. Metab.* **2010**, *7*, 18. [CrossRef] [PubMed]
443. Pereira, C.P.M.; Souza, A.C.R.; Vasconcelos, A.R.; Prado, P.S.; Name, J.J. Antioxidant and anti-inflammatory mechanisms of action of astaxanthin in cardiovascular diseases (Review). *Int. J. Mol. Med.* **2021**, *47*, 37–48. [CrossRef] [PubMed]
444. Donoso, A.; González-Durán, J.; Muñoz, A.A.; González, P.A.; Agurto-Muñoz, C. Therapeutic uses of natural astaxanthin: An evidence-based review focused on human clinical trials. *Pharmacol. Res.* **2021**, *166*, 105479. [CrossRef] [PubMed]
445. Xu, S.; Chaudhary, O.; Rodríguez-Morales, P.; Sun, X.; Chen, D.; Zappasodi, R.; Xu, Z.; Pinto, A.F.M.; Williams, A.; Schulze, I.; et al. Uptake of oxidized lipids by the scavenger receptor CD36 promotes lipid peroxidation and dysfunction in CD8+ T cells in tumors. *Immunity* **2021**, *54*, 1561–1577.e7. [CrossRef] [PubMed]
446. Eggersdorfer, M.; Wyss, A. Carotenoids in human nutrition and health. *Arch. Biochem. Biophys.* **2018**, *652*, 18–26. [CrossRef]
447. Yu, R.X.; Hu, X.M.; Xu, S.Q.; Jiang, Z.J.; Yang, W. Effects of fucoxanthin on proliferation and apoptosis in human gastric adenocarcinoma MGC-803 cells via JAK/STAT signal pathway. *Eur. J. Pharmacol.* **2011**, *657*, 10–19. [CrossRef]
448. Yu, R.X.; Yu, R.T.; Liu, Z. Inhibition of two gastric cancer cell lines induced by fucoxanthin involves downregulation of Mcl-1 and STAT3. *Hum. Cell* **2018**, *31*, 50–63. [CrossRef]
449. Zhu, Y.; Cheng, J.; Min, Z.; Yin, T.; Zhang, R.; Zhang, W.; Hu, L.; Cui, Z.; Gao, C.; Xu, S.; et al. Effects of fucoxanthin on autophagy and apoptosis in SGC-7901cells and the mechanism. *J. Cell Biochem.* **2018**, *119*, 7274–7284. [CrossRef]
450. Long, Y.; Cao, X.; Zhao, R.; Gong, S.; Jin, L.; Feng, C. Fucoxanthin treatment inhibits nasopharyngeal carcinoma cell proliferation through induction of autophagy mechanism. *Environ. Toxicol.* **2020**, *35*, 1082–1090. [CrossRef]
451. Lopes-Costa, E.; Abreu, M.; Gargiulo, D.; Rocha, E.; Ramos, A.A. Anticancer effects of seaweed compounds fucoxanthin and phloroglucinol, alone and in combination with 5-fluorouracil in colon cells. *J. Toxicol. Environ. Heal. A* **2017**, *80*, 776–787. [CrossRef] [PubMed]
452. Kawee-Ai, A.; Kim, S.M. Application of microalgal fucoxanthin for the reduction of colon cancer risk: Inhibitory activity of fucoxanthin against beta-glucuronidase and DLD-1 cancer cells. *Nat. Prod. Commun.* **2014**, *9*, 921–924.
453. Tamura, S.; Narita, T.; Fujii, G.; Miyamoto, S.; Hamoya, T.; Kurokawa, Y.; Takahashi, M.; Miki, K.; Matsuzawa, Y.; Komiya, M.; et al. Inhibition of NF-kappaB transcriptional activity enhances fucoxanthinol-induced apoptosis in colorectal cancer cells. *Genes Environ.* **2019**, *41*, 1. [CrossRef] [PubMed]
454. Sui, Y.; Gu, Y.; Lu, Y.; Yu, C.; Zheng, J.; Qi, H. Fucoxanthin@polyvinylpyrrolidone nanoparticles promoted oxidative stress-induced cell death in Caco-2 human colon cancer cells. *Mar. Drugs* **2021**, *19*, 92. [CrossRef] [PubMed]
455. Ravi, H.; Kurrey, N.; Manabe, Y.; Sugawara, T.; Baskaran, V. Polymeric chitosan-glycolipid nanocarriers for an effective delivery of marine carotenoid fucoxanthin for induction of apoptosis in human colon cancer cells (Caco-2 cells). *Mater. Sci. Eng. C* **2018**, *91*, 785–795. [CrossRef]
456. Liu, C.L.; Lim, Y.P.; Hu, M.L. Fucoxanthin enhances cisplatin-induced cytotoxicity via NF-κB-mediated pathway and downregulates DNA repair gene expression in human hepatoma HepG2 cells. *Mar. Drugs* **2013**, *11*, 50–66. [CrossRef] [PubMed]
457. Foo, S.C.; Yusoff, F.M.; Imam, M.U.; Foo, J.B.; Ismail, N.; Azmi, N.H.; Tor, Y.S.; Khong, N.M.H.; Ismail, M. Increased fucoxanthin in *Chaetoceros calcitrans* extract exacerbates apoptosis in liver cancer cells via multiple targeted cellular pathways. *Biotechnol. Rep.* **2018**, *21*, e00296. [CrossRef]
458. Rwigemera, A.; Mamelona, J.; Martin, L.J. Inhibitory effects of fucoxanthinol on the viability of human breast cancer cell lines MCF-7 and MDA-MB-231 are correlated with modulation of the NF-kappaB pathway. *Cell Biol. Toxicol.* **2014**, *30*, 157–167. [CrossRef] [PubMed]
459. Wang, J.; Ma, Y.; Yang, J.; Jin, L.; Gao, Z.; Xue, L.; Hou, L.; Sui, L.; Liu, J.; Zou, X. Fucoxanthin inhibits tumour-related lymphangiogenesis and growth of breast cancer. *J. Cell. Mol. Med.* **2019**, *23*, 2219–2229. [CrossRef]
460. Hou, L.; Gao, C.; Chen, L.; Hu, G.; Xie, S. Essential role of autophagy in fucoxanthin-induced cytotoxicity to human epithelial cervical cancer HeLa cells. *Acta Pharmacol. Sin.* **2013**, *34*, 1403–1410. [CrossRef]
461. Ye, G.; Wang, L.; Yang, K.; Wang, C. Fucoxanthin may inhibit cervical cancer cell proliferation via downregulation of HIST1H3D. *J. Int. Med. Res.* **2020**, *48*, 300060520964011. [CrossRef] [PubMed]

462. Jin, Y.; Qiu, S.; Shao, N.; Zheng, J. Fucoxanthin and tumor necrosis factor-related apoptosis-inducing ligand (TRAIL) synergistically promotes apoptosis of human cervical cancer cells by targeting PI3K/Akt/NF-κB signaling pathway. *Med. Sci. Monit.* **2018**, *24*, 11–18. [CrossRef]
463. Wang, L.; Zeng, Y.; Liu, Y.; Hu, X.; Li, S.; Wang, Y.; Li, L.; Lei, Z.; Zhang, Z. Fucoxanthin induces growth arrest and apoptosis in human bladder cancer T24 cells by up-regulation of p21 and down-regulation of mortalin. *Acta Biochim. Biophys. Sin.* **2014**, *46*, 877–884. [CrossRef] [PubMed]
464. Garg, S.; Afzal, S.; Elwakeel, A.; Sharma, D.; Radhakrishnan, N.; Dhanjal, J.K.; Sundar, D.; Kaul, S.C.; Wadhwa, R. Marine carotenoid fucoxanthin possesses anti-metastasis activity: Molecular evidence. *Mar. Drugs* **2019**, *17*, 338. [CrossRef] [PubMed]
465. Rokkaku, T.; Kimura, R.; Ishikawa, C.; Yasumoto, T.; Senba, M.; Kanaya, F.; Mori, N. Anticancer effects of marine carotenoids, fucoxanthin and its deacetylated product, fucoxanthinol, on osteosarcoma. *Int. J. Oncol.* **2013**, *43*, 1176–1186. [CrossRef] [PubMed]
466. Chung, T.W.; Choi, H.J.; Lee, J.Y.; Jeong, H.S.; Kim, C.H.; Joo, M.; Choi, J.Y.; Han, C.W.; Kim, S.Y.; Choi, J.S.; et al. Marine algal fucoxanthin inhibits the metastatic potential of cancer cells. *Biochem. Biophys. Reses. Commun.* **2013**, *439*, 580–585. [CrossRef]
467. Yang, Y.; Yang, I.; Cao, M.; Su, Z.; Wu, R.; Fang, M.; Kong, A.; Drugs, B.; District, C.L.; City, T. Fucoxanthin elicits epigenetic modifications, Nrf2 activation and blocking transformation in mouse skin JB6 P+ cells. *AAPS J.* **2018**, *20*, 32. [CrossRef] [PubMed]
468. Lopes, F.G.; Oliveira, K.A.; Lopes, R.G.; Poluceno, G.G.; Simioni, C.; Pescador, G.D.S.; Bauer, C.M.; Maraschin, M.; Derner, R.B.; Garcez, R.C.; et al. Anti-cancer effects of fucoxanthin on human glioblastoma cell line. *Anticancer Res.* **2020**, *40*, 6799–6815. [CrossRef]
469. Pruteanu, L.L.; Kopanitsa, L.; Módos, D.; Kletnieks, E.; Samarova, E.; Bender, A.; Gomez, L.D.; Bailey, D.S. Transcriptomics predicts compound synergy in drug and natural product treated glioblastoma cells. *PLoS ONE* **2020**, *15*, e0239551. [CrossRef] [PubMed]
470. Wu, H.L.; Fu, X.Y.; Cao, W.Q.; Xiang, W.Z.; Hou, Y.J.; Ma, J.K.; Wang, Y.; Fan, C.D. Induction of apoptosis in human glioma cells by fucoxanthin via triggering of ROS-mediated oxidative damage and regulation of MAPKs and PI3K-AKT pathways. *J. Agric. Food Chem.* **2019**, *67*, 2212–2219. [CrossRef] [PubMed]
471. Tafuku, S.; Ishikawa, C.; Yasumoto, T.; Mori, N. Anti-neoplastic effects of fucoxanthin and its deacetylated product, fucoxanthinol, on Burkitt's and Hodgkin's lymphoma cells. *Oncol. Rep.* **2012**, *28*, 1512–1518. [CrossRef]
472. Yamamoto, K.; Ishikawa, C.; Katano, H.; Yasumoto, T.; Mori, N. Fucoxanthin and its deacetylated product, fucoxanthinol, induce apoptosis of primary effusion lymphomas. *Cancer Lett.* **2011**, *300*, 225–234. [CrossRef] [PubMed]
473. Kim, K.N.; Heo, S.J.; Kang, S.M.; Ahn, G.; Jeon, Y.J. Fucoxanthin induces apoptosis in human leukemia HL-60 cells through a ROS-mediated Bcl-xL pathway. *Toxicol. Vitr.* **2010**, *24*, 1648–1654. [CrossRef]
474. Almeida, T.P.; Ferreira, J.; Vettorazzi, A.; Azqueta, A.; Rocha, E.; Ramos, A.A. Cytotoxic activity of fucoxanthin, alone and in combination with the cancer drugs imatinib and doxorubicin, in CML cell lines. *Environmen. Toxicol. Pharmacol.* **2018**, *59*, 24–33. [CrossRef] [PubMed]
475. Millán, C.S.; Soldevilla, B.; Martín, P.; Gil-Calderón, B.; Compte, M.; Pérez-Sacristán, B.; Donoso, E.; Peña, C.; Romero, J.; Granado-Lorencio, F.; et al. β-Cryptoxanthin synergistically enhances the antitumoral activity of oxaliplatin through ΔNP73 negative regulation in colon cancer. *Clin. Cancer Res.* **2015**, *21*, 4398–4409. [CrossRef]

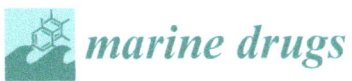

Review

Molecular Mechanisms of Astaxanthin as a Potential Neurotherapeutic Agent

Eshak I. Bahbah [1], Sherief Ghozy [2], Mohamed S. Attia [3], Ahmed Negida [4], Talha Bin Emran [5], Saikat Mitra [6], Ghadeer M. Albadrani [7], Mohamed M. Abdel-Daim [8], Md. Sahab Uddin [9,10,*] and Jesus Simal-Gandara [11,*]

1. Faculty of Medicine, Al-Azhar University, Damietta 34511, Egypt; isaacbahbah@gmail.com
2. Faculty of Medicine, Mansoura University, Mansoura 35516, Egypt; sherief_ghozy@yahoo.com
3. Department of Pharmaceutics, Faculty of Pharmacy, Zagazig University, Zagazig 44519, Egypt; mosalahnabet@gmail.com
4. Faculty of Medicine, Zagazig University, Zagazig 44519, Egypt; ahmed.said.negida@gmail.com
5. Department of Pharmacy, BGC Trust University Bangladesh, Chittagong 4381, Bangladesh; talhabmb@bgctub.ac.bd
6. Department of Pharmacy, Faculty of Pharmacy, University of Dhaka, Dhaka 1000, Bangladesh; saikatmitradu@gmail.com
7. Department of Biology, College of Science, Princess Nourah bint Abdulrahman University, Riyadh 11474, Saudi Arabia; gmalbadrani@pnu.edu.sa
8. Pharmacology Department, Faculty of Veterinary Medicine, Suez Canal University, Ismailia 41522, Egypt; abdeldaim.m@vet.suez.edu.eg
9. Department of Pharmacy, Southeast University, Dhaka 1213, Bangladesh
10. Pharmakon Neuroscience Research Network, Dhaka 1207, Bangladesh
11. Nutrition and Bromatology Group, Department of Analytical and Food Chemistry, Faculty of Food Science and Technology, University of Vigo—Ourense Campus, E32004 Ourense, Spain
* Correspondence: msu-neuropharma@hotmail.com (M.S.U.); jsimal@uvigo.es (J.S.-G.); Tel.: +880-1710-220110 (M.S.U.); +34-988-387000 (J.S.-G.)

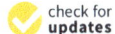

Citation: Bahbah, E.I.; Ghozy, S.; Attia, M.S.; Negida, A.; Emran, T.B.; Mitra, S.; Albadrani, G.M.; Abdel-Daim, M.M.; Uddin, M.S.; Simal-Gandara, J. Molecular Mechanisms of Astaxanthin as a Potential Neurotherapeutic Agent. *Mar. Drugs* **2021**, *19*, 201. https://doi.org/10.3390/md19040201

Academic Editors: Elena Talero and Javier Ávila-Román

Received: 27 February 2021
Accepted: 28 March 2021
Published: 3 April 2021

Publisher's Note: MDPI stays neutral with regard to jurisdictional claims in published maps and institutional affiliations.

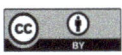

Copyright: © 2021 by the authors. Licensee MDPI, Basel, Switzerland. This article is an open access article distributed under the terms and conditions of the Creative Commons Attribution (CC BY) license (https://creativecommons.org/licenses/by/4.0/).

Abstract: Neurological disorders are diseases of the central and peripheral nervous system that affect millions of people, and the numbers are rising gradually. In the pathogenesis of neurodegenerative diseases, the roles of many signaling pathways were elucidated; however, the exact pathophysiology of neurological disorders and possible effective therapeutics have not yet been precisely identified. This necessitates developing multi-target treatments, which would simultaneously modulate neuroinflammation, apoptosis, and oxidative stress. The present review aims to explore the potential therapeutic use of astaxanthin (ASX) in neurological and neuroinflammatory diseases. ASX, a member of the xanthophyll group, was found to be a promising therapeutic anti-inflammatory agent for many neurological disorders, including cerebral ischemia, Parkinson's disease, Alzheimer's disease, autism, and neuropathic pain. An effective drug delivery system of ASX should be developed and further tested by appropriate clinical trials.

Keywords: astaxanthin; neuroprotective agent; oxidative stress; neuroinflammation; neurological diseases

1. Introduction

Marine carotenoids are highly antioxidant, reparative, antiproliferative, and anti-inflammatory and can be applied as photo-protective skin to inhibit harmful ultraviolet radiation effects [1,2]. Non-photosynthetic marine species are unable to produce carotenoids de novo, except for marine autotrophic organisms [3]. Several studies have already reported that marine animals may either accumulate carotenoids directly from food or partially modify them through the metabolic pathways [4,5]. Consequently, carotenoids obtained from several marine species act on various pathways, including the conversion of metal derivatives into harmless molecules, converting hydroperoxides into more stable compounds, acting as quenchers of singlet molecular oxygen, and preventing the formation of free radicals through the block of free radical oxidation reactions and inhibition of the auto-oxidation chain reaction [3,6,7].

Astaxanthin (ASX) is one of the marine carotenoids, which was originally isolated by Kuhn and Sorensen from a lobster [8]. ASX exists everywhere in nature; however, it particularly presents as a red-orange pigment in several marine animals, including salmonids, shrimp, and crayfish [9,10]. While plants, microbes, and microalgae may also produce ASX, the *Haematococcus pluvialis* chlorophyte algae are known to have the highest potential to accumulate ASX [11–14]. Nowadays, there are many synthetics ASX; nevertheless, health concerns have arisen concerning the use of synthetic ASX for medical purposes. ASX is closely related to other carotenoids, including zeaxanthin, lutein, and β-carotene; therefore, it shares many similar biological functions [3,15,16]. Previously, it has been reported that ASX is biologically more active than the aforementioned carotenoids [17–19]. ASX has been previously reported to have therapeutic anticancer, antidiabetic, anti-inflammatory, and antioxidant activities, and neuro-, cardiovascular, ocular, and skin-protective effects [20].

In terms of neurological protective effects, many studies have mentioned the role of ASX in neurological disorders, including cerebral ischemia, Parkinson's disease (PD), Alzheimer's disease (AD), autism, and neuropathic pain, which we will discuss in the following sections [21–23]. In this review, we aimed to explore the potential therapeutic use of ASX in neurological and neuroinflammatory diseases.

2. Bioavailability and Pharmacokinetics of Astaxanthin

The administration of ASX with dietary oils, particularly fish oil, may promote the absorption of ASX and enhance the neutrophil's phagocytic activity [19,24]. Studies showed enhanced bioavailability and antioxidant effects of ASX when administered alongside olive oil in rats [25,26]. Moreover, Otton and his colleagues [27] reported that ASX administration with fish oil reduced the production of nitric oxide (NO) and increased the release of calcium, superoxide dismutase (SOD), catalase, and glutathione peroxidase (GPx). Owing to the lipophilic nature of ASX, it was thought that ASX transforms metabolically in the rats' tissues before it is extracted [28].

It was observed that a high-cholesterol diet might improve the absorption of ASX in humans, which is transported into the liver via the lymphatic system. Matrix dissolution and mixed micelles integration are two essential steps leading up to membrane absorption [24]. It should be incorporated with chylomicrons after absorbing it by intestinal mucosal cells to be transported to the liver. After that, ASX is integrated and transferred to the tissues by lipoproteins [29]. Okada et al. [30] reported that smoking could significantly reduce the half-life of ASX, indicating that smoking enhances the metabolism and elimination of ASX. This finding was confirmed by many investigators who demonstrated that the half-life of carotenoids is significantly affected by smoking [31,32]. The reported half-life of plasma ASX ranged between 16 and 21 h [28,33]. In terms of tolerability, Odeberg et al. [34] reported that a single dose of 40 mg for healthy volunteers was well-tolerated.

3. Astaxanthin for Neurological Disorders

3.1. Alzheimer's Disease

AD is a chronic and serious neurodegenerative disease characterized by impairment of memory and cognitive function. In recent decades, the prevalence of AD has risen significantly [35,36]. It may have a huge effect and obstacles on the well-being and the ability to lead a healthy life by the affected patients [37,38]. The excessive accumulation of β-amyloid protein (Aβ) in the cerebral cortex and hippocampus is one of AD's main features [39]. Aβ contributes to oxidative stress production by forming reactive oxygen and nitrogen species [40]. Many adverse effects are related to oxidative stress production, including the formation of neurofibrillary tangles, inflammation, apoptosis, protein oxidation, and lipid peroxidation [41,42]. As a result of these disturbances, a reduction in cognitive functions can be developed in response to the significant damage of neural connections between the cerebral cortex and the hippocampus [43]. Many researchers have proposed antioxidants supplementation to prevent oxidative stress' adverse effects by enhancing the endogenous oxidative defense [44–46]. Previous studies have demonstrated the potential effective role that ASX might have in the management of AD. A previous study by Taksima et al. [47], where the authors used ASX powder obtained from shrimp shells (*Litopenaeus vannamei*), showed that Wistar rats with AD had significantly improved levels of their cognitive abilities. ASX has significantly enhanced spatial and non-spatial memory and reduced neurodegeneration, assessed by the object recognition test and Aβ plaque level [47]. It was thought that ASX might improve GPx activity, which was observed to be suppressed due to mitochondrial dysfunction and Aβ accumulation [47,48].

Moreover, ASX participates in reducing protein carbonyl and malondialdehyde (MDA) levels, which result from the destruction of polyunsaturated fatty acids by the reactive oxygen species (ROS) and act on inducing neuronal deterioration [49,50]. Likewise, the role of ASX in the elimination of superoxide anion has been reported [51]. In AD, many reports have linked the production of ROS and neuronal death due to the formation of senile plaques [52,53]. Compared to the vehicle-AD group, it has demonstrated a significant reduction in hippocampal and cortical neuronal loss in the oral ASX group [47,54]. In the same context, Che et al. [55] reported that after application of synthesized ASX, their double transgenic mice (APP/PS1) showed improved cognitive abilities by reducing neuroinflammation and the related oxidative distress, which is a major cause that can inaugurate the mechanism and impact the prognosis of AD [56,57]. A study has shown that the number of references and working memory errors has significantly reduced in APP/PS1 treated with ASX. Moreover, ASX has improved the APP/PS1 behavior, reduced the hippocampal and cortical Aβ numbers, and decreased the soluble and insoluble Aβ 40 and Aβ 42 levels [55]. These changes were accompanied by a significant elevation in the level of superoxide dismutase (SOD) and a significant decline in the nitric oxide (NO) and nitric oxide synthase (NOS) levels. Interestingly, it was reported that ASX might induce a significant suppression of p-Tau expression; however, it did not affect the regulation of p-GSK-3β expression [58]. ASX possesses a powerful anti-inflammatory activity that abolishes the expression of inflammatory mediators, including TNF-α, PGE2, and IL-1β, and inhibits the development of nitric oxide (NO) as well as the NF-κB-dependent signaling pathway [36,59].

Other studies have described similar anti-inflammatory effects of astaxanthin via using different laboratory models. ASX, at a dose of 50 μM, declined the release of inflammatory mediators in activated microglial (BV-2 cell line) cells via the regulation of NF-κB cascade factors (e.g., p-IKKα, p-IκBα, and p-NF-κB p65, IL-6, and MAPK) [60].

In terms of cytokines, ASX sub-retinally reduced the level of TNF-α but not IL-1β [55,61]. Furthermore, ASX has been reported to be effective in terms of apoptosis suppression in APP/PS1 mice, as it suppresses the expression of caspase-9 and caspase-3 proteins [55]. The favorable effects of ASX in decreasing any potentially present oxidative stress are owed to the capability to pass the blood–brain barrier, enabling it to perform its favorable effects. The exact mechanism explaining the anti-inflammatory actions of ASX is not well understood. However, many studies have reported some observations that might help understand it. A previous investigation by Wang et al. [62] reported that ASX significantly reduced oxidative stress and reduced the present ischemia, which occurred secondary to brain injury. Via the ERK1/2 pathway, ASX also induced the expression of the Ho-1 enzyme (which has antioxidant properties), reducing cell death and protecting neuroblastoma cells that were susceptible to injury [62]. The favorable effects of ASX were also demonstrated by Wen et al. [63], that showed the neuroprotective role that this compound plays in the hippocampal HT22 cells of their mice also by increasing the expression of Ho-1 antioxidant activities. Another mechanism for enhancing the cognitive ability in rats with AD is the inhibition of glutathione-induced cell death, which has been previously reported to take part in the prognosis and AD severity [64,65]. Moreover, ASX demonstrated the protective effects on mitochondria's double membrane system with boosting efficient energy production [9,66]. Specifically, ASX protected the mitochondria of cultured nerve cells from toxic attacks and increased mitochondrial activity through enhanced oxygen consumption without increased reactive oxygen species production [66–68], indicating its potential efficacy in the management and possible prevention of neurodegenerative diseases and neuroinflammation [9,69].

Hongo et al. [58] used a new AD model, the App^{NL-G-F} mice model, which is associated with mild memory decline, microglial formation, increased level of p-Tau, and accumulation of Aβ_{42} in the hippocampus. Their findings indicated that ASX significantly reduced the Aβ_{42} deposition, p-Tau, and Iba1 fraction. On the other hand, it increased the glutathione biosynthesis, leading to an increase in the hippocampal parvalbumin-positive-positive neuron density, which plays a significant role in gamma oscillation production [70]. According to a recent study, gamma oscillations' optogenetic or sensory activation led to the decline of Aβ peptides in the hippocampus of the AD mouse model (5XFAD mouse) due to microglial activation and the resulting increase in Aβ microglial uptake [71]. A reduction in the Iba1 fraction may be attributed to reducing Aβ42 precipitation in ASX-fed AppNL-G-F mice as microglia accumulate around Aβ deposition [72]. Regarding the effect of ASX on p-Tau, two pathways were suggested: the amyloid cascade theory and the autophagy-mediated degradation [73]. The p-Tau fraction was positively correlated with the Aβ42 fraction, which supports the amyloid cascade theory [58]. The promotion of nuclear factor erythroid 2-related factor 2 (Nrf2)/antioxidant response element (ARE) by ASX, resulting in reducing p-Tau, suggested the effect of ASX on the autophagy [74]. In AD-like model rats, which were induced using hydrated aluminum chloride (AlCl3.6H2O) solution, Hafez and her colleagues showed that ASX significantly reduced the disposition of Aβ1-42, the level of MDA, the activity of acetylcholinesterase and monoamine oxidase, and the expression of β-site amyloid precursor protein cleaving enzyme 1 (BACE1). Moreover, ASX significantly elevated the miRNA-124 expression, Nrf2 upregulation, and the content of serotonin and acetylcholine [75]. Figure 1 summarizes the aforementioned mechanisms of ASX in AD.

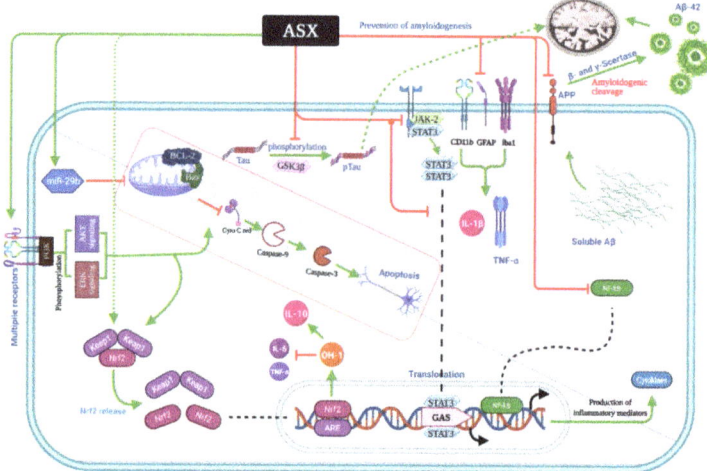

Figure 1. Astaxanthin mechanism of action in Alzheimer's disease. Aβ: Amyloid beta, APP: β-amyloid precursor protein, ASX: Astaxanthin, NF-κB: Nuclear factor-kappa B, TNF-α: Tumor necrosis factor-alpha, IL: Interleukin, Iba1: Ionized calcium-binding adaptor molecule 1, GFAP: Glial fibrillary acidic protein, STAT3: Signal transducer and activator of transcription 3, JAK2: Janus Kinase 2, GSK3β: Glycogen synthase kinase 3 beta, p-Tau: Phosphorylated tau, Bcl-2: B-cell lymphoma 2, Bax: Bcl-2-associated X protein, Nrf2: Nuclear factor erythroid 2-related factor 2, GAS: Glyoxylate, anapleurotic and succinyl CoA, OH: Hydroxide, Keap1: Kelch-like ECH-associated protein 1, Akt: Protein kinase B.

3.2. Parkinson's Disease

PD is the second most common neurodegenerative disorder [76]. It is age-related and is caused by oxidative stress and neuroinflammation [77]. The global prevalence of PD is estimated to be 0.1–0.2%, which increases with age (>80 years old) up to 3% [78,79]. PD occurs mainly due to the motor and non-motor dysfunctional disorders, which are attributable to loss of the dopaminergic neurons, the devastation of the non-dopaminergic ones, and the accumulation of the alpha-synuclein, which is the major component of Lewy bodies and plays a significant role in the development and progression of PD [80,81]. There are strong evidences that firstly, it affects the vagus nerve motor nucleus, the olfactory bulbs, and the nucleus, then the locus coeruleus, and thus, finally, the substantia nigra. Cortical regions of the brain at a later point are impaired. Damages to these particular neural structures are the result of numerous pathophysiological alterations that not only affect the engine system, but also neurological and neuropsychological systems [82]. Although many treatment modalities are currently approved for PD management, many adverse events have been associated, and therefore, many approaches have been made to discover novel multi-targeting modalities to treat PD properly. In the last decade, numerous miRNAs have been recognized and suggested as key gene expression regulators in human cells [83].

Almost all genes related to PD have been observed to be mediated by miRNAs, including alpha-synuclein (SNCA), LRRK2, and several transcription and growth factors [84]. MiR-7 was found to influence the SNCA accumulation and engaged with the PD etiology [85]. MiR-7 decreasing of the SN area was known as a therapeutic indicator of PD, not only involving SNCA accumulation but also dopaminergic neuron loss and miR-7 replacement therapy [86]. This was indicated by Shen et al. [87], who reported that ASX could decrease the previously induced stress in the endoplasmic reticulum by acting on the miR-7/SNCA axis to reduce the potential nerve damage that may be caused by PD. SNCA is the main gene that is usually responsible for the development and early initiation of PD. During the initiation and development of multiple neurodegenerative disorders like PD, miRNAs are presented spatially and temporally, suggesting that miRNAs play a key role in PD pathogenesis. In vivo, they also found that ASX has a potential protective effect against the neuron injury induced by 1-methyl-4-phenyl-1,2,3,6-tetrahydropyridine (MPTP) via a miR-7/SNCA axis. On the other hand, the favorable events of ASX were not reported in the animal study by Grimmig et al. [88] that reported that the compound's efficacy was limited in aged animals with PD as it was not able to counteract the toxicity of MPTP. However, they found that in both young and aged mice, the neuronal damage in the substantial nigra was prevented by ASX. Therefore, they suggested that any clinical recommendations for PD should take aging as an important factor. Previous studies have investigated the potential effects that modified ASX compounds might have on PD. These compounds include the docosahexaenoic acid (DHA)-acylated ASX ester and ASX in combination with the non-esterified ASX and DHA.

Evidence shows that the first compound's efficacy was significantly better than the latter one in reducing the development of MPTP-induced PD in mice [89]. Wang et al. [89] also proved that DHA-ASX could significantly reduce the progression of PD by reducing the apoptotic phenomena of the dopamine neurons by acting through the P38 MAPK and JNK pathway (Figure 2). Although the three ASX-derived compounds showed favorable events in reducing oxidative stress, DHA-ASX was the only significant compound that can limit PD progression by reducing cell apoptosis. A previous study also indicated ASX's ability to inhibit the activities of the mitogen-activated protein kinase and P13K/AKT, which might favor its actions on many neurological diseases, such as PD [90]. Moreover, it has been indicated that ASX also has anti-oxidative stress that is attributable to MPP mechanisms in PC12 cells by acting through the NOX2/HO-1 and NR1/SP1 pathways [91,92]. Previous studies indicated the favorable events of ASX that showed that ASX administration is associated with decreased reactive oxygen species synthesis, reduced mitochondrial dysfunction, and reduced cellular apoptosis [93,94].

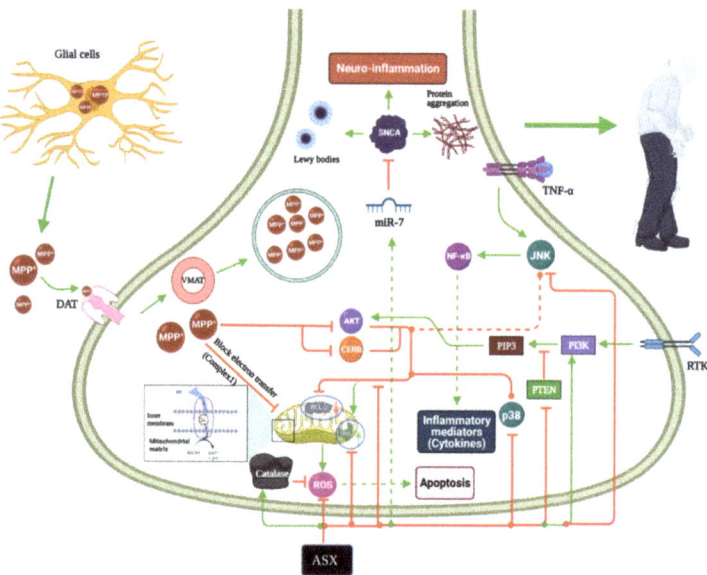

Figure 2. Astaxanthin mechanism of action in Parkinson's disease. NF-κB: Nuclear factor-kappa B, TNF-α: Tumor necrosis factor-alpha, Akt: Protein kinase B, ASX: Astaxanthin, ROS: Reactive oxygen species, RTK: Receptor tyrosine kinase, PIP3: Phosphatidylinositol-3,4,5-triphosphate, PI3K: Phosphatidylinositol 3-kinase, JNK: c-Jun N-terminal kinase, CREB: cAMP Response Element-Binding Protein, PTEN: Phosphatase and tensin homolog deleted on chromosome 10, MPTP: 1-methyl-4-phenyl-1,2,3,6-tetrahydropyridine, VMAT: Vesicular monoamine transporter, DAT: Dopamine transporter, SNCA: Alpha-synuclein.

3.3. Neuropathic Pain and Central Nervous System Injuries

Neuropathic pain develops when a disorder or an injury occurs within the somatosensory pathway, stimulating the underlying affected neurons [95]. Neuropathic pain development was previously explained by many mechanisms and pathways, mainly dependent on the effector mediator. Many inflammatory mediators, such as prostaglandins, cytokines, and reactive oxygen species, in addition to the neuromodulators, which mainly include glutamate, have been frequently observed in such painful events [96–99]. These factors can cause pain through apoptosis, neuron firing, and impacting many structures and processes, such as microglia, astrocytes, and ion currents [100]. Although many treatment modalities can be used to manage neuropathic pain, approaching to obtain favorable modalities that may have more advantages is essential to enhance the quality of care. One of the treatment modalities that has shown successful results recently is counteracting the neuroinflammatory process. Gugliandolo et al. [101] found that reversing the neuroinflammation was protective against peripheral nerve injury and neuropathic pain in an experimental study. In terms of experimental studies on ASX, Keudo et al. [51] reported that favorable effects of reducing pain in carrageenan-induced pain and edema in mice were significantly associated with ASX that was also obtained from *Litopenaeus vannamei* and was efficacious in reducing the painful sensations and inflammation. Sharma et al. [102] supported this by concluding that ASX reduced the oxidative stress that resulted in behavioral and chemical alternations in vivo and in vitro experiments, where the objects suffered from induced neuropathic pain.

Moreover, the effective anti-inflammatory effects of ASX were further proven by its ability to reduce chronic pain by reducing the potential thermal hyperalgesia and the possible presence of depressive symptoms in the affected mice [103]. Another report by Fakhri et al. [104] showed that ASX is able to significantly inhibit ERK1/2 and activate protein kinase B (AKT), which, in turn, are responsible for initiating chemical and thermal painful sensations. Another potential mechanism of ASX actions is that it blocks the inflammatory signaling and reduces the associated mediators as glutamatergic-phospo-p38-mitogen-activated protein kinase (p-p38MAPK) and NR2B [105]. Long-standing exposure of neurons to glutamate contributes to cell death [106]. There are many adverse effects attributed to the neuronal exposure to glutamate, including neuronal damage triggered by L-glutamate, retinal ganglion cells death due to glutamate stress, and cytotoxicity of HT22 cells, which is mediated by mitochondrial dysfunction, inactivation of caspase, and dysregulation of the AKT/GSK-3b signaling pathway [107–110]. Fortunately, ASX provides neuroprotective effects against all of these adverse effects. In cases of spinal cord injury (SCI), it is known that NMDARs subunits like NMDARs 2B (NR2B) and glutamate participate in the neuropathy pain pathway [99,111]. NR2B is a cation channel that is essential for many forms of synaptic plasticity and mediates the neurotransmission of glutamate and many other aspects of development and synaptic transmission in neuropathy pain [112].

However, NR2B activation can be toxic for the spinal cord. It has been proposed that ASX participates in reducing neuropathic pain by inhibiting the glutamate-initiated signaling pathway through decreasing the expression of NR2B and p-p38MAPK [2,105,113]. Moreover, ASX inhibits the MIF, p-p38MAPK, p-ERK, and AKT pathways and stimulates the p-AKT and ERK pathways [114]. MIF upregulates NR2B; therefore, it can be considered a major mediator of neuropathic pain, and it has been shown by several cell lines in the peripheral and central nervous system, especially within cells located in sensory transmission regions [115]. Furthermore, in response to tissue damage and stress, it is dramatically elevated, often reaching concentrations about 1000 times higher than other cytokines causing pain [116]. In general, in view of its antioxidant, anti-inflammation, and anti-apoptotic mechanisms, ASX may be considered a new prospect for lowering neuropathic pain in animal models. The reduction of NR2B and MIF, which are very significant in the occurrence of neuropathic pain after SCI, may be partly involved (Figure 3).

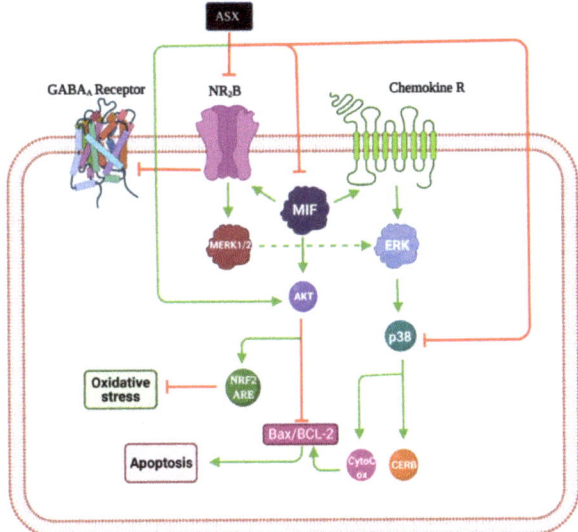

Figure 3. Astaxanthin mechanism of action in neuropathic pain. Bcl-2: B-cell lymphoma 2, Bax: Bcl-2-associated X protein, Nrf2: Nuclear factor erythroid 2-related factor 2, Akt: Protein kinase B, ASX: astaxanthin, CREB: cAMP Response element-binding protein, MERK: Mitogen-extracellular signal-regulated kinases, MIF: Macrophage migration inhibitory factor, NR2B: N-methyl D-aspartate receptor subtype 2B, GABA: Gamma-aminobutyric acid.

3.4. Autism

The prevalence of autism has recently increased, with many social, behavioral, and communicational burdens over the affected patients and the surrounding individuals [117–119]. In addition to having many neurodegenerative events being involved in its mechanism [120–122], autism is also associated with increased levels and frequencies of synthesis and release of various proinflammatory mediators [123]. Gastrointestinal (GI) symptoms are common among autism patients. The gut microbiota regulates neuropsychological functions, intestinal homeostasis, and functional GI disturbances through the microbiota-gut-brain axis [124]. Moreover, previous studies have suggested that patients with autism might have an underlying degree of oxidative stress [125–128]. Consequently, previous studies have demonstrated that ASX might have a potential role in reducing the inflammatory state and oxidative stress that might be present in autistic patients [129,130]. Furthermore, it was believed that ASX could significantly reduce bacterial loads and attenuate gastric inflammation in mice infected with H. pylori, and increase the production of IgA antibody-secreting cells in the small intestine of mice. Therefore, ASX could have a potential in the prevention or treatment of dysbiosis and its associated diseases like autism, AD, and PD [131].

Fernández et al. [132] previously suggested the administration of carotenoids as routine food in patients with autism to reduce the potential oxidative stress and inflammatory state. Al-Amin et al. [133] also reported that ASX reduced the actions of catalase activities, restricted lipid peroxidation, and reduced the levels of nitric oxide, which are involved in developing oxidative stress. This has led to a significant enhancement in the assessed behavioral parameters and a significant increase in the assessed paw withdrawal latency in the studied mice that suffered from autism, secondary to valproic-acid induction [133].

3.5. Cerebral Ischemia

Prolonged cerebral ischemia can lead to the development of irreversible adverse events. Previous investigations demonstrated a potential impact of ASX carotenoid for reducing the severity of cerebral ischemia and potentiating the chances of brain tissue recovery. Xue et al. [134] reported that ASX was significantly able to reduce ischemia and improve the cognitive and learning abilities in their model of mice that were subjected to repeated cerebral ischemia by reducing apoptosis and hippocampal damage. Some mechanisms can explain the prevention of brain disorders by ASX by enhancing reperfusion rates following ischemia. These include activation of the Nrf2–ARE pathway, reducing the reactive oxygen species levels, reducing apoptosis, and enhancing nerve regeneration [135].

Moreover, evidence shows that ASX possesses an essential role in providing the necessary oxygenation for the apoptotic brain tissue through the GSK3β/PI3K/Nrf2/Akt pathways [136]. Wang et al. [135] confirmed this by indicating that ASX was able to enhance the prognosis and motor functions through the cAMP/protein kinase A (PKA)/cAMP response element-binding protein (CREB). Previous studies also showed that ASX has protective roles in acute cerebral infarctions and brain injury [137,138].

4. Potential of Astaxanthin in Counteracting Neuroinflammation

A huge body of literature supports the role of ASX in preventing neuroinflammation, which makes it a potential candidate for further testing in various neurological disorders, where neuroinflammation plays a key role in disease pathology and progression, including AD, PD, nerve injury, cerebral ischemia, and autism.

For example, Che et al. [55] reported improved cognitive abilities in AD transgenic mice by reducing neuroinflammation and the related oxidative distress [56,57], and Kidd et al. [9] reported similar favorable results on the mitochondria and microcirculation [69]. Gugliandolo et al. [101] also reported that reversing the neuroinflammation was effective in protecting against peripheral nerve injury and neuropathic pain. Similarly, counteracting the neuroinflammation has recently been shown to improve recovery in Parkinson's disease experimental models [139]. Impellizzeri et al. also reported that reversing the neuroinflammation was an alternative strategy for the treatment of cerebral ischemia and particularly for vascular dementia.

Based on the aforementioned ASX mechanisms of actions, the promising findings in experimental studies, and the fact that neuroinflammation plays a key role in AD, PD, nerve injury, cerebral ischemia, and autism, we support the advancement of this neurotherapeutic candidate to further testing in clinical trials.

5. Safety of Astaxanthin

Many studies reported that ASX is safe and has no side effects or toxic effects when accumulating in animal or human tissues [26]. However, excessive consumption of ASX may lead to altering the pigmentation of the skin of animals [24]. The accumulation of ASX was also observed in the eyes of the rats [140]. Administration of ASX was associated with increased antioxidant enzymes and reduced blood pressure in hypertensive rats [141]. As a feed additive, the United States Food and Drug Administration (FDA) approved ASX at up to 80 mg/kg, while the European Food Safety Authority (EFSA) approved up to 100 mg/kg [142].

In terms of daily intake, it was reported that 0.034 mg/kg/day of natural ASX is the acceptable daily intake in humans [143]. However, recent clinical trials reported favorable outcomes with higher doses up to 8 mg per day or even higher [144,145]. In a safety report, the investigators have assessed more than 80 clinical trials to detect the side effects and safety concerns of ASX [146]. Their findings highlighted that there were no serious adverse effects reported in any one of the evaluated studies, even in the studies that administrated high doses of ASX (up to 45 mg) [147]. Some mild adverse events such as increased frequency of bowel movements were reported [148]. Moreover, there was no detectable change in the liver parameters [149].

6. Conclusions

ASX, a ketocarotenoid extracted from marine carotenoids, provides various health benefits in a wide variety of diseases. As a multi-target neuroprotective agent, ASX tackles neurodegenerative diseases' pathophysiology through antioxidant, anti-inflammatory, and anti-apoptotic mechanisms. Moreover, through its fat-soluble properties, ASX would be able to effectively pass through the blood–brain barrier. Therefore, ASX seems to be an excellent candidate for more evaluation of the neuroprotective properties, which would eventually result in ASX becoming a novel neurotherapeutic agent. Although the current evidence supports the neuroprotective pharmacological effects of ASX, there is a lack of an effective drug delivery system in the previous studies. Therefore, future clinical trials should be conducted to examine the possible delivery methods. Moreover, there is a need to further investigate the precise pathophysiological pathways involved in neurodegeneration and the possible neuroprotective mechanisms of ASX in humans.

Author Contributions: This work was carried out in collaboration with all authors. All authors have read and agreed to the published version of the manuscript.

Funding: This work was funded by the Deanship of Scientific Research at Princess Nourah bint Abdulrahman University, through the Fast-track Research Funding Program.

Acknowledgments: This work was funded by the Deanship of Scientific Research at Princess Nourah bint Abdulrahman University, through the Fast-track Research Funding Program. Authors are also thankful to BioRender for making figures.

Conflicts of Interest: The authors declare no conflict of interest.

References

1. Maoka, T. Carotenoids in marine animals. *Mar. Drugs* **2011**, *9*, 278–293. [CrossRef]
2. Attal, N.; Cruccu, G.; Baron, R.; Haanpää, M.; Hansson, P.; Jensen, T.S.; Nurmikko, T. EFNS guidelines on the pharmacological treatment of neuropathic pain: 2010 revision. *Eur. J. Neurol.* **2010**, *17*, e1113–e1188. [CrossRef]

3. Galasso, C.; Corinaldesi, C.; Sansone, C. Carotenoids from Marine Organisms: Biological Functions and Industrial Applications. *Antioxidants* **2017**, *6*. [CrossRef]
4. Chuyen, H.V.; Eun, J.B. Marine carotenoids: Bioactivities and potential benefits to human health. *Crit. Rev. Food Sci. Nutr.* **2017**, *57*, 2600–2610. [CrossRef]
5. Maoka, T.; Akimoto, N.; Tsushima, M.; Komemushi, S.; Mezaki, T.; Iwase, F.; Takahashi, Y.; Sameshima, N.; Mori, M.; Sakagami, Y. Carotenoids in marine invertebrates living along the Kuroshio current coast. *Mar. Drugs* **2011**, *9*, 1419–1427. [CrossRef] [PubMed]
6. Brotosudarmo, T.H.P.; Limantara, L.; Setiyono, E.; Heriyanto. Structures of Astaxanthin and Their Consequences for Therapeutic Application. *Int. J. Food Sci.* **2020**, *2020*, 2156612. [CrossRef]
7. Phaniendra, A.; Jestadi, D.B.; Periyasamy, L. Free radicals: Properties, sources, targets, and their implication in various diseases. *Indian J. Clin. Biochem. IJCB* **2015**, *30*, 11–26. [CrossRef] [PubMed]
8. Davinelli, S.; Nielsen, M.E.; Scapagnini, G. Astaxanthin in Skin Health, Repair, and Disease: A Comprehensive Review. *Nutrients* **2018**, *10*, 522. [CrossRef] [PubMed]
9. Kidd, P. Astaxanthin, cell membrane nutrient with diverse clinical benefits and anti-aging potential. *Altern. Med. Rev. A J. Clin. Ther.* **2011**, *16*, 355–364.
10. Mezzomo, N.; Ferreira, S.R.S. Carotenoids Functionality, Sources, and Processing by Supercritical Technology: A Review. *J. Chem.* **2016**, *2016*, 3164312. [CrossRef]
11. Zhang, C.; Chen, X.; Too, H.P. Microbial astaxanthin biosynthesis: Recent achievements, challenges, and commercialization outlook. *Appl. Microbiol. Biotechnol.* **2020**, *104*, 5725–5737. [CrossRef]
12. Mularczyk, M.; Michalak, I.; Marycz, K. Astaxanthin and other Nutrients from *Haematococcus pluvialis*-Multifunctional Applications. *Mar. Drugs* **2020**, *18*. [CrossRef] [PubMed]
13. Khoo, K.S.; Lee, S.Y.; Ooi, C.W.; Fu, X.; Miao, X.; Ling, T.C.; Show, P.L. Recent advances in biorefinery of astaxanthin from Haematococcus pluvialis. *Bioresour. Technol.* **2019**, *288*, 121606. [CrossRef] [PubMed]
14. Shah, M.M.; Liang, Y.; Cheng, J.J.; Daroch, M. Astaxanthin-Producing Green Microalga Haematococcus pluvialis: From Single Cell to High Value Commercial Products. *Front. Plant Sci.* **2016**, *7*, 531. [CrossRef] [PubMed]
15. Higuera-Ciapara, I.; Félix-Valenzuela, L.; Goycoolea, F.M. Astaxanthin: A review of its chemistry and applications. *Crit. Rev. Food Sci. Nutr.* **2006**, *46*, 185–196. [CrossRef]
16. Martín, J.F.; Gudiña, E.; Barredo, J.L. Conversion of beta-carotene into astaxanthin: Two separate enzymes or a bifunctional hydroxylase-ketolase protein? *Microb. Cell Factories* **2008**, *7*, 3. [CrossRef]
17. Sztretye, M.; Dienes, B.; Gönczi, M.; Czirják, T.; Csernoch, L.; Dux, L.; Szentesi, P.; Keller-Pintér, A. Astaxanthin: A Potential Mitochondrial-Targeted Antioxidant Treatment in Diseases and with Aging. *Oxid. Med. Cell. Longev.* **2019**, *2019*, 3849692. [CrossRef]
18. Fakhri, S.; Abbaszadeh, F.; Dargahi, L.; Jorjani, M. Astaxanthin: A mechanistic review on its biological activities and health benefits. *Pharmacol. Res.* **2018**, *136*, 1–20. [CrossRef] [PubMed]
19. Ambati, R.R.; Phang, S.M.; Ravi, S.; Aswathanarayana, R.G. Astaxanthin: Sources, extraction, stability, biological activities and its commercial applications–a review. *Mar. Drugs* **2014**, *12*, 128–152. [CrossRef]
20. Yuan, J.P.; Peng, J.; Yin, K.; Wang, J.H. Potential health-promoting effects of astaxanthin: A high-value carotenoid mostly from microalgae. *Mol. Nutr. Food Res.* **2011**, *55*, 150–165. [CrossRef]
21. Wang, M.; Deng, X.; Xie, Y.; Chen, Y. Astaxanthin Attenuates Neuroinflammation in Status Epilepticus Rats by Regulating the ATP-P2X7R Signal. *Drug Des. Dev. Ther.* **2020**, *14*, 1651–1662. [CrossRef] [PubMed]
22. Xu, L.; Zhu, J.; Yin, W.; Ding, X. Astaxanthin improves cognitive deficits from oxidative stress, nitric oxide synthase and inflammation through upregulation of PI3K/Akt in diabetes rat. *Int. J. Clin. Exp. Pathol.* **2015**, *8*, 6083–6094.
23. Lu, Y.; Wang, X.; Feng, J.; Xie, T.; Si, P.; Wang, W. Neuroprotective effect of astaxanthin on newborn rats exposed to prenatal maternal seizures. *Brain Res. Bull.* **2019**, *148*, 63–69. [CrossRef] [PubMed]
24. Barros, M.P.; Marin, D.P.; Bolin, A.P.; de Cássia Santos Macedo, R.; Campoio, T.R.; Fineto, C., Jr.; Guerra, B.A.; Polotow, T.G.; Vardaris, C.; Mattei, R.; et al. Combined astaxanthin and fish oil supplementation improves glutathione-based redox balance in rat plasma and neutrophils. *Chem. Biol. Interact.* **2012**, *197*, 58–67. [CrossRef] [PubMed]
25. Ranga Rao, A.; Raghunath Reddy, R.L.; Baskaran, V.; Sarada, R.; Ravishankar, G.A. Characterization of microalgal carotenoids by mass spectrometry and their bioavailability and antioxidant properties elucidated in rat model. *J. Agric. Food Chem.* **2010**, *58*, 8553–8559. [CrossRef] [PubMed]
26. Rao, A.R.; Sindhuja, H.N.; Dharmesh, S.M.; Sankar, K.U.; Sarada, R.; Ravishankar, G.A. Effective inhibition of skin cancer, tyrosinase, and antioxidative properties by astaxanthin and astaxanthin esters from the green alga Haematococcus pluvialis. *J. Agric. Food Chem.* **2013**, *61*, 3842–3851. [CrossRef]
27. Otton, R.; Marin, D.P.; Bolin, A.P.; De Cássia Santos Macedo, R.; Campoio, T.R.; Fineto, C., Jr.; Guerra, B.A.; Leite, J.R.; Barros, M.P.; Mattei, R. Combined fish oil and astaxanthin supplementation modulates rat lymphocyte function. *Eur. J. Nutr.* **2012**, *51*, 707–718. [CrossRef]
28. Page, G.I.; Davies, S.J. Astaxanthin and canthaxanthin do not induce liver or kidney xenobiotic-metabolizing enzymes in rainbow trout (Oncorhynchus mykiss Walbaum). *Comp. Biochem. Physiology. Toxicol. Pharmacol. CBP* **2002**, *133*, 443–451. [CrossRef]
29. Olson, J.A. Absorption, transport and metabolism of carotenoids in humans. *Pure Appl. Chem.* **1994**, *66*, 1011–1016. [CrossRef]

30. Okada, Y.; Ishikura, M.; Maoka, T. Bioavailability of astaxanthin in Haematococcus algal extract: The effects of timing of diet and smoking habits. *Biosci. Biotechnol. Biochem.* **2009**, *73*, 1928–1932. [CrossRef]
31. Kelly, G.S. The interaction of cigarette smoking and antioxidants. Part I: Diet and carotenoids. *Altern. Med. Rev. A J. Clin. Ther.* **2002**, *7*, 370–388.
32. Kvaavik, E.; Totland, T.H.; Bastani, N.; Kjøllesdal, M.K.; Tell, G.S.; Andersen, L.F. Do smoking and fruit and vegetable intake mediate the association between socio-economic status and plasma carotenoids? *Eur. J. Public Health* **2014**, *24*, 685–690. [CrossRef]
33. Østerlie, M.; Bjerkeng, B.; Liaaen-Jensen, S. Plasma appearance and distribution of astaxanthin E/Z and R/S isomers in plasma lipoproteins of men after single dose administration of astaxanthin. *J. Nutr. Biochem.* **2000**, *11*, 482–490. [CrossRef]
34. Mercke Odeberg, J.; Lignell, A.; Pettersson, A.; Höglund, P. Oral bioavailability of the antioxidant astaxanthin in humans is enhanced by incorporation of lipid based formulations. *Eur. J. Pharm. Sci. Off. J. Eur. Fed. Pharm. Sci.* **2003**, *19*, 299–304. [CrossRef]
35. Karlawish, J.; Jack, C.R., Jr.; Rocca, W.A.; Snyder, H.M.; Carrillo, M.C. Alzheimer's disease: The next frontier-Special Report. *Alzheimer's Dement.* **2017**, *13*, 374–380. [CrossRef]
36. Uddin, M.S.; Kabir, M..T.; Rahman, M..S.; Behl, T.; Jeandet, P.; Ashraf, G.M.; Najda, A.; Bin-Jumah, M.N.; El-Seedi, H.R.; Abdel-Daim, M.M. Revisiting the Amyloid Cascade Hypothesis: From Anti-Aβ Therapeutics to Auspicious New Ways for Alzheimer's Disease. *Int. J. Mol. Sci.* **2020**, *21*, 5858. [CrossRef]
37. Sayed, A.; Bahbah, E.I.; Kamel, S.; Barreto, G.E.; Ashraf, G.M.; Elfil, M. The neutrophil-to-lymphocyte ratio in Alzheimer's disease: Current understanding and potential applications. *J. Neuroimmunol.* **2020**, *349*, 577398. [CrossRef] [PubMed]
38. Bahbah, E.I.; Fathy, S.; Negida, A. Is Alzheimer's disease linked to Herpes simplex virus type 1 infection? A mini-review of the molecular correlation and the possible disease connections. *Clin. Exp. Neuroimmunol.* **2019**, *10*, 192–196. [CrossRef]
39. Uddin, M.S.; Kabir, M.T.; Tewari, D.; Mamun, A.A.; Mathew, B.; Aleya, L.; Barreto, G.E.; Bin-Jumah, M.N.; Abdel-Daim, M.M.; Ashraf, G.M. Revisiting the role of brain and peripheral Aβ in the pathogenesis of Alzheimer's disease. *J. Neurol. Sci.* **2020**, *416*, 116974. [CrossRef]
40. Butterfield, D.A.; Swomley, A.M.; Sultana, R. Amyloid β-peptide (1-42)-induced oxidative stress in Alzheimer disease: Importance in disease pathogenesis and progression. *Antioxid. Redox Signal.* **2013**, *19*, 823–835. [CrossRef]
41. Elhelaly, A.E.; AlBasher, G.; Alfarraj, S.; Almeer, R.; Bahbah, E.I.; Fouda, M.M.A.; Bungau, S.G.; Aleya, L.; Abdel-Daim, M.M. Protective effects of hesperidin and diosmin against acrylamide-induced liver, kidney, and brain oxidative damage in rats. *Environ. Sci. Pollut Res. Int.* **2019**, *26*, 35151–35162. [CrossRef] [PubMed]
42. Abdel-Daim, M.M.; Abushouk, A.I.; Bahbah, E.I.; Bungau, S.G.; Alyousif, M.S.; Aleya, L.; Alkahtani, S. Fucoidan protects against subacute diazinon-induced oxidative damage in cardiac, hepatic, and renal tissues. *Env. Sci. Pollut. Res. Int.* **2020**, *27*, 11554–11564. [CrossRef]
43. Bui, T.T.; Nguyen, T.H. Natural product for the treatment of Alzheimer's disease. *J. Basic Clin. Physiol. Pharmacol.* **2017**, *28*, 413–423. [CrossRef] [PubMed]
44. Nakajima, A.; Ohizumi, Y. Potential Benefits of Nobiletin, A Citrus Flavonoid, against Alzheimer's Disease and Parkinson's Disease. *Int. J. Mol. Sci.* **2019**, *20*. [CrossRef]
45. Hatziagapiou, K.; Kakouri, E.; Lambrou, G.I.; Bethanis, K.; Tarantilis, P.A. Antioxidant Properties of Crocus Sativus L. and Its Constituents and Relevance to Neurodegenerative Diseases; Focus on Alzheimer's and Parkinson's Disease. *Curr. Neuropharmacol.* **2019**, *17*, 377–402. [CrossRef]
46. Wojsiat, J.; Zoltowska, K.M.; Laskowska-Kaszub, K.; Wojda, U. Oxidant/Antioxidant Imbalance in Alzheimer's Disease: Therapeutic and Diagnostic Prospects. *Oxidative Med. Cell. Longev.* **2018**, *2018*, 6435861. [CrossRef] [PubMed]
47. Taksima, T.; Chonpathompikunlert, P.; Sroyraya, M.; Hutamekalin, P.; Limpawattana, M.; Klaypradit, W. Effects of Astaxanthin from Shrimp Shell on Oxidative Stress and Behavior in Animal Model of Alzheimer's Disease. *Mar. Drugs* **2019**, *17*. [CrossRef]
48. Shichiri, M. The role of lipid peroxidation in neurological disorders. *J. Clin. Biochem. Nutr.* **2014**, *54*, 151–160. [CrossRef]
49. Hritcu, L.; Noumedem, J.A.; Cioanca, O.; Hancianu, M.; Kuete, V.; Mihasan, M. Methanolic extract of Piper nigrum fruits improves memory impairment by decreasing brain oxidative stress in amyloid beta(1-42) rat model of Alzheimer's disease. *Cell. Mol. Neurobiol.* **2014**, *34*, 437–449. [CrossRef]
50. Dalle-Donne, I.; Rossi, R.; Giustarini, D.; Milzani, A.; Colombo, R. Protein carbonyl groups as biomarkers of oxidative stress. *Clin. Chim. Acta Int. J. Clin. Chem.* **2003**, *329*, 23–38. [CrossRef]
51. Kuedo, Z.; Sangsuriyawong, A.; Klaypradit, W.; Tipmanee, V.; Chonpathompikunlert, P. Effects of Astaxanthin from Litopenaeus Vannamei on Carrageenan-Induced Edema and Pain Behavior in Mice. *Molecules* **2016**, *21*, 382. [CrossRef] [PubMed]
52. Zhang, Y.Y.; Fan, Y.C.; Wang, M.; Wang, D.; Li, X.H. Atorvastatin attenuates the production of IL-1β, IL-6, and TNF-α in the hippocampus of an amyloid β1-42-induced rat model of Alzheimer's disease. *Clin. Interv. Aging* **2013**, *8*, 103–110. [PubMed]
53. Asadbegi, M.; Yaghmaei, P.; Salehi, I.; Komaki, A.; Ebrahim-Habibi, A. Investigation of thymol effect on learning and memory impairment induced by intrahippocampal injection of amyloid beta peptide in high fat diet- fed rats. *Metab. Brain Dis.* **2017**, *32*, 827–839. [CrossRef] [PubMed]
54. Rahman, S.O.; Panda, B.P.; Parvez, S.; Kaundal, M.; Hussain, S.; Akhtar, M.; Najmi, A.K. Neuroprotective role of astaxanthin in hippocampal insulin resistance induced by Aβ peptides in animal model of Alzheimer's disease. *Biomed. Pharmacother. Biomed. Pharmacother.* **2019**, *110*, 47–58. [CrossRef]

55. Che, H.; Li, Q.; Zhang, T.; Wang, D.; Yang, L.; Xu, J.; Yanagita, T.; Xue, C.; Chang, Y.; Wang, Y. Effects of Astaxanthin and Docosahexaenoic-Acid-Acylated Astaxanthin on Alzheimer's Disease in APP/PS1 Double-Transgenic Mice. *J. Agric. Food Chem.* **2018**, *66*, 4948–4957. [CrossRef]
56. Kim, H.A.; Miller, A.A.; Drummond, G.R.; Thrift, A.G.; Arumugam, T.V.; Phan, T.G.; Srikanth, V.K.; Sobey, C.G. Vascular cognitive impairment and Alzheimer's disease: Role of cerebral hypoperfusion and oxidative stress. *Naunyn-Schmiedeberg's Arch. Pharmacol.* **2012**, *385*, 953–959. [CrossRef]
57. Padurariu, M.; Ciobica, A.; Lefter, R.; Serban, I.L.; Stefanescu, C.; Chirita, R. The oxidative stress hypothesis in Alzheimer's disease. *Psychiatr. Danub.* **2013**, *25*, 401–409.
58. Hongo, N.; Takamura, Y.; Nishimaru, H.; Matsumoto, J.; Tobe, K.; Saito, T.; Saido, T.C.; Nishijo, H. Astaxanthin Ameliorated Parvalbumin-Positive Neuron Deficits and Alzheimer's Disease-Related Pathological Progression in the Hippocampus of App(NL-G-F/NL-G-F) Mice. *Front. Pharmacol.* **2020**, *11*, 307. [CrossRef]
59. Solomonov, Y.; Hadad, N.; Levy, R. The Combined Anti-Inflammatory Effect of Astaxanthin, Lyc-O-Mato and Carnosic Acid In Vitro and In Vivo in a Mouse Model of Peritonitis. *J. Nutr. Food Sci.* **2018**, *8*. [CrossRef]
60. Kim, Y.H.; Koh Hk Fau-Kim, D.-S.; Kim, D.S. Down-regulation of IL-6 production by astaxanthin via ERK-, MSK-, and NF-κB-mediated signals in activated microglia. *Int. Immunopharmacol.* **2010**, *10*, 1560–1572. [CrossRef]
61. Landon, R.; Gueguen, V.; Petite, H.; Letourneur, D.; Pavon-Djavid, G.; Anagnostou, F. Impact of Astaxanthin on Diabetes Pathogenesis and Chronic Complications. *Mar. Drugs* **2020**, *18*, 357. [CrossRef]
62. Wang, H.Q.; Sun, X.B.; Xu, Y.X.; Zhao, H.; Zhu, Q.Y.; Zhu, C.Q. Astaxanthin upregulates heme oxygenase-1 expression through ERK1/2 pathway and its protective effect against beta-amyloid-induced cytotoxicity in SH-SY5Y cells. *Brain Res.* **2010**, *1360*, 159–167. [CrossRef] [PubMed]
63. Wen, X.; Huang, A.; Hu, J.; Zhong, Z.; Liu, Y.; Li, Z.; Pan, X.; Liu, Z. Neuroprotective effect of astaxanthin against glutamate-induced cytotoxicity in HT22 cells: Involvement of the Akt/GSK-3β pathway. *Neuroscience* **2015**, *303*, 558–568. [CrossRef] [PubMed]
64. Kim, G.H.; Kim, J.E.; Rhie, S.J.; Yoon, S. The Role of Oxidative Stress in Neurodegenerative Diseases. *Exp. Neurobiol.* **2015**, *24*, 325–340. [CrossRef]
65. Zhang, Y.; Wang, W.; Hao, C.; Mao, X.; Zhang, L. Astaxanthin protects PC12 cells from glutamate-induced neurotoxicity through multiple signaling pathways. *J. Funct. Foods* **2015**, *16*, 137–151. [CrossRef]
66. Wolf, A.M.; Asoh, S.; Hiranuma, H.; Ohsawa, I.; Iio, K.; Satou, A.; Ishikura, M.; Ohta, S. Astaxanthin protects mitochondrial redox state and functional integrity against oxidative stress. *J. Nutr. Biochem.* **2010**, *21*, 381–389. [CrossRef] [PubMed]
67. Lu, Y.P.; Liu, S.Y.; Sun, H.; Wu, X.M.; Li, J.J.; Zhu, L. Neuroprotective effect of astaxanthin on H(2)O(2)-induced neurotoxicity in vitro and on focal cerebral ischemia in vivo. *Brain Res.* **2010**, *1360*, 40–48. [CrossRef]
68. Kim, J.H.; Choi, W.; Lee, J.H.; Jeon, S.J.; Choi, Y.H.; Kim, B.W.; Chang, H.I.; Nam, S.W. Astaxanthin inhibits H2O2-mediated apoptotic cell death in mouse neural progenitor cells via modulation of P38 and MEK signaling pathways. *J. Microbiol. Biotechnol.* **2009**, *19*, 1355–1363. [CrossRef] [PubMed]
69. Barros, M.P.; Poppe, S.C.; Bondan, E.F. Neuroprotective properties of the marine carotenoid astaxanthin and omega-3 fatty acids, and perspectives for the natural combination of both in krill oil. *Nutrients* **2014**, *6*, 1293–1317. [CrossRef]
70. Nakamura, T.; Matsumoto, J.; Takamura, Y.; Ishii, Y.; Sasahara, M.; Ono, T.; Nishijo, H. Relationships among parvalbumin-immunoreactive neuron density, phase-locked gamma oscillations, and autistic/schizophrenic symptoms in PDGFR-β knock-out and control mice. *PLoS ONE* **2015**, *10*, e0119258. [CrossRef]
71. Iaccarino, H.F.; Singer, A.C.; Martorell, A.J.; Rudenko, A.; Gao, F.; Gillingham, T.Z.; Mathys, H.; Seo, J.; Kritskiy, O.; Abdurrob, F.; et al. Gamma frequency entrainment attenuates amyloid load and modifies microglia. *Nature* **2016**, *540*, 230–235. [CrossRef] [PubMed]
72. Hellwig, S.; Masuch, A.; Nestel, S.; Katzmarski, N.; Meyer-Luehmann, M.; Biber, K. Forebrain microglia from wild-type but not adult 5xFAD mice prevent amyloid-β plaque formation in organotypic hippocampal slice cultures. *Sci. Rep.* **2015**, *5*, 14624. [CrossRef]
73. Zhu, X.; Chen, Y.; Chen, Q.; Yang, H.; Xie, X. Astaxanthin Promotes Nrf2/ARE Signaling to Alleviate Renal Fibronectin and Collagen IV Accumulation in Diabetic Rats. *J. Diabetes Res.* **2018**, *2018*, 6730315. [CrossRef]
74. Jo, C.; Gundemir, S.; Pritchard, S.; Jin, Y.N.; Rahman, I.; Johnson, G.V. Nrf2 reduces levels of phosphorylated tau protein by inducing autophagy adaptor protein NDP52. *Nat. Commun.* **2014**, *5*, 3496. [CrossRef]
75. Hafez, H.A.; Kamel, M.A.; Osman, M.Y.; Osman, H.M.; Elblehi, S.S.; Mahmoud, S.A. Ameliorative effects of astaxanthin on brain tissues of alzheimer's disease-like model: Cross talk between neuronal-specific microRNA-124 and related pathways. *Mol. Cell. Biochem.* **2021**. [CrossRef]
76. Shalash, A.S.; Hamid, E.; Elrassas, H.; Bahbah, E.I.; Mansour, A.H.; Mohamed, H.; Elbalkimy, M. Non-motor symptoms in essential tremor, akinetic rigid and tremor-dominant subtypes of Parkinson's disease. *PLoS ONE* **2021**, *16*, e0245918. [CrossRef]
77. Elfil, M.; Bahbah, E.I.; Attia, M.M.; Eldokmak, M.; Koo, B.B. Impact of Obstructive Sleep Apnea on Cognitive and Motor Functions in Parkinson's Disease. *Mov. Disord.* **2021**, *36*, 570–580. [CrossRef]
78. Strickland, D.; Bertoni, J.M. Parkinson's prevalence estimated by a state registry. *Mov. Disord. Off. J. Mov. Disord. Soc.* **2004**, *19*, 318–323. [CrossRef] [PubMed]
79. Tysnes, O.B.; Storstein, A. Epidemiology of Parkinson's disease. *J. Neural Transm.* **2017**, *124*, 901–905. [CrossRef] [PubMed]

80. Archibald, N.; Miller, N.; Rochester, L. Neurorehabilitation in Parkinson disease. *Handb. Clin. Neurol.* **2013**, *110*, 435–442. [CrossRef] [PubMed]
81. Shtilbans, A.; Henchcliffe, C. Biomarkers in Parkinson's disease: An update. *Curr. Opin. Neurol.* **2012**, *25*, 460–465. [CrossRef]
82. Kwan, L.C.; Whitehill, T.L. Perception of Speech by Individuals with Parkinson's Disease: A Review. *Parkinsons Disease* **2011**, *2011*, 389767. [CrossRef]
83. Ge, H.; Yan, Z.; Zhu, H.; Zhao, H. MiR-410 exerts neuroprotective effects in a cellular model of Parkinson's disease induced by 6-hydroxydopamine via inhibiting the PTEN/AKT/mTOR signaling pathway. *Exp. Mol. Pathol.* **2019**, *109*, 16–24. [CrossRef] [PubMed]
84. Leggio, L.; Vivarelli, S.; L'Episcopo, F.; Tirolo, C.; Caniglia, S.; Testa, N.; Marchetti, B.; Iraci, N. microRNAs in Parkinson's Disease: From Pathogenesis to Novel Diagnostic and Therapeutic Approaches. *Int. J. Mol. Sci.* **2017**, *18*, 2698. [CrossRef] [PubMed]
85. McMillan, K.J.; Murray, T.K.; Bengoa-Vergniory, N.; Cordero-Llana, O.; Cooper, J.; Buckley, A.; Wade-Martins, R.; Uney, J.B.; O'Neill, M.J.; Wong, L.F.; et al. Loss of MicroRNA-7 Regulation Leads to α-Synuclein Accumulation and Dopaminergic Neuronal Loss In Vivo. *Mol. Ther. J. Am. Soc. Gene Ther.* **2017**, *25*, 2404–2414. [CrossRef] [PubMed]
86. Titze-de-Almeida, R.; Titze-de-Almeida, S.S. miR-7 Replacement Therapy in Parkinson's Disease. *Curr. Gene Ther.* **2018**, *18*, 143–153. [CrossRef] [PubMed]
87. Shen, D.F.; Qi, H.P.; Ma, C.; Chang, M.X.; Zhang, W.N.; Song, R.R. Astaxanthin suppresses endoplasmic reticulum stress and protects against neuron damage in Parkinson's disease by regulating miR-7/SNCA axis. *Neurosci. Res.* **2020**. [CrossRef]
88. Grimmig, B.; Daly, L.; Subbarayan, M.; Hudson, C.; Williamson, R.; Nash, K.; Bickford, P.C. Astaxanthin is neuroprotective in an aged mouse model of Parkinson's disease. *Oncotarget* **2018**, *9*, 10388–10401. [CrossRef]
89. Wang, C.C.; Shi, H.H.; Xu, J.; Yanagita, T.; Xue, C.H.; Zhang, T.T.; Wang, Y.M. Docosahexaenoic acid-acylated astaxanthin ester exhibits superior performance over non-esterified astaxanthin in preventing behavioral deficits coupled with apoptosis in MPTP-induced mice with Parkinson's disease. *Food Funct.* **2020**, *11*, 8038–8050. [CrossRef] [PubMed]
90. Wang, X.J.; Chen, W.; Fu, X.T.; Ma, J.K.; Wang, M.H.; Hou, Y.J.; Tian, D.C.; Fu, X.Y.; Fan, C.D. Reversal of homocysteine-induced neurotoxicity in rat hippocampal neurons by astaxanthin: Evidences for mitochondrial dysfunction and signaling crosstalk. *Cell Death Discov.* **2018**, *4*, 50. [CrossRef]
91. Ye, Q.; Zhang, X.; Huang, B.; Zhu, Y.; Chen, X. Astaxanthin suppresses MPP(+)-induced oxidative damage in PC12 cells through a Sp1/NR1 signaling pathway. *Mar. Drugs* **2013**, *11*, 1019–1034. [CrossRef]
92. Ye, Q.; Huang, B.; Zhang, X.; Zhu, Y.; Chen, X. Astaxanthin protects against MPP(+)-induced oxidative stress in PC12 cells via the HO-1/NOX2 axis. *BMC Neurosci.* **2012**, *13*, 156. [CrossRef]
93. Liu, X.; Shibata, T.; Hisaka, S.; Osawa, T. Astaxanthin inhibits reactive oxygen species-mediated cellular toxicity in dopaminergic SH-SY5Y cells via mitochondria-targeted protective mechanism. *Brain Res.* **2009**, *1254*, 18–27. [CrossRef] [PubMed]
94. Ikeda, Y.; Tsuji, S.; Satoh, A.; Ishikura, M.; Shirasawa, T.; Shimizu, T. Protective effects of astaxanthin on 6-hydroxydopamine-induced apoptosis in human neuroblastoma SH-SY5Y cells. *J. Neurochem.* **2008**, *107*, 1730–1740. [CrossRef] [PubMed]
95. Finnerup, N.B.; Haroutounian, S.; Kamerman, P.; Baron, R.; Bennett, D.L.H.; Bouhassira, D.; Cruccu, G.; Freeman, R.; Hansson, P.; Nurmikko, T.; et al. Neuropathic pain: An updated grading system for research and clinical practice. *Pain* **2016**, *157*, 1599–1606. [CrossRef] [PubMed]
96. Kramer, J.L.; Minhas, N.K.; Jutzeler, C.R.; Erskine, E.L.; Liu, L.J.; Ramer, M.S. Neuropathic pain following traumatic spinal cord injury: Models, measurement, and mechanisms. *J. Neurosci. Res.* **2017**, *95*, 1295–1306. [CrossRef]
97. Lampert, A.; Hains, B.C.; Waxman, S.G. Upregulation of persistent and ramp sodium current in dorsal horn neurons after spinal cord injury. *Exp. Brain Res.* **2006**, *174*, 660–666. [CrossRef] [PubMed]
98. Naseri, K.; Saghaei, E.; Abbaszadeh, F.; Afhami, M.; Haeri, A.; Rahimi, F.; Jorjani, M. Role of microglia and astrocyte in central pain syndrome following electrolytic lesion at the spinothalamic tract in rats. *J. Mol. Neurosci. Mn* **2013**, *49*, 470–479. [CrossRef] [PubMed]
99. D'Angelo, R.; Morreale, A.; Donadio, V.; Boriani, S.; Maraldi, N.; Plazzi, G.; Liguori, R. Neuropathic pain following spinal cord injury: What we know about mechanisms, assessment and management. *Eur. Rev. Med. Pharmacol. Sci.* **2013**, *17*, 3257–3261.
100. Finnerup, N.B.; Otto, M.; McQuay, H.J.; Jensen, T.S.; Sindrup, S.H. Algorithm for neuropathic pain treatment: An evidence based proposal. *Pain* **2005**, *118*, 289–305. [CrossRef]
101. Gugliandolo, E.; D'amico, R.; Cordaro, M.; Fusco, R.; Siracusa, R.; Crupi, R.; Impellizzeri, D.; Cuzzocrea, S.; Di Paola, R. Effect of PEA-OXA on neuropathic pain and functional recovery after sciatic nerve crush. *J. Neuroinflamm.* **2018**, *15*, 264. [CrossRef] [PubMed]
102. Sharma, K.; Sharma, D.; Sharma, M.; Sharma, N.; Bidve, P.; Prajapati, N.; Kalia, K.; Tiwari, V. Astaxanthin ameliorates behavioral and biochemical alterations in in-vitro and in-vivo model of neuropathic pain. *Neurosci. Lett.* **2018**, *674*, 162–170. [CrossRef] [PubMed]
103. Jiang, X.; Yan, Q.; Liu, F.; Jing, C.; Ding, L.; Zhang, L.; Pang, C. Chronic trans-astaxanthin treatment exerts antihyperalgesic effect and corrects co-morbid depressive like behaviors in mice with chronic pain. *Neurosci. Lett.* **2018**, *662*, 36–43. [CrossRef] [PubMed]
104. Fakhri, S.; Dargahi, L.; Abbaszadeh, F.; Jorjani, M. Effects of astaxanthin on sensory-motor function in a compression model of spinal cord injury: Involvement of ERK and AKT signalling pathway. *Eur. J. Pain* **2019**, *23*, 750–764. [CrossRef] [PubMed]
105. Fakhri, S.; Dargahi, L.; Abbaszadeh, F.; Jorjani, M. Astaxanthin attenuates neuroinflammation contributed to the neuropathic pain and motor dysfunction following compression spinal cord injury. *Brain Res. Bull.* **2018**, *143*, 217–224. [CrossRef]

106. Marvizón, J.C.; McRoberts, J.A.; Ennes, H.S.; Song, B.; Wang, X.; Jinton, L.; Corneliussen, B.; Mayer, E.A. Two N-methyl-D-aspartate receptors in rat dorsal root ganglia with different subunit composition and localization. *J. Comp. Neurol.* **2002**, *446*, 325–341. [CrossRef]
107. Gorman, A.L.; Yu, C.G.; Ruenes, G.R.; Daniels, L.; Yezierski, R.P. Conditions affecting the onset, severity, and progression of a spontaneous pain-like behavior after excitotoxic spinal cord injury. *J. Pain* **2001**, *2*, 229–240. [CrossRef]
108. Yu, C.G.; Fairbanks, C.A.; Wilcox, G.L.; Yezierski, R.P. Effects of agmatine, interleukin-10, and cyclosporin on spontaneous pain behavior after excitotoxic spinal cord injury in rats. *J. Pain* **2003**, *4*, 129–140. [CrossRef]
109. Hains, B.C.; Waxman, S.G. Sodium channel expression and the molecular pathophysiology of pain after SCI. *Prog. Brain Res.* **2007**, *161*, 195–203. [CrossRef]
110. Ji, R.R.; Woolf, C.J. Neuronal plasticity and signal transduction in nociceptive neurons: Implications for the initiation and maintenance of pathological pain. *Neurobiol. Dis.* **2001**, *8*, 1–10. [CrossRef]
111. Lerch, J.K.; Puga, D.A.; Bloom, O.; Popovich, P.G. Glucocorticoids and macrophage migration inhibitory factor (MIF) are neuroendocrine modulators of inflammation and neuropathic pain after spinal cord injury. *Semin. Immunol.* **2014**, *26*, 409–414. [CrossRef] [PubMed]
112. Baastrup, C.; Finnerup, N.B. Pharmacological management of neuropathic pain following spinal cord injury. *CNS Drugs* **2008**, *22*, 455–475. [CrossRef] [PubMed]
113. Fakhri, S.; Aneva, I.Y.; Farzaei, M.H.; Sobarzo-Sánchez, E. The Neuroprotective Effects of Astaxanthin: Therapeutic Targets and Clinical Perspective. *Molecules* **2019**, *24*, 2640. [CrossRef] [PubMed]
114. Yamagishi, R.; Aihara, M. Neuroprotective effect of astaxanthin against rat retinal ganglion cell death under various stresses that induce apoptosis and necrosis. *Mol. Vis.* **2014**, *20*, 1796–1805.
115. Ikonomidou, C.; Bosch, F.; Miksa, M.; Bittigau, P.; Vöckler, J.; Dikranian, K.; Tenkova, T.I.; Stefovska, V.; Turski, L.; Olney, J.W. Blockade of NMDA receptors and apoptotic neurodegeneration in the developing brain. *Science* **1999**, *283*, 70–74. [CrossRef]
116. Alexander, J.K.; Cox, G.M.; Tian, J.B.; Zha, A.M.; Wei, P.; Kigerl, K.A.; Reddy, M.K.; Dagia, N.M.; Sielecki, T.; Zhu, M.X.; et al. Macrophage migration inhibitory factor (MIF) is essential for inflammatory and neuropathic pain and enhances pain in response to stress. *Exp. Neurol.* **2012**, *236*, 351–362. [CrossRef]
117. Islam, M.S.; Kanak, F.; Iqbal, M.A.; Islam, K.F.; Al-Mamun, A.; Uddin, M.S. Analyzing the Status of the Autism Spectrum Disorder Amid Children with Intellectual Disabilities in Bangladesh. *Biomed. Pharmacol. J.* **2018**, *11*, 689–701. [CrossRef]
118. Boyle, C.A.; Boulet, S.; Schieve, L.A.; Cohen, R.A.; Blumberg, S.J.; Yeargin-Allsopp, M.; Visser, S.; Kogan, M.D. Trends in the prevalence of developmental disabilities in US children, 1997-2008. *Pediatrics* **2011**, *127*, 1034–1042. [CrossRef] [PubMed]
119. Kern, J.K.; Geier, D.A.; Sykes, L.K.; Geier, M.R. Evidence of neurodegeneration in autism spectrum disorder. *Transl. Neurodegener.* **2013**, *2*, 17. [CrossRef] [PubMed]
120. Kemper, T.L.; Bauman, M. Neuropathology of infantile autism. *J. Neuropathol. Exp. Neurol.* **1998**, *57*, 645–652. [CrossRef]
121. Lee, M.; Martin-Ruiz, C.; Graham, A.; Court, J.; Jaros, E.; Perry, R.; Iversen, P.; Bauman, M.; Perry, E. Nicotinic receptor abnormalities in the cerebellar cortex in autism. *Brain A J. Neurol.* **2002**, *125*, 1483–1495. [CrossRef]
122. Courchesne, E.; Pierce, K.; Schumann, C.M.; Redcay, E.; Buckwalter, J.A.; Kennedy, D.P.; Morgan, J. Mapping early brain development in autism. *Neuron* **2007**, *56*, 399–413. [CrossRef] [PubMed]
123. Li, X.; Chauhan, A.; Sheikh, A.M.; Patil, S.; Chauhan, V.; Li, X.M.; Ji, L.; Brown, T.; Malik, M. Elevated immune response in the brain of autistic patients. *J. Neuroimmunol.* **2009**, *207*, 111–116. [CrossRef]
124. Sabit, H.; Tombuloglu, H.; Rehman, S.; Almandil, N.B.; Cevik, E.; Abdel-Ghany, S.; Rashwan, S.; Abasiyanik, M.F.; Yee Waye, M.M. Gut microbiota metabolites in autistic children: An epigenetic perspective. *Heliyon* **2021**, *7*, e06105. [CrossRef]
125. Granot, E.; Kohen, R. Oxidative stress in childhood–in health and disease states. *Clin. Nutr.* **2004**, *23*, 3–11. [CrossRef]
126. Evans, T.A.; Siedlak, S.L.; Lu, L.; Fu, X.; Wang, Z.; McGinnis, W.R.; Fakhoury, E.; Castellani, R.J.; Hazen, S.L.; Walsh, W.J. The autistic phenotype exhibits a remarkably localized modification of brain protein by products of free radical-induced lipid oxidation. *Am. J. Biochem. Biotechnol.* **2008**, *4*, 61–72. [CrossRef]
127. Sajdel-Sulkowska, E.; Lipinski, B.; Windom, H.; Audhya, T.; McGinnis, W. Oxidative stress in autism: Elevated cerebellar 3-nitrotyrosine levels. *Am. J. Biochem. Biotechnol.* **2008**, *4*, 73–84.
128. Sajdel-Sulkowska, E.M.; Xu, M.; McGinnis, W.; Koibuchi, N. Brain region-specific changes in oxidative stress and neurotrophin levels in autism spectrum disorders (ASD). *Cerebellum* **2011**, *10*, 43–48. [CrossRef]
129. Krajcovicova-Kudlackova, M.; Valachovicova, M.; Mislanova, C.; Hudecova, Z.; Sustrova, M.; Ostatnikova, D. Plasma concentrations of selected antioxidants in autistic children and adolescents. *Bratisl Lek Listy* **2009**, *110*, 247–250. [PubMed]
130. Ornoy, A.; Weinstein-Fudim, L.; Ergaz, Z. Prevention or Amelioration of Autism-Like Symptoms in Animal Models: Will it Bring Us Closer to Treating Human ASD? *Int. J. Mol. Sci.* **2019**, *20*, 1074. [CrossRef] [PubMed]
131. Lyu, Y.; Wu, L.; Wang, F.; Shen, X.; Lin, D. Carotenoid supplementation and retinoic acid in immunoglobulin A regulation of the gut microbiota dysbiosis. *Exp. Biol. Med. (Maywood)* **2018**, *243*, 613–620. [CrossRef]
132. Fernández, M.J.F.; Valero-Cases, E.; Rincon-Frutos, L. Food Components with the Potential to be Used in the Therapeutic Approach of Mental Diseases. *Curr. Pharm. Biotechnol.* **2019**, *20*, 100–113. [CrossRef] [PubMed]
133. Al-Amin, M.M.; Rahman, M.M.; Khan, F.R.; Zaman, F.; Mahmud Reza, H. Astaxanthin improves behavioral disorder and oxidative stress in prenatal valproic acid-induced mice model of autism. *Behav. Brain Res.* **2015**, *286*, 112–121. [CrossRef] [PubMed]

134. Xue, Y.; Qu, Z.; Fu, J.; Zhen, J.; Wang, W.; Cai, Y.; Wang, W. The protective effect of astaxanthin on learning and memory deficits and oxidative stress in a mouse model of repeated cerebral ischemia/reperfusion. *Brain Res. Bull.* **2017**, *131*, 221–228. [CrossRef] [PubMed]
135. Wang, Y.L.; Zhu, X.L.; Sun, M.H.; Dang, Y.K. Effects of astaxanthin on axonal regeneration via cAMP/PKA signaling pathway in mice with focal cerebral infarction. *Eur. Rev. Med. Pharmacol. Sci.* **2019**, *23*, 135–143. [CrossRef] [PubMed]
136. Zhang, J.; Ding, C.; Zhang, S.; Xu, Y. Neuroprotective effects of astaxanthin against oxygen and glucose deprivation damage via the PI3K/Akt/GSK3β/Nrf2 signalling pathway in vitro. *J. Cell. Mol. Med.* **2020**, *24*, 8977–8985. [CrossRef] [PubMed]
137. Nai, Y.; Liu, H.; Bi, X.; Gao, H.; Ren, C. Protective effect of astaxanthin on acute cerebral infarction in rats. *Hum. Exp. Toxicol.* **2018**, *37*, 929–936. [CrossRef]
138. Cakir, E.; Cakir, U.; Tayman, C.; Turkmenoglu, T.T.; Gonel, A.; Turan, I.O. Favorable Effects of Astaxanthin on Brain Damage due to Ischemia- Reperfusion Injury. *Comb. Chem. High Throughput Screen.* **2020**, *23*, 214–224. [CrossRef]
139. Carelli, S.; Giallongo, T.; Gombalova, Z.; Rey, F.; Gorio, M.C.F.; Mazza, M.; Di Giulio, A.M. Counteracting neuroinflammation in experimental Parkinson's disease favors recovery of function: Effects of Er-NPCs administration. *J. Neuroinflamm.* **2018**, *15*, 333. [CrossRef]
140. Stewart, J.S.; Lignell, A.; Pettersson, A.; Elfving, E.; Soni, M.G. Safety assessment of astaxanthin-rich microalgae biomass: Acute and subchronic toxicity studies in rats. *Food Chem. Toxicol. Int. J. Publ. Br. Ind. Biol. Res. Assoc.* **2008**, *46*, 3030–3036. [CrossRef]
141. Hussein, G.; Nakamura, M.; Zhao, Q.; Iguchi, T.; Goto, H.; Sankawa, U.; Watanabe, H. Antihypertensive and neuroprotective effects of astaxanthin in experimental animals. *Biol. Pharm. Bull.* **2005**, *28*, 47–52. [CrossRef]
142. EFSA Panel on Dietetic Products, N. Allergies. Scientific Opinion on the safety of astaxanthin-rich ingredients (AstaREAL A1010 and AstaREAL L10) as novel food ingredients. *EFSA J.* **2014**, *12*, 3757.
143. Additives, E.P.O.; Feed, P.O.S.U.I.A. Scientific Opinion on the safety and efficacy of synthetic astaxanthin as feed additive for salmon and trout, other fish, ornamental fish, crustaceans and ornamental birds. *EFSA J.* **2014**, *12*, 3724.
144. Imai, A.; Oda, Y.; Ito, N.; Seki, S.; Nakagawa, K.; Miyazawa, T.; Ueda, F. Effects of Dietary Supplementation of Astaxanthin and Sesamin on Daily Fatigue: A Randomized, Double-Blind, Placebo-Controlled, Two-Way Crossover Study. *Nutrients* **2018**, *10*, 281. [CrossRef] [PubMed]
145. Mashhadi, N.S.; Zakerkish, M.; Mohammadiasl, J.; Zarei, M.; Mohammadshahi, M.; Haghighizadeh, M.H. Astaxanthin improves glucose metabolism and reduces blood pressure in patients with type 2 diabetes mellitus. *Asia Pac. J. Clin. Nutr.* **2018**, *27*, 341–346. [CrossRef] [PubMed]
146. Brendler, T.; Williamson, E.M. Astaxanthin: How much is too much? A safety review. *Phytother. Res.* **2019**, *33*, 3090–3111. [CrossRef]
147. Kajita, M.; Kato, T.; Yoshimoto, T.; Masuda, K. Study on the safety of high-dose administration of astaxanthin. *Folia Jpn. Ophthalmol. Clin.* **2010**, *3*, 365–370.
148. Kupcinskas, L.; Lafolie, P.; Lignell, A.; Kiudelis, G.; Jonaitis, L.; Adamonis, K.; Andersen, L.P.; Wadström, T. Efficacy of the natural antioxidant astaxanthin in the treatment of functional dyspepsia in patients with or without Helicobacter pylori infection: A prospective, randomized, double blind, and placebo-controlled study. *Phytomedicine Int. J. Phytother. Phytopharm.* **2008**, *15*, 391–399. [CrossRef] [PubMed]
149. Katsumata, T.; Ishibashi, T.; Kyle, D. A sub-chronic toxicity evaluation of a natural astaxanthin-rich carotenoid extract of Paracoccus carotinifaciens in rats. *Toxicol. Rep.* **2014**, *1*, 582–588. [CrossRef]

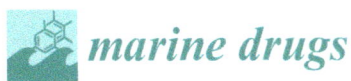

Review

Xanthophylls from the Sea: Algae as Source of Bioactive Carotenoids

Antia G. Pereira [1,2], Paz Otero [1], Javier Echave [1], Anxo Carreira-Casais [1], Franklin Chamorro [1], Nicolas Collazo [1], Amira Jaboui [1], Catarina Lourenço-Lopes [1], Jesus Simal-Gandara [1,*] and Miguel A. Prieto [1,2,*]

1. Nutrition and Bromatology Group, Analytical and Food Chemistry Department, Faculty of Food Science and Technology, Ourense Campus, University of Vigo, E-32004 Ourense, Spain; antia.gonzalez.pereira@uvigo.es (A.G.P.); paz.otero@uvigo.es (P.O.); javier.echave@uvigo.es (J.E.); anxocc@uvigo.es (A.C.-C.); chamorro1984@gmail.com (F.C.); nicolascollazojimenez@gmail.com (N.C.); jarb.amira@gmail.com (A.J.); lopes@uvigo.es (C.L.-L.)
2. Centro de Investigação de Montanha (CIMO), Instituto Politécnico de Bragança, Campus de Santa Apolonia, 5300-253 Bragança, Portugal
* Correspondence: jsimal@uvigo.es (J.S.-G.); mprieto@uvigo.es (M.A.P.)

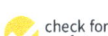

Citation: Pereira, A.G.; Otero, P.; Echave, J.; Carreira-Casais, A.; Chamorro, F.; Collazo, N.; Jaboui, A.; Lourenço-Lopes, C.; Simal-Gandara, J.; Prieto, M.A. Xanthophylls from the Sea: Algae as Source of Bioactive Carotenoids. *Mar. Drugs* **2021**, *19*, 188. https://doi.org/10.3390/md19040188

Academic Editors: Elena Talero and Javier Ávila-Román

Received: 28 February 2021
Accepted: 25 March 2021
Published: 27 March 2021

Publisher's Note: MDPI stays neutral with regard to jurisdictional claims in published maps and institutional affiliations.

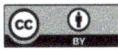

Copyright: © 2021 by the authors. Licensee MDPI, Basel, Switzerland. This article is an open access article distributed under the terms and conditions of the Creative Commons Attribution (CC BY) license (https://creativecommons.org/licenses/by/4.0/).

Abstract: Algae are considered pigment-producing organisms. The function of these compounds in algae is to carry out photosynthesis. They have a great variety of pigments, which can be classified into three large groups: chlorophylls, carotenoids, and phycobilins. Within the carotenoids are xanthophylls. Xanthophylls (fucoxanthin, astaxanthin, lutein, zeaxanthin, and β-cryptoxanthin) are a type of carotenoids with anti-tumor and anti-inflammatory activities, due to their chemical structure rich in double bonds that provides them with antioxidant properties. In this context, xanthophylls can protect other molecules from oxidative stress by turning off singlet oxygen damage through various mechanisms. Based on clinical studies, this review shows the available information concerning the bioactivity and biological effects of the main xanthophylls present in algae. In addition, the algae with the highest production rate of the different compounds of interest were studied. It was observed that fucoxanthin is obtained mainly from the brown seaweeds *Laminaria japonica*, *Undaria pinnatifida*, *Hizikia fusiformis*, *Sargassum* spp., and *Fucus* spp. The main sources of astaxanthin are the microalgae *Haematococcus pluvialis*, *Chlorella zofingiensis*, and *Chlorococcum* sp. Lutein and zeaxanthin are mainly found in algal species such as *Scenedesmus* spp., *Chlorella* spp., *Rhodophyta* spp., or *Spirulina* spp. However, the extraction and purification processes of xanthophylls from algae need to be standardized to facilitate their commercialization. Finally, we assessed factors that determine the bioavailability and bioaccesibility of these molecules. We also suggested techniques that increase xanthophyll's bioavailability.

Keywords: carotenoids; xanthophylls; natural compounds; algae; bioactive; health

1. Introduction

In recent years, consumer demand for naturally sourced products to promote health and reduce disease has grown steadily [1]. This demand has entailed an increased interest in new natural sources of food, pharmaceutical, and cosmetic products [2,3]. In this context, the marine environment has been considered a potential reservoir of natural compounds [4]. Among the organisms present in this environment, it is worth highlighting algae. Algae constitute a polyphyletic group of photosynthetic primary producers organisms, which represent an interesting source of chemical components with high-value biological activities. [5]. Although the total number of algal species is unknown, it is thought to vary between one and ten million [6].

The high value of algal extracts is due to their large number of molecules such as carbohydrates, proteins, peptides, lipids (including oils and polyunsaturated fatty acids, PUFAs), minerals, iodine, phenols (polyphenols, tocopherols), alkaloids, terpenes, and pigments (as chlorophylls, carotenoids, and phycobilins) [7,8]. Within these compounds, one of the groups with greater interest are pigments due to the concentrations in which they are present, these being higher than that of other compounds such as phenolic compounds. In fact, algae are considered pigment-producing organisms. They have a great variety of pigments, which can be classified into three large groups: chlorophylls, carotenoids, and phycobilins. Therefore, different carotenoids (CA) profiles can be used as a medium for algal classification [9]. In this way, a first classification of the algae allows us to make a division according to the size of the algae (microalgae or macroalgae) and the following divisions according to their tones, among other characteristics. As a result, the first group comprises greenish algae (Cyanophyceae), green algae (Chlorophyceae), diatoms (Bacillariophyceae), and golden algae (Chrysophyceae), among others. Meanwhile, the macroalgae family includes red (Rhodophyta), brown (Ochrophyta), and green algae (Chlorophyta) [10–12]. This diversity of species and, therefore, of its chemical compositions is interesting, since once compounds are properly isolated or extracted from algae, they may show a diverse range of biological activities, such as antioxidant, antimicrobial, anticancer, anti-allergic, antiviral, and anticoagulant activities, among others [7,8]. This diversity of biological activities implies that there is also a significant variety of potential applications in human health, agriculture, and in food and cosmetic industries [4], in which its application depends on its chemical composition.

On an industrial scale, the most interesting species are those that produce high percentages of CA. CA are usually located in chloroplasts or stored in vesicles and a cytoplasmic matrix of plants, algae, photosynthetic bacteria, and some fungi [9]. All CA are tetraterpenes, which are compounds that have a skeleton composed of 40 carbon atoms conjugated in polyene chains [9]. They are classified into two main groups: (i) compounds that have a hydrocarbon long chain known as carotenes and (ii) compounds that have an oxygen atom in its structure, known as xanthophylls. The first group includes α-carotene, β-carotene, lycopene, and phytoene, among others. The most representative molecules of the second group are fucoxanthin, astaxanthin, lutein, zeaxanthin, and β-cryptoxanthin. This difference in its structure makes xanthophylls more polar than carotenes due to the presence of oxygen in the form of methoxy, hydroxy, keto, carboxy, and epoxy positions. However, except for lutein, they are still non-polar compounds [13]. Its structure with alternating double bonds is responsible for many of its biological functions, being the main function in photosynthetic organisms to act as accessory pigments for the capture of light in photosynthesis, and to protect photosynthetic machinery against self-oxidation [14]. However, despite the wide diversity of molecules in the carotenoid family, with more than 700 compounds currently known, only about 30 CA have a significant role in photosynthesis [13]. In recent years, numerous studies have highlighted CA multiple effects on human health due to their antioxidant properties, preventing the damage caused by oxidative stress and therefore declining the risk of chronic diseases [14,15]. However, the biological properties of CA are not limited to their antioxidant properties. The scientific literature has shown CA actions as anti-tumor [16–18], anti-inflammatory [19,20], neuroprotective, antimicrobial, antidiabetic, and antiobesity [21,22]. Therefore, algae have several CA with market interest (β-carotene, fucoxanthin, astaxanthin, lutein, zeaxanthin, and violaxanthin), representing a natural and sustainable source of these compounds [9].

Among the xanthophylls of interest is fucoxanthin, which is one of the most abundant marine CA, accounting for approximately 10% of the total production of natural CA [23]. It is found in abundant concentrations in the chloroplasts of several brown seaweeds, such as *Laminaria japonica*, *Undaria pinnatifida*, *Sargassum fusiformis*, in several species belonging to the genera *Sargassum* (*Sargassum horneri*) and *Fucus* (*Fucus serratus*, *Fucus vesiculosus*) and in diatoms (*Bacillariophyta*) [9,24–26]. Another xanthophyll of interest is astaxanthin (AS), which is a red pigment. AS is considered a potent antioxidant as it has about ten times more antioxidant activity than other CA [27]. The main natural sources of this pigment are the microalgae *Haematococcus pluvialis*, *Chlorella zofingiensis*, and *Chlorococcum* sp. [28]. *H. pluvialis* is a single-celled green freshwater alga. It is the richest source of natural AS and is already produced on an industrial scale [26]. Procedures have been technologically advanced to grow *Haematococcus* containing 1.5–3.0% AS dry weight [27,29]. The richest source of β-carotene is the halotolerant green microalgae *Dunaliella salina*, accumulating up to 10% of it based on the dry weight of the microalgae [30,31]. When *H. pluvialis* and *D. salina* are cultivated in extreme conditions (such as high salinity, high luminosity, or lack of nutrients), AS and β-carotene, respectively, can reach more than 90% of the total carotenoids [7]. Lutein and zeaxanthin are pigments found in algal species such as *Scenedesmus* spp., *Chlorella* spp., *Rhodophyta* spp., or *Spirulina* spp. respectively [32]. Esteban et al., 2009 [33], reported that red algae (*Rhodophyta*) show a common carotenoid pattern of β-carotene and one to three xanthophylls: lutein, zeaxanthin, or anteraxanthin. *Corallina elongata* and *Jania rubenseran* were the only algae that contained anteraxanthin as the main xanthophyll. *Spirulina platensis* (strain pacifica) microalgae is a source of β-cryptoxantine, β-carotene, and zeaxanthin. β-cryptoxantine is a pigment that can also be found in plants [34]. The siphonaxanthin content in green algae such as *Umbraulva japonica*, *Caulerpa lentillifera*, and *Codium fragile* constitutes about 0.03%–0.1% of the dry weight [35]. The cyanobacteria *Synechococcus* sp. strain PCC7002 produces a monocyclic myxoxanthophyll, which is identified as Myxol-2 Fucoside (Myxoxanthophyll), in addition to producing other CA such as β-carotene, zeaxanthin, and sinecoxanthin [36]. The CA composition in cyanobacteria is very different from that of other algae, including for example β-carotene, zeaxanthin, myxol pentosides, and echineone [32].

Animals should get all these CA through the diet, as they are unable to synthesize them. CA are commonly incorporated as dietary supplements, feed additives, and food colorants in several sorts of food, such as dairy products and beverages, and also in the pharmaceutical and cosmetic industries [37]. As shown in Figure 1, CA have a high repertoire of commercial applications due to their multiple biological properties. Among the most notable applications are cosmetic, nutraceuticals, pharmaceutical purposes, and other human applications.

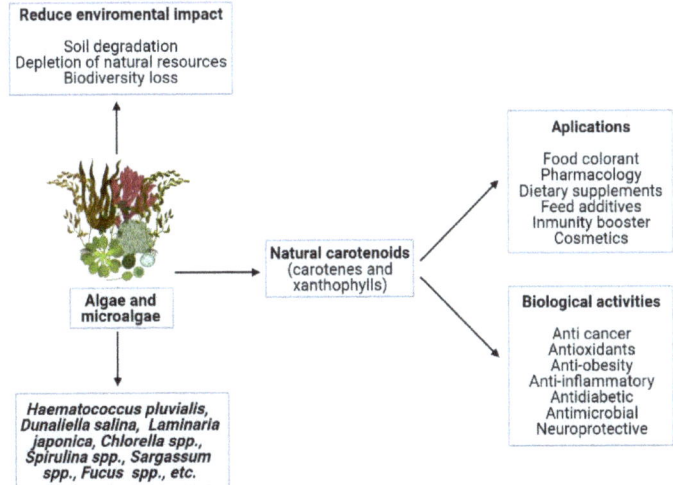

Figure 1. Positive effects on human health and industrial applications of carotenoids from natural sources.

Attributable to the various positive activities on human health and the multiple industrial applications of CA, global demand continues to increase. It is estimated that in 2026, the CA market will grow to USD 2.0 billion, registering an annual growth rate for CA of 4.2% [38]. The most relevant and important pigments on the market today are β-carotene and AS, followed by lutein, lycopene, and canthaxanthin [13,31]. So far, most commercial

CA are artificially produced. However, the strong global interest in food of natural origin that is safe, healthy, and environmentally friendly has increased the demand for natural sources of CA [22]. Algae and algal extracts are a sustainable option for CA and have numerous benefits in comparison to alternative natural sources. For instance, its cultivation and production is cheap, easy, and ecological, its removal has higher yields and is simple, and raw materials are not scarce, nor are there seasonal limitations [32,39,40]. In order to obtain high concentrations of a certain compound, culture conditions and environmental stress can be modified to manipulate the biochemical composition of microalgae [39]. However, under optimal growth conditions, the concentration of CA pigments is often too low to produce microalgal-based pigments, making it economically unviable [13,40]. To improve its economic viability, it is vital to explore and understand how environmental factors and the integration of nutrients into the environment affect the production of compounds. Understanding how the metabolic pathways of species vary according to the culture conditions, the co-production and accumulation of multiple compounds in microalgae will be improved [41]. The purpose of this review is to highlight the impact of xanthophylls from algae on human health, and to study the factors affecting the feasibility of their production and use as a sustainable alternative source of CA in the coming years.

2. Main Xanthophylls Present in Algae

From examining the findings, algae are a raw material of interest due to their pigment content and the potential bioactivities they possess. However, at present, relatively few species are used for such purposes since their exploitation at an industrial level is scarce. Table 1 lists some cases on algae exploitation to obtain high value xanthophylls. It includes information about the main algae species producing xanthophylls and their applications together with the main extraction techniques used to obtain the high-value molecules. The amount obtained in each case provides necessary information to estimate whether the process is viable.

Table 1. Xanthophylls in algae: mass production, concentration, and application.

Mol.	Algae	Extraction	Concentration	Applications	Ref.
FU	Fucus vesiculosus	Enzyme-assisted extraction	0.66 mg/g DW	Development of value-added nutraceutical products from seaweed	[42]
	Fucus serratus	Supercritical fluid extraction	2.18 mg/g DW	Obtaining high-purity fucoxanthin	[43]
	Laminaria japonica	Microwave-assisted extraction	0.04 mg/g DW	Obtaining high-purity fucoxanthin	[44]
	Laminaria japonica	Maceration	0.10 mg/g DW	Drug against chronic kidney disease	[45]
	Undaria pinnatifida	Microwave-assisted extraction	0.90 mg/g DW	Obtention of high-purity fucoxanthin	[44]
	Undaria pinnatifida	Maceration	3.09 mg/g DW	Scones	[46]
	Undaria pinnatifida	Supercritical fluid extraction	0.99 mg/g DW	Carotenoid isolation	[3]
	Undaria pinnatifida	Maceration	2.67 mg/g DW	Drug development	[47]
	Padina tetrastromatica	Ultrasonic-assisted extraction	0.75 mg/g DW	Nutraceuticals and biomedical applications	[48]
	Cystoseira hakodatensis	Maceration	3.47 mg/g DW	Optimization of the environmental conditions	[49]
	Himanthalia elongata	Maceration	18.60 mg/g DW	Commercial fucoxanthin production	[50]
	Tisochrysis lutea	Ultrasonic-assisted extraction	0.25 mg/g DW	Nutraceutical, cosmetic and pharmaceutical applications, such as for the treatment of metastatic melanoma	[51]

Table 1. Cont.

Mol.	Algae	Extraction	Concentration	Applications	Ref.
	Pavlova luthcri	Ultrasonic-assisted extraction	0.03 mg/g DW	Yogurt	[52]
	Phaeodactylum tricornutum	Maceration	0.1 mg/g DW	Milk	[53]
AS	Haematococcus pluvialis	Conventional extraction	900 kg/2 ha/year		[54]
	Haematococcus pluvialis	Two-stage system	3.8% dw	Antioxidant, anti-tumor, anti-inflammatory, ocular protective effect, antidiabetic, coloring agent	[55]
	Haematococcus pluvialis	Enzyme	3.6% dw		[56]
	Haematococcus pluvialis	Conventional extraction	2–3% dw		[57]
	Haematococcus pluvialis	Pressurized extraction	99% of total AS		[58]
LU	Chlorella protothecoides	Maceration	83.8 mg/L		[59]
	Chlorella protothecoides	Mechanical	83.8 mg/L		[60]
	Chlorella protothecoideswas	Mechanical	4.92 mg/g	Antioxidant, light-filtering, eye protection, colorant, potential therapeutic use against several chronic diseases, lower risk of cancer, anti-inflammatory benefits	[61]
	Chlorella vulgaris	Heptane–ethanol–water extraction	30 mg/g		[62]
	Scenedesmus almeriensis	-	0.54% wt		[63]
	Dunaliella salina	Conventional extraction	15.4 mg m^{-2} d^{-1}		[64]
ZEA	Nannochloropsis oculata	Supercritical fluids extraction	13.17 mg/g		[65]
	Chlorella ellipsoidea	Pressurized liquid extraction	4.26 mg/g	Antioxidant, anti-inflammatory, eyes and UV light protection, prevention of coronary syndromes, anti-tumoral, anti-cardiovascular diseases, and structural actions in neural tissue	[66]
	Synechocystis sp	Pulse electric field	1.64 mg/g		[1]
	Himanthalia elongata	Pulse electric field	0.13 mg/g		[1]
	Heterochlorella luteoviridis	Moderate electric field	244 µg/g		[9]
CRY	Spirulina platensis	Supercritical fluid extraction	7.5 mg/100 g	Antioxidant, anti-inflammatory, anticancer (lung, oral, pharyngeal), improves respiratory function, stimulation of bone formation and protection, modulation response to phytosterols in post-menopausal women, decreases risk of degenerative diseases	[34,67]
	Palisada perforata	Conventional extraction	14.2% total carotenoids		[68]
	Gracilaria gracilis	Conventional extraction	10.2% total carotenoids		[68]
	Pandorina morum	Maceration	2.38 µg/g DW		[69]
	Nanochlorum eucaryotum	Enzyme extraction	-		[70]
SIP	Codium fragile	Maceration	16 mg/kg fresh algae	Anti-angiogenic, antioxidant, cancer-preventing action; inhibit adipogenesis	[71]
	Caulerpa lentillifera	Maceration	0.1% DW		[72]
	Umbraulva japonica	Maceration	0.1% DW		[35]
DIAD	Phaeodactylum tricornutum	MeOH extraction	19% of total pigments		[73]
	Phaeodactylum tricornutum	MeOH extraction	-	Antioxidant	[74]
	Odontella aurita	EtOH extraction	10% total carotenoids		[75]
	Phaeodactylum tricornutum	Whole	14 µg/L		[76]
DIAT	Phaeodactylum tricornutum	MeOH extraction	17% of total pigments	Antioxidant	[73]

Mol: Molecules/compounds; FU: Fucoxanthin; AS: Astaxanthin; LU: Lutein; ZEA: Zeaxanthin; CRY: β-cryptoxanthin; SIP: Siphonaxanthin; DIAD: Diadinoxanthin; DIAT: Diatoxanthin. dw: Dry weight.

2.1. Fucoxanthin

Fucoxanthin (FU) (Figure 2) is produced by many algae as a secondary metabolite. It is present in the chloroplasts of eukaryotic algae and is involved in the process of photosynthesis performed by algae, which is thought to be more efficient than the photosynthesis of plants [77]. This molecule is considered one of the most abundant pigments in brown algae, and it represents up to 10% of the total CA found in nature [78]. It has been studied primarily in microalgae and brown macroalgae from several families such as *Undaria*, *Laminaria*, *Sargassum*, *Eisenia*, *Himathalia*, *Alaria*, or *Cystoseira* [79,80]. FU has a chemical structure derived from carotene but with an oxygenated backbone. In addition, this compound has several different functional groups such as hydroxyl, carboxyl, epoxy, and carbonyl moieties, and it also has an allenic bond [25]. FU is orange to brown in color, and it is responsible for the coloration of algae from the Phaeophyceae family. This lipophilic pigment absorbs light in a range from 450 to 540 nm, which translates in the blue-green to yellow-green part of the visible spectrum, and it behaves as the primary light-harvesting CA for many algae transferring energy to the chlorophyll–protein complexes with high efficiency thanks to its unique CA structure [81].

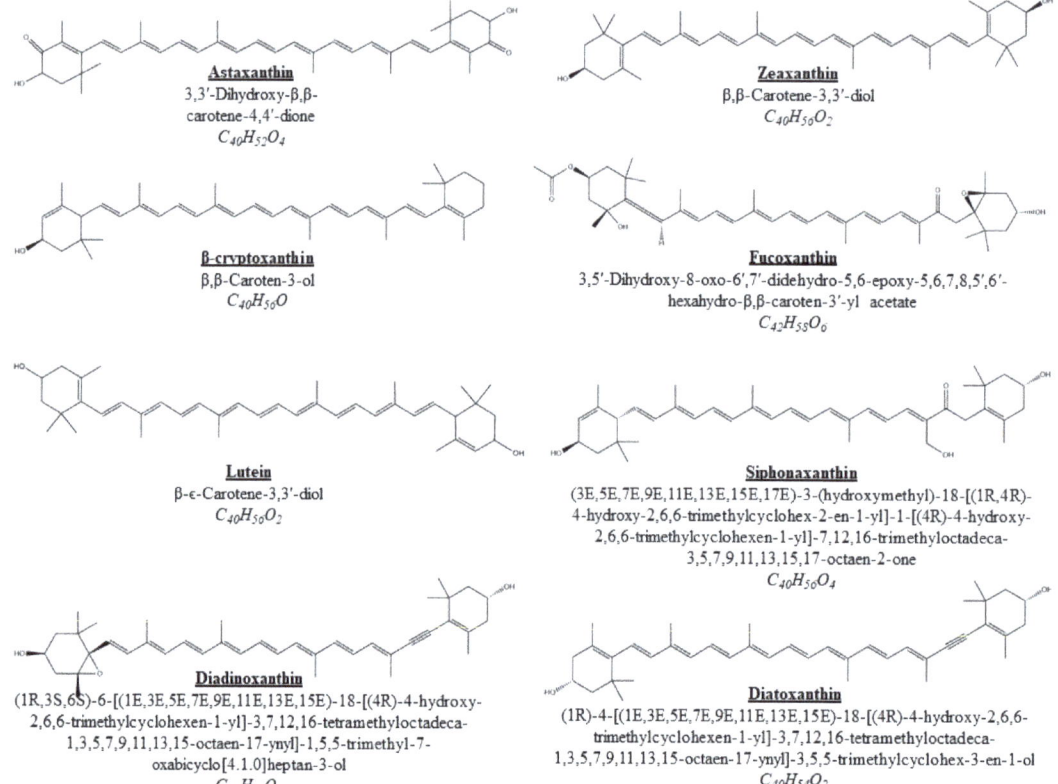

Figure 2. Chemical structure of the main xanthophylls present in algae [82].

Many bioactivities have been reposted regarding FU. Several articles have been published about its antioxidant, anticancer, anti-inflammatory, antimicrobial, antihypertensive, anti-obesity, antidiabetic, and anti-angiogenic activities, and also its photoprotective and neuroprotective effects (Table 1) [79,83–91]. Considering all these properties, FU has a great potential for applications in all sectors, from supplements and enriched foods to anti-aging cosmetics and to the pharmaceutical sector in the development of new innovative drugs for all kinds of pathologies including different types of cancer. For all these reasons, the FU market is expected to keep growing and reach 120 million dollars by 2022 [92].

Even though the artificial laboratory synthesis of FU is possible, it is a very expensive process that makes the extraction of FU from algae so appealing. However, the extraction and purification processes of FU from algae need to be standardized to facilitate its future commercialization and incorporation to new profitable products on the market [48]. Nevertheless, some companies already overcame these problems, and valuable products with FU have reached the market. For example, food supplements with FU intended to contribute to the loss of weight and improve eye, brain, liver, and joint health, are being sold with the commercial name of ThinOgen® and Fucovital®. These products can be found in the form of oils or microencapsulated powders [93]. Furthermore, FU is being studied to help combat cancer-related diseases, showing different anticancer mechanisms of action, such as inhibition of cell proliferation, induction of apoptosis, cell cycle arrest, an increase of intracellular reactive oxygen species, and anti-angiogenic effects [84,88,94–97]. Many studies have been made applying FU extracts to human cell lines, such as human bronchopulmonary carcinoma cell line NSCLC-N6, erythromyeloblastoid leukemia cell line K562, and the human lymphoblastoid cell line TK6, all with positive results [98]. Similar results were observed in prostate cancer (PC-3) cells, leukemia cells (HL-60), and cervical adenocarcinoma cells (HeLa). In addition, in vivo studies were also performed. For example, in mice, the administration of FU suppressed tumor growth of primary effusion lymphoma, sarcomas, and osteosarcoma [51,55,96]. Due to its anti-inflammatory activity, FU is also being tested to prevent and treat inflammatory-related diseases, thanks to fucoxanthin's strong antioxidant capacity and gut microbiota regulation [99], and its capacity to inhibit the production of nitric oxide, which is one of the determinants of inflammation in cells [100]. Some examples of FU incorporations in several food matrixes can already be found in the literature such as fortified yogurt [52] and milk [53], enriched canola oil [101], baked products such as scones [46], and even ground chicken breast meat [102].

2.2. Astaxanthin

Astaxanthin (AS) is a ketocarotenoid that fits in the group of terpenes and is formed from five carbon precursors, isopentenyl diphosphate, and dimethylallyl diphosphate. It is produced by a restricted number of algae (mainly microalgae), plants, bacteria, and fungi [103]. In microalgae, this compound is a secondary CA, which means that its accumulation in cytosolic lipid bodies ensues exclusively beneath environmental stress or adverse culture conditions, such as high light, high salinity, and nutrient deprivation. Despite this, algae represent the most important natural source of this compound in the aquatic food chain [104].

The commercial manufacture of this pigment has conventionally been executed by chemical synthesis. However, current studies proved that some microalgae might be the most capable source for its industrial biological production [105]. The best known and most used microalgae for its production are *Haematococcus pluvialis* and *Chlorella zofingiensis* [106]. *Haematococcus pluvialis* is one of the organisms with the highest concentrations of AS; thus, it is the main industrial source for the natural production of this compound [107]. It is common to reach yields of 38–40 g/kg (3.8–4%) of dried algae, and its scale at an industrial level is possible due to the high reproduction rate of this microalga [78,79]. The amount of AS found in cells corresponds to 85–95% of the total CA content; thus, it is relatively easy to purify it from the remaining CA [108]. Other species such as *C. zofingiensis* have also been studied, but the content of AS found was 50% AS of total CA, being the other main CA canthaxanthin and adonixanthin [109]. The extraction of AS, which is a lipophilic compound, can be carried out with organic solvents and oils, and it is common to combine its extraction with solvents with other types of extractions such as enzymatic or microwave extraction [107].

This compound is known as one of the most potent antioxidants; its capacity is due to the large amount of conjugated double bonds (thirteen). Different studies confirm that its antioxidant capacity is 65 times more potent than that produced by ascorbic acid; 10 times stronger than β-carotene, canthaxanthin, lutein, and zeaxanthin; and 100 times more effective than α-tocopherol, all of which are antioxidants used routinely [108]. For this reason, various products containing AS are already available on the market in various forms including oils, tablets, capsules, syrups, soft, creams, biomass, or ground [107]. An example is AstaPure® (Algatech LTD) produced from the microalgae *H. pluvialis*. Moreover, the consumption as a supplement does not represent any risk of toxicity, since the human body is not capable of transforming AS into vitamin A [107]. In 2019, the European Food Safety Authority (EFSA) has established an acceptable daily intake of 0.2 mg per kg body weight [110]. However, in order to be used as a food additive, more studies are still required due to stability, conservation, handling, and storage problems in this type of matrix [111].

AS has also anti-inflammatory activity, which is mainly due to its antioxidant properties and has been concerned in meliorate lifestyle-related illnesses and dealing health. AS additionally has anti-aging activity [105]. These beneficial effects have been demonstrated for both animals and humans [107].

2.3. Lutein

Chemically, lutein (LU) is a polyisoprenoid with 40 carbon atoms and cyclic structures at each end of its conjugated chain. Therefore, it has a similar structure to zeaxanthin (explaining below), differing from it in the site of the double bond in one ring, giving three chiral centers compared to the two of zeaxanthin [112]. LU is already used regularly in sectors such as cosmetics, pharmaceuticals, and food, which is mainly due to its color and bioactivities, and its anticancer properties are worth noting [61]. In fact, different studies demonstrate the antitumor effects of LU. For example, it was found that oral LU supplementation reduced the influence of ultraviolet irradiation by diminishing acute inflammatory responses and hyperproliferative rebound induced by ultraviolet rays [113]. In addition, this compound is widely known for its preventative effects against age-related macular degeneration and cataracts [62]. These health-promoting properties of LU along with its potential as a natural food colorant have led to improved research on the potential of LU as a high-value nutraceutical ingredient [114].

In general terms and for healthy people, food is a proper source of LU, and it does not require being added in a balanced diet, as it is safe to consume 60 mg/day for an adult of 60 kg [115]. This dietary contribution of LU is mainly due to the consumption of vegetables. However, algae is being considered as a new reservoir of lutein [59]. Among them, the best source at the commercial level is microalgae, especially those belonging to the *Chlorella* genus. This alga is an effective source of LU production, and it is safer than that of chemical origin whose use remains questionable. For this reason, the growth optimization studies of this alga are gaining interest owing to the high growth rates of the alga, along with their high pigment content. Several studies analyze the effect of LU production under different microalgae growth conditions in bioreactors. In most of them, the optimized parameters are the concentration of nitrate, ammonium, and urea in the batch [60,61]. However, the cultivation conditions of other newer species such as *Scenedesmus almeriensis* have also been optimized to increase their LU production. In this case, the contribution of nutrients has a lesser effect due to the high tolerance of this microalga to varied ranges of temperature, pH, salinity, and nutrient concentration [63]. Other widely studied species for its high content of LU are *D. salina* and *Galdieria sulphuraria* [59]. Mostly, it is still necessary to reduce costs regarding the growth and extraction process of LU from microalgae to be profitable. For this, it is not only necessary to optimize the consumption of nutrients, but also to analyze the subsequent processes such as harvesting and drying that entail large energy costs. In this regard, the currently available studies seem to indicate that the best option may be tubular photobioreactors [114,116].

2.4. Zeaxanthin

Zeaxanthin (ZEA) is a structural isomer of LU. Both isomers are usually found in various foods, being mainly present in green leafy vegetables and algae [117]. It is formed by a polyene chain with 11 conjugated double bonds and ionone rings. The ionone rings have a hydroxyl group that can attach to the fatty acids during esterification [118]. This compound, as well as some derivatives (meso-zeaxanthin), has a high antioxidant effect due to its chemical structure and distribution of the bonds. Furthermore, it also has a powerful anti-inflammatory effect attributable to the down-regulated expression of several inflammatory mediator genes. Consequently, these compounds may also be used in cancer prevention, as tumors are considered inflammatory diseases. Therefore, their use in chemotherapy may be of great interest [119]. Other bioactivities include photoprotection as well as the prevention and treatment of some eye diseases such as progress of macular degeneration and cataracts [120,121]. Moreover, ZEA has been proved to possess anti-tyrosinase activity, an enzyme associated with the production of melanin. Therefore, the inhibition effect of ZEA on this enzyme may avoid the formation of skin spots, which point to the use of this pigment as a whitening agent [122]. Hence, ZEA is a CA with promising nutraceutical implications.

Humans are not able to synthetize ZEA, as there is no biosynthetic pathway for this compound; thus, it has to be obtained from the diet. For this reason, its extraction from natural sources including vegetables, plants, macroalgae, cyanobacteria, and microalgae is of great interest [123]. There are several species of microalgae that produce this pigment. One of them is *Dunaliella salina*, which has also been genetically modified to increase its yield under all growth conditions, reaching 6 mg ZEA per gram of algae [124]. Other species that synthesize ZEA include *Spirulina, Corallina officinalis, Cyanophora paradoxa* and *Glaucocystis nostochinearum* [117]. These organisms can accumulate ZEA in a concentration up to nine times higher than traditional sources of this compound such as red peppers. This is the case of *Chlorella ellipsoidea*. In addition, algae have the advantage over plant matrices that the ZEA present in algae is in free form, while in plants, it is present as mono and diesters of ZEA [66]. As a consequence, numerous studies show the development of protocols to obtain ZEA from microalgae on a large scale [125]. Moreover, the production of this compound can be increased by varying the conditions in which algae cultivation takes place. One option is to increase photosynthetic irradiance over that required for the saturation of photosynthesis [117].

2.5. Minor Carotenoids

In addition to FU, AS, LU, and ZEA, algae can synthetize low amounts of other CA that belong to the xanthophyll group. In this section, we assessed these minor molecules also susceptible to be exploited by the nutraceutical industry. These include β-cryptoxanthin, siphonaxanthin, saproxanthin, myxol, diatoxanthin, and diadinoxanthin. They are only present in some bacteria and marine algae.

2.5.1. β-Cryptoxanthin

β-cryptoxanthin is an oxygenated CA with a chemical structure close to that of β-carotene, being the most important difference the higher polarity of β-cryptoxanthin. The interest of this compound shows a positive correlation between the intake of β-cryptoxanthin and the prevention of several diseases. In fact, this molecule is characterized by having provitamin A activity, anti-obesity effects, antioxidant activities, and anti-inflammatory, and anti-tumor activity [126]. Furthermore, the influence of β-cryptoxanthin on some inflammatory markers is probably stronger than other CA [127]. This compound is much less common than β-carotene, and it can only be found in a small number of foods. Some of them are fruits and vegetables such as tangerines, red peppers, and pumpkin [128]. It is also possible to find this compound in algae, mainly in red algae due to its hue [68]. Its concentration on each product will depend on environmental factors such as season, processing techniques, and storage temperatures [126].

2.5.2. Siphonaxanthin

Siphonaxanthin is a specific keto-carotenoid current in comestible green algae such as *Codium fragile, Caulerpa lentillifera*, and *Umbraulva japonica*, constituting around 0.1% of their dry weight [35]. This compound is present mainly in species belonged to the Siphonales order, which is characterized by grouping green algae inhabiting deep waters from both freshwater and marine environments [67].

Some studies have been carried out with this molecule, showing the potential beneficial effects on health, including anticancer activities and its suitability in the treatment of leukemia, with even better results than those obtained with FU [35]. This greater capacity to produce an apoptosis-inducing effect may be due to the fact that siphonaxanthin, unlike FU, does not have an epoxide or an allenic bond in its structure, but it does contain an additional hydroxyl group at carbon 19 that might be responsible for this activity [129]. Other activities include anti-angiogenic, antioxidant and anti-inflammatory. The anti-inflammatory effect is due to the suppression of mast cell degranulation in vivo as it alters the functions of lipid rafts by localizing in the cell membrane and inhibiting the translocation of immunoglobulin E (IgE) / IgE receptor (FcεRI) to lipid rafts [130].

2.5.3. Saproxanthin

Saproxanthin is an uncommon and recently described natural CA found in algae, bacteria, and archaea [131], being bacteria the main source. Chemically, it is a tetraterpene with a CA β-cycle additionally hydroxylated at C3 as one end group and simple hydration of the most distant double bond at the other termination of the compound [132]. Therefore, this compound is also a xanthophyll. It was initially reported and described by Aasen and Jensen in *Saprospira grandis* [67]. This compound is a potent antioxidant. It is produced by algae with the aim to protect itself from the activated oxygen produced by light [133]. In vitro studies have shown its pure form pose high antioxidant activity against lipid peroxidation in the rat brain homogenate model and a neuroprotective effect of L-glutamate toxicity [133,134].

2.5.4. Myxol

Myxol is a derivative of γ-carotene and is present in different forms in nature (free or combined with fucosides or nitrogen groups). Nevertheless, in the free state, it is found primarily in marine environments [67]. It should be noted that this pigment is glycosylated in the 2′-OH position instead of the usual position (1′-OH) of the molecule [36]. The main group of organisms that produce this compound are cyanobacteria [135]. Cyanobacteria were previously called myxophyceae, which is named after the characteristic molecule of this family [36]. Some cyanobacteria in which this pigment has been characterized are Anabaena and Nostoc [136]. Nonetheless, algae not only contain free myxol; thus, it is also possible to quantify some combined forms of myxol. One study detected the presence of pro-glyoxylate derivative compounds such as pro-2′-O-methyl-methylpentoside and 4-keto-myxol-2′-methylpentoside in freshwater algae *Oscillatoria limosa* [137]. All variants of this molecule have been proved to have antioxidant properties. In fact, its antioxidant activity is greater than that of other frequently used antioxidant molecules such as ZEA and β-carotene [138]. For example, one study was able to demonstrate significant antioxidant activities against lipid peroxidation in the rat brain homogenate model and a neuroprotective effect of L-glutamate toxicity [134]. Other in vitro studies have concluded that myxol might also be effective in strengthening biological membranes, reducing permeability to oxygen. Nonetheless, these novel and rare CA require meticulous assessments before their execution [138].

2.5.5. Diatoxanthin

Diatoxanthin, a ZEA analogue, is a type of xanthophyll found in phytoplankton and diatoms. Diatoms are often called golden brown microalgae, due to their content of pigments, mainly CA, comprising FU, diadinoxanthin, and diatoxanthin [139]. These compounds have the function of serving as a protection system for algae against the harmful effects of light saturation. Thanks to its presence, the algae are able to quickly acclimatize to the difference in the amount of light received and therefore continue to carry out their vital functions without alterations [140]. Therefore, an effective way to increase the production of this compound, and hence its performance, is to increase the blue-light irradiation; 300 µmol photons m^{-2}·s^{-1} is enough for *Euglena gracilis* [141].

2.5.6. Diadinoxanthin

Similar to diatoxanthin, diadinoxanthin is present only in limited algal groups, including diatoms. In fact, these pigments might be considered as diatom-specific CA [73]. Both compounds are interrelated, since diadinoxanthin is the inactive precursor of diatoxanthin, and it can be transferred to the active compound very quickly when subjected to high light stress [140]. Diadinoxanthin, together with FU, can be obtained from neoxanthin. For this, it is necessary to have a simple isomerization of one of the allenic double bonds of neoxanthin molecule [74]. Its antioxidant activity is based on deepoxidized diadinoxanthin to diatoxanthin, which leads to reduction of the singlet oxygen inside the cell, avoiding cellular damage [142].

3. Mechanism of Action of Xanthophylls

3.1. Metabolism

The mechanism of action of xanthophylls is the specific binding through which the molecule produces its pharmacological effect. This effect will depend on the absorption, distribution, and metabolism of the compound, which are critical parameters of the pharmacokinetics of the xanthophylls. This can be seen in various studies that show the low presence of this type of compound in human tissues, which directly depends on their metabolism and intestinal absorption, and therefore, its bioavailability [143]. The metabolism of xanthophylls is poorly studied, especially for those that do not have provitamin A activity. Hence, more studies are needed to understand its metabolism and, therefore, be able to develop different applications according to the mechanism by which its biological activities occur.

In turn, this would allow the development of safe and effective applications in humans as well as increase its bioavailability [144]. For example, studies on FU metabolism revealed that this compounds itself is not present in plasma but rather its metabolites due to oxidative reactions that take place on FU in mammals. This reaction transforms both compounds into ketocarotenoids [145]. In addition, when FU is administered orally, it undergoes a process of hydrolysis at the intestinal level, giving rise to fucoxanthinol, while liver metabolization results in other active metabolites such as amarouciaxanthin A [146,147]. In fact, it was reported that dietary FU accumulated in the heart and liver as fucoxanthinol and in adipose tissue as amarouciaxanthin A, the latter being non-detectable by HPLC in human serum [148]. Therefore, the oral administration of this compound may only provide some bioactive metabolites, as it is completely metabolized. To release products that maintain its biological activities, it is necessary to develop alternatives that prolong its biological half-life [146], such as emulsions or encapsulations (Table 2).

Table 2. Delivery systems used to increase marine carotenoids' bioavailability.

Mol.	Delivery System	Assay	Benefits	Results	Use	Ref.
FU	Palm stearin solid lipid core	In vitro	Increase stability during storage	Release of FU of 22.92% during 2 h in SGF and 56.55% during 6 h SIF	Oral supplements	[149]
	Nanoparticles of zein	ABTS DPPH	Increase antioxidant activity	More antioxidant than free FU	Foods and beverages	[150]
	Nanoemulsion	In vitro	Increase stability during storage; antiobesity	95% of FU remains in the emulsion after 4 weeks	Food, beverages, nutraceutics	[151]
	Nanoemulsion (LCT)	In vitro digestion and bioability assays in rats	Increase stability	Increase FU level in serum blood (LCT > MCT)	Functional foods and nutraceutics	[152]
	Chitosan–glycolipid nanogels	In vitro	Significant increase in bioavailability	Lpx levels (nmol MDA/mL) higher in control (30.9) than in emulsions (17.0–12.15)	Foods and nutraceutics	[153]
AS	Fish oil	In vitro	Useful for supplementation	Better antioxidant effect	Oral supplements	[154]
	Encapsulation	TBARS Peroxide enzymes	Increase stability	Better antioxidant effect	Foods	[155]
	Pectin–chitosan multilayer	Stability Assays	Increase stability	Better stability than monolayer	Nutraceuticals, functional, medical foods	[156]
	L-lacic acid	Release and stability test	Increase stability	Enhance stability	Functional foods and nutraceutics	[157]
	Ascobyl palmitate emulsion	Stability assay	Sublingual delivery	Enhance sports performance, skin protection, cardioprotective	Dietetic supplementation in sports	[158]
LU	β-CD	In vitro	Increase stability	More stable against oxidating agents	Foods	[159]
	Glycyrrhizic acid, arabinogalactan	In vitro	Solubility enhancement	Prevention of H-aggregates formation, increase of photostability	Foods	[159]
ZEA	Sea Buckthorn oil and water emulsion	Stability and digestive assays	Increase bioaccesibility	Increase 64.55%	Functional foods and nutraceutics	[160]
	High-pressure treatment	Stability and digestive assays		Improve *Nannochloropsis* sp. ZEA disponibility	Foods	[161]
	Glycyrrhizic acid, arabinogalactan	In vitro	Solubility enhancement	Prevention of H-aggregates formation, increase of photostability	Foods	[159]

SGF: Simulated gastric fluid; SIF: Simulated intestinal fluid; LCT: Long-chain triglycerides; MCT: Medium-chain triglycerides.

A study carried out on rats reported that the pharmacokinetic parameters of AS only depend on the dose when it is administered intravenously due to the metabolism that takes place in the liver as a result of saturation of hepatic metabolism of AS [162]. As for AS metabolites described in humans, these are fundamentally 3-hydroxy-4-oxo-β-ionone and 3-hydroxy-4-oxo-7,8-dihydro-β-ionone [163]. The metabolization of AS after oral intake leads to 3-hydroxy-4-oxo-7,8-dihydro-β-ionol and 3-hydroxy-4-oxo-7,8-dihydro-β-ionone, being both compounds detected in plasma [164]. Several researchers hypothesize that the rate at which these reactions take place is determined by the structure of the ring, as well as by the length of the fatty acyl residue formed. Moreover, several enzymes, such as for example diacylglycerol acyltransferase 1, can catalyze the synthesis of AS esters in some strain. This is the case of the microalga *Haematococcus pluvialis* [165].

As for LU and its structural isomer, ZEA, studies carried out in humans have shown that both undergo an in vivo oxidation process that gives rise to several metabolites [166]. LU gives rise to a series of compounds (3′-epilutein, 3′-oxolutein) due to the presence of the enzyme that also mediated the conversion of fucoxanthinol to amarouciaxanthin A [167]. Other compounds such as 3-hydroxy-3′,4′-didehydro-β,γ-carotene and 3-hydroxy-2′,3′-didehydro-β,ε-carotene appear as result of acid hydrolysis in the stomach [168]. However, this compound is capable of remaining intact in its intact form in human ocular tissue due to the inability of the enzyme β-carotene-9′,10′-oxygenase to act on said organ. In this way, there is an extraordinary accumulation of these compounds in the ocular tissue, serving as a mechanism for the prevention of ocular diseases [169]. ZEA, being an isomer of LU, will undergo similar processes to LU. However, it is a much less studied molecule. In this way, ZEA will also be accumulated in the ocular tissue due to the inactivity of the enzymes responsible for the metabolism of ZEA in the organs of sight [170]. Therefore, to determine the bioavailability of LU it is necessary to quantify said metabolites, which also may have different bioactivities, with complementary studies.

3.2. Bioavailability and Bioaccessibility

Xanthophylls have been subjected to numerous studies due to its antioxidant activity and protective effect against several diseases [171]. In recent years, different studies have been carried out comparing the properties of synthetic CA with those of natural origin [172], noting that some of them can only be obtained from natural sources, where there is much more diversity. In addition, these CA obtained from algae can be co-extracted with other bioactive components such as polysaccharides or fatty acids. Therefore, the idea of incorporating CA in foods, nutraceuticals, or cosmetic products is of increasing interest due to their effective bioactive properties [173]. However, to develop and evaluate the viability of any food or cosmetic products that maintain these activities, it is necessary to know its bioactivity, bioavailability, and bioaccesibility [174]. These three parameters are influenced by several factors such as the food matrix; the type of cooking; the time of cooking; the CA involved; the presence of fats, fibers, proteins, and other nutrients in the diet; and the health or nutritional status in humans [175–179].

In humans, once CA are ingested, they are released from the food matrix through the action of gastric enzymes and must be emulsified with lipids in order to improve their absorption [180]. Moreover, its absorption mechanism will be determined by the concentration in which the compound is present. At low concentrations, absorption is mainly due to the action of type 1 class B scavenger receptor, which also captures high-density lipoproteins, platelet glycoprotein 4, and NPC1-like intracellular cholesterol transporter 1 [181]. At high concentrations, the main mechanism is passive diffusion through mucosa [182]. Enzymes released in the duodenum will also play an important role in the absorption, since in this part of the small intestine, pancreatic lipase is released. This enzyme assists the formation of mixed micelles of emulsified droplets with CA. This process depends on the concentration of bile acids among others [183]. Once the micelles are formed, they pass into the blood. Then, micelles are taken up by enterocytes, in which metabolization takes places due to the presence of the enzyme β-carotene oxygenase. The non-metabolized CA, such as LU and ZEA, are incorporated into chylomicrons or low-density lipoproteins (LDL) and are transported to the liver where they can be eliminated by the bile or metabolized and secreted in very low-density lipoprotein (VLDL) or high-density lipoproteins (HDL) to the peripheral tissues, as it can be seen in Figure 3 [180,184].

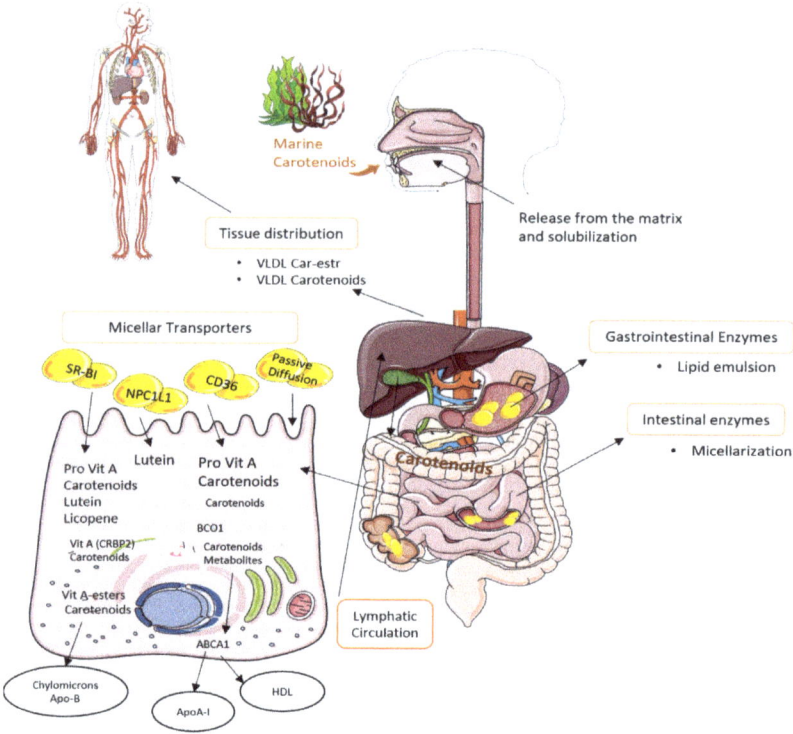

Figure 3. Uptake, transport, and secretion pathways of marine carotenoids in the human body.

All these absorption processes involve passing through membranes, which will be determined by the polarity of the membrane and the compounds. CA are frequently esterified with fatty acids, which decreases the polarity, so except for lutein, they are considered non-polar molecules. Among CA, xanthophylls have a bit higher polarity than carotenes. This is due to the small number of oxygen atoms in their structure (Figure 2). In addition, the polar groups of the molecules are at opposite ends of the molecule, so their forces cancel out. Therefore, the presence of hydroxyl groups makes them a bit more polar than carotenes, which do not contain oxygen but are still considered non-polar molecules [185]. CA polarity and flexibility seem to be correlate with bioaccessibility and uptake efficiency. This may be due to the fact that this type of CA presents a better affinity for lipid transporters and/or for plasma membranes, which would increase absorption [186]. Therefore, these compounds may be the CA with highest bioavailability. Different mechanisms have also been developed to increase the bioavailability of these compounds, of which the most common are the elaboration of emulsions or encapsulations.

3.2.1. Fucoxanthin

Different in vitro, in vivo, and clinical studies show that FU digestion and absorption gives rise to metabolites such as fucoxanthinol. In a study carried out with mice, FU was transformed into fucoxanthinol in the gastrointestinal mucosa by deacetylation due to the action of lipase and cholesterol esterase enzymes. Then, the fucoxanthinol that reached the liver was transformed to amarouciaxanthin by deoxidation. As a result, fucoxanthinol could be detected in the heart, spleen, liver, and lung, and amarouciaxanthin could be found in adipose tissue [145,148]. During all this process, pH is a limiting factor since, as it was observed in an in vitro simulated digestion study, enzymes can be inactivated due to low pH and, consequently, FU would remain intact [187]. A study of the colonic fermentation of FU reported that 50% of FU can be metabolized by action of the human microbiota, ensuring that the compound is bioaccessible [187]. However, the absorption of FU is lower than the rest of the CA despite achieving better accumulation [188]. This may be due to digestion of the compound. In fact, FU supplementation in adults correlated with fucoxanthinol increase in serum [189]. A human trial carried out with FU extracted from *Undaria pinnatifida* concluded that after the supplementation of an extract with 6.1 mg of FU, FU could not be detected in blood, and the metabolite fucoxanthinol was at very low concentration, which confirms the limited intestinal absorption of FU [190]. In order to improve its absorption, different mechanisms have been developed, of which the most common encapsulation is in micelles or liposomes [149]. The best results are obtained when long or medium-chain triglycerides are used to carry out the encapsulation [152]. Encapsulation can also be done with chitosan-glycolipid nanogels, which increase FU bioavailability by 68% according to in vitro studies [153]. Other options include encapsulation with proteins such as zein and caseinate, which provide better stability to FU and enhance its antioxidant and anti-tumor activity compared to free FU [150]. Yet, human studies are scarce and contradictory, since numerous factors that influence bioavailability are reported, such as the dietary fiber of the food matrix; the interaction with other nutrients such as lipids and proteins; the solubility of the molecule; or the affinity with intestinal transporters.

3.2.2. Astaxanthin

AS is considered the compound with the highest bioavailability among CA, followed by lutein, β-carotene, and lycopene [185]. However, its bioavailability depends on the type of matrix and on the stresses of this molecule in colonic Caco-2/TC7 cells [191]. A study carried out in an in vitro digestion model with human intestinal Caco-2 cells of three geometric isomers of AS conclude that the isomerization occurs at a gastrointestinal level, with the 13-cis-astaxanthin isomer showing the greater bioaccessibility and the higher concentrations in blood [192]. In human plasma, AS increases in a dose-dependent manner, achieving stimulation of the immune system, and decreasing oxidative stress and inflammation [193]. High doses (100 mg) present maximum levels of absorption at 11.5 h, while low doses (10 mg) reach them at 6.5 h [194]. Moreover, the bioavailability of said compound can be improved by emulsion with lipids, becoming between 1.7 and 3.7 times better compared to the reference formulation [195]. Other options include encapsulation with lipoprotein aggregates, maltodextrin, pectin, or chitosan [155]. Newer encapsulation methods have also been developed such as oleic acid–bovine serum albumin complexes nanoparticles [196], which are able to find products that, for example, use nanoemulsions with ascorbyl palmitate in sublingual application to favor the absorption and bioavailability of AS [158]. Nevertheless, as AS may be easily degraded by digestive acids, intake after digestion has shown increased levels of absorption [197]. Moreover, the consumption of AS in synergy with fish oil increased the lipid-lowering effects and increased phagocytic activity compared to the consumption of free AS [154]. On the contrary, sociological factors such as smoking habits also play an important role in bioavailability, since tobacco inhibits the bioavailability of AS [194]. AS has already been studied as dietary supplements in Europe, Japan, and the United States, demonstrating their safety in human clinical trials of up to 40 mg/day. Based on these data, the US Food and Drug Administration has approved AS from *H. pluvialis* for human consumption at 12 mg per day and up 24 mg per day for no more than 30 days [194].

3.2.3. β-Cryptoxanthin

The bioaccesibility of various xanthophylls has been demonstrated in numerous studies. In this regard, an in vitro gastric simulation study proved that all-trans-β-cryptoxanthin has 31.87% of bioaccessibility that could be improved by modifying the nature of the matrix [198]. Additional studies suggest a mechanism for the digestion and intestinal absorption of β-cryptoxanthin in its free and esterified forms. The study was made in a digestion model with Caco-2 cells and intestinal cells clone Caco-2 TC7, reporting that β-cryptoxanthin is more bioaccessible than β-carotene, but having worse uptake with Caco-2 TC7 cells [199]. At present, this lack of knowledge makes this compound subject to controversy, since there are studies with disparate results. For example, some of the sources that were consulted state that serum β-cryptoxanthin bioavailability is greater than β-carotene measured in humans after dietary intake [200].

3.2.4. Zeaxanthin

ZEA constitutes one of the three macular pigments, and it is characterized by having a preventive effect in age-related eye diseases [201]; consequently, its consumption is important, as humans are not able to synthesize it or store it at the ocular level [202]. In this sense, the bioavailability and bioavailability of this compound is essential to meet its beneficial effects on health [202]. However, in the case of the ZEA, temperature plays a fundamental role, since thermal processing promotes ZEA release and solubilization in the gastric environment [67]. In addition, its consumption associated with diets or foods rich in fat favors the formation of micelles. These micelles will increase the absorption of the compound at the intestinal level [203]. This is the reason why foods such as sea buckthorn, with a carotenoid-rich oil, possess high bioavailability of ZEA [160]. Thanks to this property, it is relatively easy to increase the bioaccesibility of ZEA, as shown by various studies. One of them endorses the use of coconut oil to increase 6% of ZEA bioaccesibility in goji berries [204]. However, despite the increase in the solubility of ZEA in lipid emulsions, it is necessary to subject the walls of the matrix to microstructural modifications, especially with microalgae, since they can influence the digestibility and bioaccesibility of CA [161]. Nevertheless, microalgae are useful as a source of ZEA in food formulations due to its good bioaccesibility and storage in studies carried out with mice [205]. Additionally, the relationship between ZEA content and bioavailability is another aspect to consider. For example, the bioaccesibility of ZEA in egg yolk is high [206], although the ZEA content is low.

3.3. Experimental Studies

The effects of CA on health have been long studied. As mentioned, some CA such as β-cryptoxanthin or β-carotene are precursors of retinol (vitamin A), while others such as fucoxanthin, lutein, or lycopene are not. As such, their intake relates to their role in retinol production, and to their antioxidant, anti-inflammatory, and anti-tumor activities [207]. In this regard, several in vitro as well as in vivo and observational or epidemiologic studies have been carried out in the last decades. Furthermore, the antioxidant role of CA has been long-known and evidenced for its use as antioxidant additive as well as antioxidant test assay [208]. The great majority of studies have assessed the intake of CA to test their effects, as it is the major ingress pathway of these molecules. As with other antioxidants of natural origin with observed health-promoting properties, it has been suggested that the potential chemopreventive effects of these molecules are derived from the synergy of their antioxidant and anti-inflammatory properties, besides their direct inhibition of certain factors involved in cell cycle and apoptosis [209]. This is due to the intimate relationship of oxidative stress as both a cause and result of inflammation and their relationship toward developing cancer [210,211]. Hence, the properties and effectiveness of CA have been tested and evaluated through various ways, both with molecular methods and relating their intake or serum levels with disease or mortality incidence. A summary of relevant findings will be addressed. Experimental designs and outcomes are shown in Table 3.

Table 3. Summary of studies and meta-analysis on the health-related properties and effects of carotenoids and observed results.

Study	Model	Dose	Experimental Design	Observations	Ref.
Fucoxanthin					
Anti-inflammatory	In vitro. RAW 264.7 macrophages with LPS-induced inflammation	15–60 μM	Expression of inflammatory mediators	D-d reduction of expression of IL6-IL-1, NO, and TNF-α	[212]
	In vitro (Apo-9′). RAW 264.7 macrophages and zebrafish model	25–100 μg/mL	Reduction of LPS-induced inflammation	D-d reduction of NO, ROS, TNF-α, and COX production	[213]
	In vitro and in vivo. RAW 264.7 and aqueous humor of rats	10 mg/kg	Reduction of LPS-induced inflammation	D-d reduction of PGE2, NO, TNF-α by inhibiting iNOS and COX-2	[214]
Anti-cancer	Ex vivo. B16F10 cell culture implanted in mice	200 μM	Growth inhibition of melanoma	D-d growth inhibition by inducing G_0/G_1 cell cycle arrest and apoptosis; inhibition production of retinoblastoma protein	[215]
	In vitro. Human leukemic HL-60 cells	15.2 μM	Inhibited the proliferation	DNA fragmentation	[216]
Astaxanthin					
Anti-inflammatory	In vitro. RAW 264.7, splenocytes, and bone-narrow macrophages	25 μM	Expression of inflammatory mediators in LPS-induced inflammation	D-d significant reduction of IL-6, IL-1β, and ROS production	[217]
	In vivo. Mice with induced acute lung injury	60 mg/kg/day for 14 days	Analysis of inflammation markers, tissue damage	Significant reduction of mortality, histological damage, inflammatory infiltration, and iNOS and NF-κβ levels	[218]
Anti-cancer	In vitro. Human colon cancer lines HCT-116, SW480, WiDr, HT-29 and LS-174	5–25 μg/mL	Growth inhibition of with *H. pluvialis* astaxanthin-rich extract	D-d cell cycle arrest and apoptosis induction by lowering expression of Bcl-2, AKT and induced expression of apoptotic MAPK	[219]
	In vivo. Chemically induced colitis and colon carcinogenesis mice	200 ppm	Analysis of inflammatory biomarkers	D-d inhibition of NF-κβ, TNF-α, IL-1β, IL-6, and COX-2 expression; lower iNOS expression at high dosage	[220]
Lutein					
Anti-inflammatory	Observational study. Early atherosclerosis patients ($n = 65$)	20 mg/day for 3 months	Differences in serum cytokines, and metabolic biomarkers	Significant reduction in serum IL-6 MCP-1 and LDL-cholesterol after 3 months of supplementation	[221]
	Observational study. Preterm infants ($n = 203$)	30 mL/kg/day until 40 weeks post-menstrual age	Differences in inflammation biomarkers	Enhanced retinal development and reduced C-reactive protein levels	[222]
Anti-cancer	In vivo. Rats	3–30 g/L	Inhibition of N-methylnitrosourea-induced colon crypt foci formation	Significantly lowered formation of aberrant crypt foci	[223]

Table 3. Cont.

Study	Model	Dose	Experimental Design	Observations	Ref.
β-cryptoxanthin					
Anti-cancer	Prospective cohort study. Smokers and non-smokers from NHANES III (n = 10,382)	Dietary contribution	20-year cohort	Higher serum levels of β-CRY were associated with lower death risk, but not for non-smokers	[224,225]
	Ex vivo. Human gastric cell lines AGS and SGC-7901 implanted in mice	0–40 μM	Growth and proliferation inhibition	D-d growth and proliferation inhibitory activity by reducing cyclins, endothelial growth factor, PKA and increasing cleaved caspases expression	[226]
	In vivo. Mice	10 mg/kg diet	Induced emphysema and lung tumorigenesis	D-d tumor mass reduction, decreased levels of IL-6 and AKT and restoration of silenced tumor-suppressor genes	[227]
	In vivo. Cigarette smoke-exposed ferrets	7.5–37.5 μg/kg/day	Inflammation biomarkers and tissue damage analysis	D-d inhibition of NF-κβ, TNF-α, AP-1 expression as well as lung tissue squamous metaplasia and inflammation	[228]
Siphonaxanthin					
Anti-cancer	In vitro. Human leukemia (HL-60) cells	5–20 μM	Analysis on cell viability and apoptosis	D-d reduction of cell viability and induction of apoptosis by increasing levels of DR5, lower expression of Bcl-2 and increase in caspase-3	[129]

D-d: Dose-dependent; LPS: Lipolypysaccharide, ROS: Reactive oxygen species, IL: Interleukin, NRF2: Nuclear factor E2-related factor 2, PKA: Protein kinase A, AKT: Protein kinase B, ERK: Extracellular signal-regulated kinase, PAI-1: Plasminogen activator inhibitor-1, MMP: Metalloproteinases, Bcl-2: B-cell lymphoma 2, PG: Prostaglandin, RR: Relative risk, CI: Confidence interval.

3.3.1. Observation In Vitro

In vitro experiments testing properties of CA are of great value to analyze the role of specific molecules and discern potential participating molecules. Their apparent results have been reinforced in multiple animals and human studies, while in some cases, results have been mixed. In fact, most experiments with CA have been made in vitro. The in vitro studies analyzed in this article can be divided into two large groups. The first corresponds to those methods that quantify the antioxidant properties of xanthophylls. The second group includes those anti-inflammatory or anti-cancer tests in cell cultures. Inflammatory models usually comprise the use of human or murine macrophage cell cultures and measure differences in the expression or translation of pro-inflammatory mediators such as cytokines (tumor necrosis factor alpha (TNF-α), interleukins (IL)-1β and IL-6), nuclear factor (NF)-κβ (which mediates the expression of these cytokines), and the production of nitric oxide (NO) or enzymes related to the inflammatory process (cyclooxygenase (COX)-2, nitric oxide synthase (iNOS)) [209]. A study on RAW 264.7 murine macrophages, splenocytes, and bone marrow-derived mice macrophages obtained from mice fed with AS reported a significant reduction of IL-1β and IL-6 and generated ROS. Moreover, the authors described that AS inhibit nuclear translocation of NF-κβ and increase the expression of nuclear factor E2-related factor (NRF)-2, which subsequently involves a lower production of reactive oxygen species (ROS) and inflammatory response [217]. Experiments involving FU or some of its metabolites such as fucoxanthinol or apo-9′-fucoxanthinone in vitro have proven anti-inflammatory activities. On murine macrophages RAW 264.7 with a lipopolysaccharide (LPS)-induced inflammation model, FU and fucoxanthin isomers such as 9′-cis or 13′-cis all displayed a significant dose-dependent inhibition of pro-inflammatory mediators IL6-IL-1, NO, and TNF-α [212]. Likewise, apo-9′-fucoxanthinone notably reduced levels of NO, ROS, TNF-α, and COX enzyme both in RAW 264.7 macrophages and zebrafish juveniles [213]. A study with different human colon and prostate cancer cell lines elucidated that besides the anti-inflammatory and antioxidant effect of β-carotene, it exerts a direct pro-apoptotic activity on cancerous cells by reducing the expression of caveolin-1 and inducing the activity of several caspases. This protein is heavily involved in cell cycle regulation, and its expression leads to increased protein kinase B levels, being both liable of cell proliferation. Conversely, caspases are signals for apoptosis. The authors were able to elucidate this significant pathway of cell growth inhibition, as this was observed in human colon and prostate cell lines that expressed caveolin-1 (HCT-116, PC-3), but not in those that do not produce it (Caco-2, LNCaP) [229].

3.3.2. Observation In Vivo

Although most of the articles studied dealt with in vitro studies, it is also possible to find various articles about in vivo studies of the activities of xanthophylls. Most of these in vivo studies have been carried out with model animals, including mice, rats, and ferrets. Regarding the results obtained, numerous studies reported that in both animals and humans, retinol levels decrease related to inflammatory responses [230]. For instance, β-cryptoxanthin displayed lower levels of TNF-α, as well as pro-inflammatory transcription factors such as NF-κβ and activator protein (AP)-1. Similarly, another study on the anticancer effect of β-cryptoxanthin on nicotin-induced lung carcinogenesis in mice reported significantly lower levels of IL-6 and AKT alongside the re-expression of tumor-suppressor genes that were silenced by nicotine administration [227]. This interaction between nicotine and β-cryptoxanthin was also analyzed in another in vivo study carried out in this case with ferrets. These ferrets were exposed to cigarette smoke for 3 months in order to induce pulmonary tissue inflammation and carcinogenesis, showing a dose-dependent reduction of both in the groups treated with β-cryptoxanthin [228]. On non-provitamin A CA, dextran sulfate sodium-induced colitis and colon carcinogenesis mice were treated with AS food supplementation. Tissue and gut mucose analysis displayed showed significantly lower NF-κβ, TNF-α, IL-1β, IL-6, iNOS, and COX-2 expression, relating these differences to the near nullification of the induced colitis and a lowered risk of colon carcinogenesis [220]. Regarding FU, which is one of the most promising xanthophylls, a study analyzed the anti-inflammatory activity of injected FU by inducing inflammation with LPS in mice and measuring pro-inflammatory mediators in their aqueous humor. FU exerted a significant reduction of prostaglandin (PG)E-2, NO, and TNF-α levels, also showing a lower infiltration of cells and proteins by the induced inflammation. The most relevant outcome of this study is that the effectiveness shown by FU was highly similar to prednisolone, which was used to establish a feasible comparison [214]. It is noteworthy that most carotenoids display anti-inflammatory and anticancer activities in a dose-dependent fashion, as in cell culture studies.

3.3.3. Observational and Epidemiological Studies

In the last decades, case-control and observational studies have also been carried out in humans to test the effectiveness of CA to extend life expectancy and other health-promoting effects such as reducing the risk of developing cancers, chronic inflammatory diseases, or cardiovascular diseases. Results on the possible chemopreventive effect of CA, especially of β-carotene, are mixed [231]. Nevertheless, this effectiveness has been reported in other studies. Various studies are available, for example, evaluating the potential health-promoting effects of LU. One of them analyzed the effect of LU supplementation in subjects from the Shanghai region with early symptoms of atherosclerosis. Albeit the study was carried out with a small sample ($n = 65$), it was observed that the levels of IL-6, MCP-1, and LDL-cholesterol were significantly lower [221]. In another study, food supplementation with β-carotene, lycopene, and lutein was provided to preterm infants. Although only C reactive was used as an inflammation marker, treated groups displayed significantly lower levels alongside improved retinal development in comparison with the control group [222]. The Alpha-Tocopherol, Beta-Carotene (ATBC) Cancer Prevention Study, which was carried out in 1994 with more than 25,000 (n = 29,133) median age male smokers, determined that intake of β-carotene and α-tocopherol supplements could increase the risk of lung cancer, after a ≤8 year follow-up [232]. Additionally, a 24-year follow-up of these subjects did not find a significant chemopreventive effect for supplementing β-carotene toward liver cancer incidence, but it did seem to exert a protective effect in diabetic subjects [233]. However, a recent prospective cohort study of a 30-year follow-up from these subjects determined a significant (p < 0.0001) correlation between CA serum levels and reduced all-cause mortality risk in the study quintiles that displayed higher CA in serum as a result of supplement intake, despite their advanced age and smoking habits [234]. These mixed results, also reported in other prospective cohort studies, show a general trend of a protective effect of CA toward cancer development and inflammation, of which research has focused extensively in β-carotene. However, the increased risks of lung cancer development observed in some studies could arguably be due to an excess of retinol in treated groups, as many studies used high-dosage CA supplements as treatment, while subjects may also intake these CA through diet [233]. Taking the case of the ATBC study, the β-carotene dose was of 20 mg, as much as three times the recommended dietary allowance of retinol [232]. Conversely, α-carotene, lycopene, and β-cryptoxanthin have been inversely correlated with developing lung cancer or at least showing a consistent chemopreventive effect [235]. Another study assessed serum CA levels from individuals from the US Third Nutrition and Health Examination Survey (NHANES III) [224], which evaluated health habits and analyzed the serum samples of the participants. In this prospective cohort study, α-carotene and β-cryptoxanthin also displayed effectiveness in lowering the risk of lung cancer development in smokers, but this effect was not apparent in non-smokers [225]. An extensive meta-analysis of human observational studies with a total sample size of more than 150,000 individuals (n = 174,067) assessed results from 13 studies, determining that provitamin A CA may exert a protective effect against cancer or cardiovascular mortality [236]. Yet, the authors noted that as mentioned, an excessive production of retinol because of supplementation may be responsible for the reported increased risks of lung cancer development in some case-control studies that considered these variables. It is noteworthy that the greatest meta-analysis up to date to our knowledge evaluated 34 observational studies with a total sample size of 592,479 participants and established correlations between intake or serum levels of α-carotene and lycopene but not β-carotene with lowered risk of developing prostate cancer [237]. These findings also noted that even if these carotenoids had an apparent chemopreventive activity, they were ineffective in preventing malignancy of prostate cancer once it was diagnosed. Altogether, albeit more extensive research with bigger sample sizes and the isolation of potential confusion factors is required, there is a great body of evidence suggesting that in controlled dose ranges, both provitamin A and non-provitamin carotenoids have chemopreventive effects on oxidative stress, inflammation, and cancer development through indirect and direct pathways.

4. Algae as Source of Carotenoids

Algae are recognized as a good source for numerous bioactive compounds of great interest, xanthophylls being among them, as reflected on this work. However, the application of these compounds is not linked only to food safety and human health, but factors such as economic costs, efficacy of the designed product, or current legislation are also of vital importance when deciding whether a product it is viable or not and, therefore, it is produced in a commercial way or not. Despite this complexity, algae have become a powerful industry due to its biotechnological applications, advancements in extraction methods, and increasing consumer demand for natural products. As a result, a wide range of products are and have been developed, ranging from nutraceuticals, food additives, or animal feed to drugs or cosmetics [67]. CA play a very important role in all these applications with even better results that their synthetic counterpart [238]. All of these progresses mean that the demand and market of CA are growing significantly, and this year is expected to reach $1.53 billion [239]. Despite this, more advances are still needed to reduce the cost of obtaining it from natural sources. It is estimated that CA derived from algae can reach the cost of $7500/kg [240], whereas synthetic CA could be obtained at roughly half the cost [241]. Nevertheless, despite the great diversity of natural and synthetic CA, only a few of them are commercially produced, including carotenes (β-carotene and lycopene) and xanthophylls (astaxanthin, lutein, zeaxanthin, canthaxanthin, and capsanthin) [242]. Some processes have been developed to increase the benefits. For example, high costs production can be reduced through the development of green technologies as they are considered more profitable, efficient, and ecological, transforming it into an environmentally friendly process [243]. Another important parameter when optimizing is the selection of algae used as source. In this regard, the genomic characterization of these species and identifying relevant target genes involved in CA synthesis and accumulation, paired with efficient culture and harvest techniques; has proven to be an efficient way to maximize CA production [116].

However, there are still barriers that must be solved for the commercialization of CA from algae, such as optimization of their extraction and purification, storage alternatives, and technologies that increase the bioaccessibility and bioavailability of the compounds present in algae [151,157,198]. Currently, different processes such as encapsulation or emulsification arise for CA to achieve their biological functions in humans. In addition, the research has provided data through in vitro and in vivo digestion studies that clarify the absorption mechanism of the different CA, which can be used by industries to improve the formulation of their products. However, more human studies of the nutritional efficiency of these CA extracted from algae are needed [203].

The lack of uniformity of legislation between the different countries makes its study complex. That is why in order to carry out the commercialization of the products obtained, it is necessary to carry out some modifications to adapt them to current legislation. In the case of the EU, as algae were not being used in a traditional or habitual way in food before 15 May 1997, they are considered as novel food as reflected in EU Regulation 2015/2283. This regulation is also applicable to all products obtained from algae such as food supplements of their bioactive components or food additives (*i.e.*, phlorotannins from *Ecklonia cava*) [244]. Therefore, its commercialization request authorization for its incorporation into the market from the European Food Safety Authority (EFSA), which requires health risk studies. These food safety analyses must also be in accordance with current legislation on food safety and food hygiene, respectively included in Regulation (EU) 178/2002 [244] and Regulation (EU) 852/2004 [245], ensuring consumer safety. Moreover, these products can be sold as nutraceuticals without scientific evidence conducted by the EFSA, which is legislated by Regulation CE No. 1924/2006 [246]. However, this same regulation dictates that the health claims alleged to these same products must be backed by proper and significant scientific evidence, which must be submitted to EFSA.

5. Conclusions

The use of algae as raw material for obtaining carotenoids, and especially xanthophylls, is an alternative that is gaining interest due to its potential and the bioactivities of the extracted compounds. Currently, CA are used commercially as food additives, feed and nutrient supplements, pigments, and, more recently, as nutraceuticals for cosmetic and pharmaceutical purposes. Despite this, there is little information on the impact of some of these xanthophylls on human health, with most of the studies focusing on FU and AS, which are compounds that also represent the main marine CA. These molecules are characterized by having a high antioxidant activity, and this may be one of the main mechanisms in their anticancer and anti-inflammatory activity. These activities will vary between the different compounds due to the nature of their terminal groups or the length of the chain, among others. However, for these proposals to be viable, it is necessary to carry out a series of advances. These advancements include increased biomass production, increased extraction, and purification performance, as well as reduced implementation costs. Some ways to solve these problems go through genetic engineering or the development of green extraction techniques.

Author Contributions: Conceptualization, A.G.P., P.O., J.E., A.C.-C., F.C., N.C., A.J., C.L.-L., J.S.-G. and M.A.P.; methodology, A.G.P., P.O. and J.E.; investigation, A.G.P., P.O., J.E., A.C.-C., F.C., N.C., A.J. and C.L.-L.; resources, A.G.P., P.O., J.E., A.C.-C., F.C., N.C., A.J. and C.L.-L.; data curation, A.G.P., P.O., J.E., A.C.-C., F.C., N.C., A.J. and C.L.-L.; writing—original draft preparation, A.G.P., P.O., J.E., A.C.-C., F.C., N.C., A.J., C.L.-L., J.S.-G. and M.A.P.; writing—review and editing, A.G.P., P.O., J.E., A.C.-C., F.C., N.C., A.J., C.L.-L., J.S.-G. and M.A.P.; visualization, A.G.P., P.O. and J.E.; supervision, J.S.-G. and M.A.P.; project administration, A.G.P., P.O. and J.E.; funding acquisition, J.S.-G. and M.A.P. All authors have read and agreed to the published version of the manuscript.

Funding: The research leading to these results was funded by Xunta de Galicia supporting the Axudas Conecta Peme, the IN852A 2018/58 NeuroFood Project and the program EXCELENCIA-ED431F 2020/12; to Ibero-American Program on Science and Technology (CYTED—AQUA-CIBUS, P317RT0003) and to the Bio Based Industries Joint Undertaking (JU) under grant agreement No 888003 UP4HEALTH Project (H2020-BBI-JTI-2019). The JU receives support from the European Union's Horizon 2020 research and innovation program and the Bio Based Industries Consortium. The project SYSTEMIC Knowledge hub on Nutrition and Food Security, has received funding from national research funding parties in Belgium (FWO), France (INRA), Germany (BLE), Italy (MIPAAF), Latvia (IZM), Norway (RCN), Portugal (FCT), and Spain (AEI) in a joint action of JPI HDHL, JPI-OCEANS and FACCE-JPI launched in 2019 under the ERA-NET ERA-HDHL (n° 696295).

Institutional Review Board Statement: Not applicable.

Informed Consent Statement: Not applicable.

Data Availability Statement: Not applicable.

Acknowledgments: The research leading to these results was supported by MICINN supporting the Ramón y Cajal grant for M.A. Prieto (RYC-2017-22891) and the FPU grant for Anxo Carreira Casais (FPU2016/06135); by Xunta de Galicia for supporting the pre-doctoral grant of Antía González Pereira (ED481A-2019/0228) and the program EXCELENCIA-ED431F 2020/12 that supports the work of F. Chamorro; by UP4HEALTH Project that supports the work of P. Otero and C. Lourenço-Lopes.

Conflicts of Interest: The authors declare no conflict of interest.

References

1. Plaza, M.; Santoyo, S.; Jaime, L.; García-Blairsy Reina, G.; Herrero, M.; Señoráns, F.J.; Ibáñez, E. Screening for Bioactive Compounds from Algae. *J. Pharm. Biomed. Anal.* **2010**, *51*, 450–455. [CrossRef]
2. Yamamoto, K.; Ishikawa, C.; Katano, H.; Yasumoto, T.; Mori, N. Fucoxanthin and Its Deacetylated Product, Fucoxanthinol, Induce Apoptosis of Primary Effusion Lymphomas. *Cancer Lett.* **2011**. [CrossRef]
3. Kanda, H.; Kamo, Y.; Machmudah, S.; Wahyudiono; Goto, M. Extraction of Fucoxanthin from Raw Macroalgae Excluding Drying and Cell Wall Disruption by Liquefied Dimethyl Ether. *Mar. Drugs* **2014**, *12*, 2383–2396. [CrossRef]
4. Alves, C.; Pinteus, S.; Simões, T.; Horta, A.; Silva, J.; Tecelão, C.; Pedrosa, R. *Bifurcaria Bifurcata*: A Key Macro-Alga as a Source of Bioactive Compounds and Functional Ingredients. *Int. J. Food Sci. Technol.* **2016**, *51*, 1638–1646. [CrossRef]
5. AGRIOS, G.N. Plant diseases caused by parasitic higher plants, invasive climbing plants, and parasitic green algae. In *Plant Pathology*; Springer: San Diego, CA, USA, 2005; pp. 705–722.
6. Ibañez, E.; Cifuentes, A. Benefits of Using Algae as Natural Sources of Functional Ingredients. *J. Sci. Food Agric.* **2013**, *93*, 703–709. [CrossRef]
7. Barkia, I.; Saari, N.; Manning, S.R. Microalgae for High-Value Products towards Human Health and Nutrition. *Mar. Drugs* **2019**, *17*, 304. [CrossRef] [PubMed]
8. Kosanić, M.; Ranković, B.; Stanojković, T. Biological Activities of Two Macroalgae from Adriatic Coast of Montenegro. *Saudi J. Biol. Sci.* **2015**, *22*, 390–397. [CrossRef] [PubMed]
9. Poojary, M.M.; Barba, F.J.; Aliakbarian, B.; Donsì, F.; Pataro, G.; Dias, D.A.; Juliano, P. Innovative Alternative Technologies to Extract Carotenoids from Microalgae and Seaweeds. *Mar. Drugs* **2016**, *14*, 1–34. [CrossRef]
10. El Gamal, A.A. Biological Importance of Marine Algae. *Saudi Pharm. J.* **2010**, *18*, 1–25. [CrossRef]
11. García, J.L.; de Vicente, M.; Galán, B. Microalgae, Old Sustainable Food and Fashion Nutraceuticals. *Microb. Biotechnol.* **2017**, *10*, 1017–1024. [CrossRef]
12. Andersen, R.A. Diversity of Eukaryotic Algae. *Biodivers. Conserv.* **1992**, *1*, 267–292. [CrossRef]

13. Gong, M.; Bassi, A. Carotenoids from Microalgae: A Review of Recent Developments. *Biotechnol. Adv.* **2016**, *34*, 1396–1412. [CrossRef] [PubMed]
14. Vílchez, C.; Forján, E.; Cuaresma, M.; Bédmar, F.; Garbayo, I.; Vega, J.M. Marine Carotenoids: Biological Functions and Commercial Applications. *Mar. Drugs* **2011**, *9*, 319–333. [CrossRef]
15. Beutner, S.; Bloedorn, B.; Frixel, S.; Blanco, I.H.; Hoffmann, T.; Martin, H.D.; Mayer, B.; Noack, P.; Ruck, C.; Schmidt, M.; et al. Quantitative Assessment of Antioxidant Properties of Natural Colorants and Phytochemicals: Carotenoids, Flavonoids, Phenols and Indigoids. The Role of β-Carotene in Antioxidant Functions. *J. Sci. Food Agric.* **2001**, *81*, 559–568. [CrossRef]
16. Saadaoui, I.; Rasheed, R.; Abdulrahman, N.; Bounnit, T.; Cherif, M.; Al Jabri, H.; Mraiche, F. Algae-Derived Bioactive Compounds with Anti-Lung Cancer Potential. *Mar. Drugs* **2020**, *18*, 197. [CrossRef]
17. Bolhassani, A. Cancer Chemoprevention by Natural Carotenoids as an Efficient Strategy. *Anticancer. Agents Med. Chem.* **2015**, *15*, 1026–1031. [CrossRef]
18. Garewal, H. Antioxidants in Oral Cancer Prevention. *Am. J. Clin. Nutr.* **1995**, *62*, 1410S–1416S. [CrossRef]
19. Kim, J.; Leite, J.; DeOgburn, R.; Smyth, J.; Clark, R.; Fernandez, M. A Lutein-Enriched Diet Prevents Cholesterol Accumulation and Decreases Oxidized LDL and Inflammatory Cytokines in the Aorta of Guinea Pigs. *J. Nutr.* **2011**, *141*, 1458–1463. [CrossRef] [PubMed]
20. Kim, K.N.; Heo, S.J.; Yoon, W.J.; Kang, S.M.; Ahn, G.; Yi, T.H.; Jeon, Y.J. Fucoxanthin Inhibits the Inflammatory Response by Suppressing the Activation of NF-KB and MAPKs in Lipopolysaccharide-Induced RAW 264.7 Macrophages. *Eur. J. Pharmacol.* **2010**, *649*, 369–375. [CrossRef]
21. Bhatt, T.; Patel, K. Carotenoids: Potent to Prevent Diseases Review. *Nat. Products Bioprospect.* **2020**, *10*, 109–117. [CrossRef] [PubMed]
22. Jain, A.; Sirisha, V.L. Algal Carotenoids: Understanding Their Structure, Distribution and Potential Applications in Human Health. *Encycl. Mar. Biotechnol.* **2020**, 33–64. [CrossRef]
23. Pangestuti, R.; Kim, S.K. Biological Activities and Health Benefit Effects of Natural Pigments Derived from Marine Algae. *J. Funct. Foods* **2011**, *3*, 255–266. [CrossRef]
24. Wang, W.J.; Wang, G.C.; Zhang, M.; Tseng, C.K. Isolation of Fucoxanthin from the Rhizoid of *Laminaria Japonica* Aresch. *J. Integr. Plant Biol.* **2005**, *47*, 1009–1015. [CrossRef]
25. Peng, J.; Yuan, J.P.; Wu, C.F.; Wang, J.H. Fucoxanthin, a Marine Carotenoid Present in Brown Seaweeds and Diatoms: Metabolism and Bioactivities Relevant to Human Health. *Mar. Drugs* **2011**, *9*, 1806–1828. [CrossRef]
26. Ojulari, O.V.; Gi Lee, S.; Nam, J.O. Therapeutic Effect of Seaweed Derived Xanthophyl Carotenoid on Obesity Management; Overview of the Last Decade. *Int. J. Mol. Sci.* **2020**, *21*, 2502. [CrossRef] [PubMed]
27. Guerin, M.; Huntley, M.E.; Olaizola, M. *Haematococcus* Astaxanthin: Applications for Human Health and Nutrition. *Trends Biotechnol.* **2003**, *21*, 210–216. [CrossRef]
28. Camacho, F.; Macedo, A.; Malcata, F. Potential Industrial Applications and Commercialization of Microalgae in the Functional Food and Feed Industries: A Short Review. *Mar. Drugs* **2019**, *17*, 312. [CrossRef] [PubMed]
29. Lorenz, R.; Cysewski, G. Commercial Potential for *Haematococcus* Microalgae as a Natural Source of Astaxanthin. *Trends Biotechnol.* **2000**, *18*, 160–167. [CrossRef]
30. Murthy, K.N.C.; Vanitha, A.; Rajesha, J.; Swamy, M.M.; Sowmya, P.R.; Ravishankar, G.A. In Vivo Antioxidant Activity of Carotenoids from *Dunaliella Salina* - A Green Microalga. *Life Sci.* **2005**, *76*, 1381–1390. [CrossRef]
31. Silva, S.C.; Ferreira, I.C.F.R.; Dias, M.M.; Barreiro, M.F. Microalgae-Derived Pigments: A 10-Year Bibliometric Review and Industry and Market Trend Analysis. *Molecules* **2020**, *25*, 3406. [CrossRef] [PubMed]
32. Christaki, E.; Bonos, E.; Giannenasa, I.; Florou-Paneria, P. Functional Properties of Carotenoids Originating from Algae. *J. Sci. Food Agric.* **2013**, *93*, 5–11. [CrossRef]
33. Esteban, R.; Martínez, B.; Fernández-Marín, B.; Becerril, J.M.; García-Plazaola, J.I. Carotenoid Composition in Rhodophyta: Insights into Xanthophyll Regulation in *Corallina Elongata*. *Eur. J. Phycol.* **2009**, *44*, 221–230. [CrossRef]
34. Careri, M.; Furlattini, L.; Mangia, A.; Musci, M.; Anklam, E.; Theobald, A.; Von Holst, C. Supercritical Fluid Extraction for Liquid Chromatographic Determination of Carotenoids in *Spirulina Pacifica* Algae: A Chemometric Approach. *J. Chromatogr. A* **2001**, *912*, 61–71. [CrossRef]
35. Sugawara, T.; Ganesan, P.; Li, Z.; Manabe, Y.; Hirata, T. Siphonaxanthin, a Green Algal Carotenoid, as a Novel Functional Compound. *Mar. Drugs* **2014**, *12*, 3660–3668. [CrossRef]
36. Graham, J.E.; Bryant, D.A. The Biosynthetic Pathway for Myxol-2′ Fucoside (Myxoxanthophyll) in the Cyanobacterium Synechococcus Sp. Strain PCC 7002. *J. Bacteriol.* **2009**, *191*, 3292–3300. [CrossRef]
37. Michalak, I.; Chojnacka, K. Algae as Production Systems of Bioactive Compounds. *Eng. Life Sci.* **2015**, *15*, 160–176. [CrossRef]
38. Joel, J. Carotenoids Market by Type (Astaxanthin, Beta-Carotene, Lutein, Lycopene, Canthaxanthin, Zeaxanthin, and Others) for Feed, Food, Supplements, Cosmetics, and Pharmaceuticals-Global Industry Perspective, Comprehensive Analysis, Size, Share, Growth, Segmen. Available online: https://www.marketsandmarkets.com/Market-Reports/carotenoid-market-158421566.html (accessed on 12 February 2021).
39. da Silva Vaz, B.; Moreira, J.B.; de Morais, M.G.; Costa, J.A.V. Microalgae as a New Source of Bioactive Compounds in Food Supplements. *Curr. Opin. Food Sci.* **2016**, *7*, 73–77. [CrossRef]

40. Mulders, K.J.M.; Lamers, P.P.; Martens, D.E.; Wijffels, R.H. Phototrophic Pigment Production with Microalgae: Biological Constraints and Opportunities. *J. Phycol.* **2014**, *50*, 229–242. [CrossRef] [PubMed]
41. Ma, R.; Wang, B.; Chua, E.T.; Zhao, X.; Lu, K.; Ho, S.H.; Shi, X.; Liu, L.; Xie, Y.; Lu, Y.; et al. Comprehensive Utilization of Marine Microalgae for Enhanced Co-Production of Multiple Compounds. *Mar. Drugs* **2020**, *18*, 467. [CrossRef] [PubMed]
42. Shannon, E.; Abu-Ghannam, N. Enzymatic Extraction of Fucoxanthin from Brown Seaweeds. *Int. J. Food Sci. Technol.* **2018**, *53*, 2195–2204. [CrossRef]
43. Heffernan, N.; Smyth, T.J.; FitzGerald, R.J.; Vila-Soler, A.; Mendiola, J.; Ibáñez, E.; Brunton, N.P. Comparison of Extraction Methods for Selected Carotenoids from Macroalgae and the Assessment of Their Seasonal/Spatial Variation. *Innov. Food Sci. Emerg. Technol.* **2016**, *37*, 221–228. [CrossRef]
44. Xiao, X.; Si, X.; Yuan, Z.; Xu, X.; Li, G. Isolation of Fucoxanthin from Edible Brown Algae by Microwave-Assisted Extraction Coupled with High-Speed Countercurrent Chromatography. *J. Sep. Sci.* **2012**, *35*, 2313–2317. [CrossRef]
45. Chen, Y.C.; Cheng, C.Y.; Liu, C.T.; Sue, Y.M.; Chen, T.H.; Hsu, Y.H.; Huang, N.J.; Chen, C.H. Combined Protective Effects of Oligo-Fucoidan, Fucoxanthin, and L-Carnitine on the Kidneys of Chronic Kidney Disease Mice. *Eur. J. Pharmacol.* **2021**, *892*, 173708. [CrossRef]
46. Sugimura, R.; Suda, M.; Sho, A.; Takahashi, T.; Sashima, T.; Abe, M.; Hosokawa, M.; Miyashita, K. Stability of Fucoxanthin in Dried Undaria Pinnatifida (Wakame) and Baked Products (Scones) Containing Wakame Powder. *Food Sci. Technol. Res.* **2012**, *18*, 687–693. [CrossRef]
47. Mori, K.; Ooi, T.; Hiraoka, M.; Oka, N.; Hamada, H.; Tamura, M.; Kusumi, T. Fucoxanthin and Its Metabolites in Edible Brown Algae Cultivated in Deep Seawater. *Mar. Drugs* **2004**, *2*, 63–72. [CrossRef]
48. Raguraman, V.; Abraham, S.L.; MubarakAli, D.; Narendrakumar, G.; Thirugnanasambandam, R.; Kirubagaran, R.; Thajuddin, N. Unraveling Rapid Extraction of Fucoxanthin from Padina Tetrastromatica: Purification, Characterization and Biomedical Application. *Process Biochem.* **2018**, *73*, 211–219. [CrossRef]
49. Nomura, M.; Kamogawa, H.; Susanto, E.; Kawagoe, C.; Yasui, H.; Saga, N.; Hosokawa, M.; Miyashita, K. Seasonal Variations of Total Lipids, Fatty Acid Composition, and Fucoxanthin Contents of Sargassum Horneri (Turner) and Cystoseira Hakodatensis (Yendo) from the Northern Seashore of Japan. *J. Appl. Phycol.* **2013**, *25*, 1159–1169. [CrossRef]
50. Rajauria, G.; Foley, B.; Abu-Ghannam, N. Characterization of Dietary Fucoxanthin from Himanthalia Elongata Brown Seaweed. *Food Res. Int.* **2017**, *99*, 995–1001. [CrossRef]
51. Gonçalves de Oliveira-Júnior, R.; Grougnet, R.; Bodet, P.E.; Bonnet, A.; Nicolau, E.; Jebali, A.; Rumin, J.; Picot, L. Updated Pigment Composition of *Tisochrysis Lutea* and Purification of Fucoxanthin Using Centrifugal Partition Chromatography Coupled to Flash Chromatography for the Chemosensitization of Melanoma Cells. *Algal Res.* **2020**, *51*, 102035. [CrossRef]
52. Robertson, R.C.; Gracia Mateo, M.R.; O'Grady, M.N.; Guihéneuf, F.; Stengel, D.B.; Ross, R.P.; Fitzgerald, G.F.; Kerry, J.P.; Stanton, C. An Assessment of the Techno-Functional and Sensory Properties of Yoghurt Fortified with a Lipid Extract from the Microalga Pavlova Lutheri. *Innov. Food Sci. Emerg. Technol.* **2016**, *37*, 237–246. [CrossRef]
53. Mok, I.K.; Yoon, J.R.; Pan, C.H.; Kim, S.M. Development, Quantification, Method Validation, and Stability Study of a Novel Fucoxanthin-Fortified Milk. *J. Agric. Food Chem.* **2016**, *64*, 6196–6202. [CrossRef]
54. Panis, G.; Carreon, J.R. Commercial Astaxanthin Production Derived by Green Alga *Haematococcus Pluvialis*: A Microalgae Process Model and a Techno-Economic Assessment All through Production Line. *Algal Res.* **2016**, *18*, 175–190. [CrossRef]
55. Aflalo, C.; Meshulam, Y.; Zarka, A.; Boussiba, S. On the Relative Efficiency of Two- vs. One-Stage Production of Astaxanthin by the Green Alga *Haematococcus Pluvialis*. *Biotechnol. Bioeng.* **2007**, *98*, 300–305. [CrossRef] [PubMed]
56. Torzillo, G.; Goksan, T.; Faraloni, C.; Kopecky, J.; Masojídek, J. Interplay between Photochemical Activities and Pigment Composition in an Outdoor Culture of *Haematococcus Pluvialis* during the Shift from the Green to Red Stage. *J. Appl. Phycol.* **2003**, *15*, 127–136. [CrossRef]
57. Ranga, R.; Sarada, A.R.; Baskaran, V.; Ravishankar, G.A. Identification of Carotenoids from Green Alga *Haematococcus Pluvialis* by HPLC and LC-MS (APCI) and Their Antioxidant Properties. *J. Microbiol. Biotechnol.* **2009**, *19*, 1333–1341. [CrossRef]
58. Molino, A.; Rimauro, J.; Casella, P.; Cerbone, A.; Larocca, V.; Chianese, S.; Karatza, D.; Mehariya, S.; Ferraro, A.; Hristoforou, E.; et al. Extraction of Astaxanthin from Microalga *Haematococcus Pluvialis* in Red Phase by Using Generally Recognized as Safe Solvents and Accelerated Extraction. *J. Biotechnol.* **2018**, *283*, 51–61. [CrossRef]
59. Sun, Z.; Li, T.; Zhou, Z.G.; Jiang, Y. Microalgae as a source of lutein: Chemistry, biosynthesis, and carotenogenesis. In *Advances in Biochemical Engineering/Biotechnology*; Springer: Heidelberg, Germany, 2016; Volume 153, pp. 37–58.
60. Shi, X.M.; Zhang, X.W.; Chen, F. Heterotrophic Production of Biomass and Lutein by *Chlorella Protothecoides* on Various Nitrogen Sources. *Enzyme Microb. Technol.* **2000**, *27*, 312–318. [CrossRef]
61. Shi, X.M.; Jiang, Y.; Chen, F. High-Yield Production of Lutein by the Green Microalga Chlorella Protothecoides in Heterotrophic Fed-Batch Culture. *Biotechnol. Prog.* **2002**, *18*, 723–727. [CrossRef]
62. Fábryová, T.; Cheel, J.; Kubáč, D.; Hrouzek, P.; Vu, D.L.; Tůmová, L.; Kopecký, J. Purification of Lutein from the Green Microalgae *Chlorella Vulgaris* by Integrated Use of a New Extraction Protocol and a Multi-Injection High Performance Counter-Current Chromatography (HPCCC). *Algal Res.* **2019**, *41*, 101574. [CrossRef]
63. Sánchez, J.F.; Fernández, J.M.; Acién, F.G.; Rueda, A.; Pérez-Parra, J.; Molina, E. Influence of Culture Conditions on the Productivity and Lutein Content of the New Strain *Scenedesmus Almeriensis*. *Process Biochem.* **2008**, *43*, 398–405. [CrossRef]

64. Serejo, M.L.; Posadas, E.; Boncz, M.A.; Blanco, S.; García-Encina, P.; Muñoz, R. Influence of Biogas Flow Rate on Biomass Composition during the Optimization of Biogas Upgrading in Microalgal-Bacterial Processes. *Environ. Sci. Technol.* **2015**, *49*, 3228–3236. [CrossRef] [PubMed]
65. Liau, B.C.; Hong, S.E.; Chang, L.P.; Shen, C.T.; Li, Y.C.; Wu, Y.P.; Jong, T.T.; Shieh, C.J.; Hsu, S.L.; Chang, C.M.J. Separation of Sight-Protecting Zeaxanthin from *Nannochloropsis Oculata* by Using Supercritical Fluids Extraction Coupled with Elution Chromatography. *Sep. Purif. Technol.* **2011**, *78*, 1–8. [CrossRef]
66. Koo, S.Y.; Cha, K.H.; Song, D.G.; Chung, D.; Pan, C.H. Optimization of Pressurized Liquid Extraction of Zeaxanthin from *Chlorella Ellipsoidea*. *J. Appl. Phycol.* **2012**, *24*, 725–730. [CrossRef]
67. Torregrosa-Crespo, J.; Montero, Z.; Fuentes, J.L.; García-Galbis, M.R.; Garbayo, I.; Vílchez, C.; Martínez-Espinosa, R.M. Exploring the Valuable Carotenoids for the Large-Scale Production by Marine Microorganisms. *Mar. Drugs* **2018**, *16*, 203. [CrossRef]
68. Schubert, N.; García-Mendoza, E.; Pacheco-Ruiz, I. Carotenoid Composition of Marine Red Algae. *J. Phycol.* **2006**, *42*, 1208–1216. [CrossRef]
69. Othman, R.; Noh, N.H.; Hatta, F.A.M.; Jamaludin, M.A. Natural Carotenoid Pigments of 6 Chlorophyta Freshwater Green Algae Species. *J. Pharm. Nutr. Sci.* **2018**, *8*, 1–5. [CrossRef]
70. Geisert, M.; Rose, T.; Bauer, W.; Zahn, R.K. Occurrence of Carotenoids and Sporopollenin in *Nanochlorum Eucaryotum*, a Novel Marine Alga with Unusual Characteristics. *BioSystems* **1987**, *20*, 133–142. [CrossRef]
71. Ricketts, T.R. The Structures of Siphonein and Siphonaxanthin from *Codium Fragile*. *Phytochemistry* **1971**, *10*, 155–160. [CrossRef]
72. Chen, X.; Sun, Y.; Liu, H.; Liu, S.; Qin, Y.; Li, P. Advances in Cultivation, Wastewater Treatment Application, Bioactive Components of *Caulerpa Lentillifera* and Their Biotechnological Applications. *PeerJ* **2019**, *2019*, e6118. [CrossRef]
73. Kuczynska, P.; Jemiola-Rzeminska, M. Isolation and Purification of All-Trans Diadinoxanthin and All-Trans Diatoxanthin from Diatom *Phaeodactylum Tricornutum*. *J. Appl. Phycol.* **2017**, *29*, 79–87. [CrossRef]
74. Dambek, M.; Eilers, U.; Breitenbach, J.; Steiger, S.; Büchel, C.; Sandmann, G. Biosynthesis of Fucoxanthin and Diadinoxanthin and Function of Initial Pathway Genes in *Phaeodactylum Tricornutum*. *J. Exp. Bot.* **2012**, *63*, 5607–5612. [CrossRef]
75. Xia, S.; Wang, K.; Wan, L.; Li, A.; Hu, Q.; Zhang, C. Production, Characterization, and Antioxidant Activity of Fucoxanthin from the Marine Diatom Odontella Aurita. *Mar. Drugs* **2013**, *11*, 2667–2681. [CrossRef] [PubMed]
76. Ragni, M.; D'Alcalà, M.R. Circadian Variability in the Photobiology of *Phaeodactylum Tricornutum*: Pigment Content. *J. Plankton Res.* **2007**, *29*, 141–156. [CrossRef]
77. Lourenço-Lopes, C.; Jiménez-López, C.; Pereira, A.G.; García-Oliveira, P.; Prieto, M.A.; Simal-Gándara, J. Fucoxanthin Extraction from Algae - Properties and Bioactivities. In Proceedings of the Iberphenol. Iberian Congress on Phenolic Compounds, Ourense, Spain, 2 October 2019.
78. Maeda, H.; Hosokawa, M.; Sashima, T.; Takahashi, N.; Kawada, T.; Miyashita, K. Fucoxanthin and Its Metabolite, Fucoxanthinol, Suppress Adipocyte Differentiation in 3T3-L1 Cells. *Int. J. Mol. Med.* **2006**, *18*, 147–152. [CrossRef]
79. Maoka, T.; Fujiwara, Y.; Hashimoto, K.; Akimoto, N. Characterization of Fucoxanthin and Fucoxanthinol Esters in the Chinese Surf Clam, Mactra Chinensis. *J. Agric. Food Chem.* **2007**. [CrossRef]
80. Willstatter, R.; Page, H. Chlorophyll. XXIV. The Pigments of the Brown Algae. *Justus Liebigs Ann. Chem.* **1914**, *404*, 237–271.
81. Kajikawa, T.; Okumura, S.; Iwashita, T.; Kosumi, D.; Hashimoto, H.; Katsumura, S. Stereocontrolled Total Synthesis of Fucoxanthin and Its Polyene Chain-Modified Derivative. *Org. Lett.* **2012**. [CrossRef]
82. Kim, S.; Chen, J.; Cheng, T.; Gindulyte, A.; He, J.; He, S.; Li, Q.; Shoemaker, B.A.; Thiessen, P.A.; Yu, B. PubChem in 2021: New data content and improved web interfaces. *Nucleic Acids Res.* **2019**, *47*, D1388–D1395. [CrossRef]
83. Soo-Jin You-Jin, H.; Seok-Chun, K.; Sung-Myung, K.; Hahk-Soo, K.; Jong-Pyung, K.; Soo-Hyun, K.; Ki-Wan, L.; Man-Gi, C. Jeon Cytoprotective Effect of Fucoxanthin Isolated from Brown Algae *Sargassum Siliquastrum* against H2O2-Induced Cell Damage. *Eur. Food Res. Technol.* **2008**, *228*, 145–151. [CrossRef]
84. Chuyen, H.V.; Eun, J.B. Marine Carotenoids: Bioactivities and Potential Benefits to Human Health. *Crit. Rev. Food Sci. Nutr.* **2017**, *57*, 2600–2610. [CrossRef]
85. Sugawara, T.; Yamashita, K.; Asai, A.; Nagao, A.; Shiraishi, T.; Imai, I.; Hirata, T. Esterification of Xanthophylls by Human Intestinal Caco-2 Cells. *Arch. Biochem. Biophys.* **2009**. [CrossRef] [PubMed]
86. Heo, S.-J.; Jeon, Y.-J. Protective Effect of Fucoxanthin Isolated from Sargassum Siliquastrum on UV-B Induced Cell Damage. *J. Photochem. Photobiol. B Biol.* **2009**, *95*, 101–107. [CrossRef] [PubMed]
87. D'Orazio, N.; Gemello, E.; Gammone, M.A.; De Girolamo, M.; Ficoneri, C.; Riccioni, G. Fucoxantin: A Treasure from the Sea. *Mar. Drugs* **2012**, *10*, 604. [CrossRef]
88. Kumar, S.R.; Hosokawa, M.; Miyashita, K. Fucoxanthin: A Marine Carotenoid Exerting Anti-Cancer Effects by Affecting Multiple Mechanisms. *Mar. Drugs* **2013**, 5130–5147. [CrossRef] [PubMed]
89. Kotake-Nara, E.; Yonekura, L.; Nagao, A. Lysoglyceroglycolipids Improve the Intestinal Absorption of Micellar Fucoxanthin by Caco-2 Cells. *J. Oleo Sci.* **2015**. [CrossRef]
90. Gao, K.; McKinley, K.R. Use of Macroalgae for Marine Biomass Production and CO_2 Remediation: A Review. *J. Appl. Phycol.* **1994**, *6*, 45–60. [CrossRef]
91. Mikami, K.; Hosokawa, M. Biosynthetic Pathway and Health Benefits of Fucoxanthin, an Algae-Specific Xanthophyll in Brown Seaweeds. *Int. J. Mol. Sci.* **2013**. [CrossRef]
92. Market Reports World. *Global Fucoxanthin Market Report 2017*; Market Reports World: Pune, India, 2017.

93. Gumus, R.; Urcar Gelen, S.; Koseoglu, S.; Ozkanlar, S.; Ceylan, Z.G.; Imik, H. The Effects of Fucoxanthin Dietary Inclusion on the Growth Performance, Antioxidant Metabolism and Meat Quality of Broilers. *Rev. Bras. Cienc. Avic.* **2018**, *20*, 487–496. [CrossRef]
94. Satomi, Y. Antitumor and Cancer-Preventative Function of Fucoxanthin: A Marine Carotenoid. *Anticancer Res.* **2017**, *1562*, 1557–1562. [CrossRef]
95. Ou, H.C.; Chou, W.C.; Chu, P.M.; Hsieh, P.L.; Hung, C.H.; Tsai, K.L. Fucoxanthin Protects against OxLDL-Induced Endothelial Damage via Activating the AMPK-Akt-CREB-PGC1α Pathway. *Mol. Nutr. Food Res.* **2019**, *63*, 1–10. [CrossRef]
96. Cianciosi, D.; Varela-Lopez, A.; Forbes-Hernandez, T.Y.; Gasparrini, M.; Afrin, S.; Reboredo-Rodriguez, P.; Zhang, J.J.; Quiles, J.L.; Nabavi, S.F.; Battino, M.; et al. Targeting Molecular Pathways in Cancer Stem Cells by Natural Bioactive Compounds. *Pharmacol. Res.* **2018**, *135*, 150–165. [CrossRef]
97. Bae, M.; Kim, M.B.; Park, Y.K.; Lee, J.Y. Health Benefits of Fucoxanthin in the Prevention of Chronic Diseases. *Biochim. Biophys. Acta - Mol. Cell Biol. Lipids* **2020**, *1865*, 158618. [CrossRef]
98. Almeida, T.P.; Ferreira, J.; Vettorazzi, A.; Azqueta, A.; Rocha, E.; Ramos, A.A. Cytotoxic Activity of Fucoxanthin, Alone and in Combination with the Cancer Drugs Imatinib and Doxorubicin, in CML Cell Lines. *Environ. Toxicol. Pharmacol.* **2018**, *59*, 24–33. [CrossRef] [PubMed]
99. Liu, M.; Li, W.; Chen, Y.; Wan, X.; Wang, J. Fucoxanthin: A Promising Compound for Human Inflammation-Related Diseases. *Life Sci.* **2020**, *255*, 1178503. [CrossRef] [PubMed]
100. Heo, S.; Yoon, W.; Kim, K.; Ahn, G.; Kang, S.; Kang, D.; Oh, C.; Jung, W.; Jeon, Y. Evaluation of Anti-Inflammatory Effect of Fucoxanthin Isolated from Brown Algae in Lipopolysaccharide-Stimulated RAW 264. 7 Macrophages. *Food Chem. Toxicol.* **2010**, *48*, 2045–2051. [CrossRef] [PubMed]
101. Zhao, D.; Kim, S.M.; Pan, C.H.; Chung, D. Effects of Heating, Aerial Exposure and Illumination on Stability of Fucoxanthin in Canola Oil. *Food Chem.* **2014**, *145*, 505–513. [CrossRef] [PubMed]
102. Sasaki, K.; Ishihara, K.; Oyamada, C.; Sato, A.; Fukushi, A.; Arakane, T.; Motoyama, M.; Yamazaki, M.; Mitsumoto, M. Effects of Fucoxanthin Addition to Ground Chicken Breast Meat on Lipid and Colour Stability during Chilled Storage, before and after Cooking. *Asian-Australasian J. Anim. Sci.* **2008**, *21*, 1067–1072. [CrossRef]
103. Hastings, J.; Owen, G.; Dekker, A. ChEBI in 2016: Improved Services and an Expanding Collection of Metabolites. *Nucleic Acids Res.* **2016**, *44*, D1214–D1219. [CrossRef]
104. Mularczyk, M.; Michalak, I.; Marycz, K. Astaxanthin and Other Nutrients from Haematococcus Pluvialis—Multifunctional Applications. *Mar. Drugs* **2020**, *18*, 459. [CrossRef]
105. Davinelli, S.; Nielsen, M.E.; Scapagnini, G. Astaxanthin in Skin Health, Repair, and Disease: A Comprehensive Review. *Nutrients* **2018**, *10*, 522. [CrossRef] [PubMed]
106. Han, D.; Li, Y.; Hu, Q. Astaxanthin in Microalgae: Pathways, Functions and Biotechnological Implications. *Algae* **2013**, *28*, 131–147. [CrossRef]
107. Ambati, R.R.; Moi, P.S.; Ravi, S.; Aswathanarayana, R.G. Astaxanthin: Sources, Extraction, Stability, Biological Activities and Its Commercial Applications - A Review. *Mar. Drugs* **2014**, *12*, 128–152. [CrossRef] [PubMed]
108. Butler, T.; Golan, Y. Astaxanthin Production from Microalgae. *Microalgae Biotechnol. Food, Heal. High Value Prod.* **2020**, 175–242. [CrossRef]
109. Liu, J.; Sun, Z.; Gerken, H.; Liu, Z.; Jiang, Y.; Chen, F. *Chlorella Zofingiensis* as an Alternative Microalgal Producer of Astaxanthin: Biology and Industrial Potential. *Mar. Drugs* **2014**, *12*, 3487–3515. [CrossRef]
110. Bampidis, V.; Azimonti, G.; Bastos, M.D.L.; Christensen, H.; Dusemund, B.; Kouba, M.; Kos Durjava, M.; López-Alonso, M.; López Puente, S.; Marcon, F.; et al. Safety and Efficacy of Astaxanthin-Dimethyldisuccinate (Carophyll®Stay-Pink 10%-CWS) for Salmonids, Crustaceans and Other Fish. *EFSA J.* **2019**, *17*. [CrossRef]
111. Martínez-Delgado, A.A.; Khandual, S.; Villanueva–Rodríguez, S.J. Chemical Stability of Astaxanthin Integrated into a Food Matrix: Effects of Food Processing and Methods for Preservation. *Food Chem.* **2017**, *225*, 23–30. [CrossRef] [PubMed]
112. Gruszecki, W.I.; Strzałka, K. Carotenoids as Modulators of Lipid Membrane Physical Properties. *Biochim. Biophys. Acta Mol. Basis Dis.* **2005**, *1740*, 108–115. [CrossRef]
113. González, S.; Astner, S.; An, W.; Goukassian, D.; Pathak, M.A. Dietary Lutein/Zeaxanthin Decreases Ultraviolet B-Induced Epidermal Hyperproliferation and Acute Inflammation in Hairless Mice. *J. Invest. Dermatol.* **2003**, *121*, 399–405. [CrossRef]
114. Saha, S.K.; Ermis, H.; Murray, P. Marine Microalgae for Potential Lutein Production. *Appl. Sci.* **2020**, *10*, 6457. [CrossRef]
115. Jia, Y.P.; Sun, L.; Yu, H.S.; Liang, L.P.; Li, W.; Ding, H.; Song, X.B.; Zhang, L.J. The Pharmacological Effects of Lutein and Zeaxanthin on Visual Disorders and Cognition Diseases. *Molecules* **2017**, *22*, 610. [CrossRef]
116. Khan, M.I.; Shin, J.H.; Kim, J.D. The Promising Future of Microalgae: Current Status, Challenges, and Optimization of a Sustainable and Renewable Industry for Biofuels, Feed, and Other Products. *Microb. Cell Fact.* **2018**, *17*, 1–21. [CrossRef] [PubMed]
117. Sajilata, M.G.; Singhal, R.S.; Kamat, M.Y. The Carotenoid Pigment Zeaxanthin—A Review. *Compr. Rev. Food Sci. Food Saf.* **2008**, *7*, 29–49. [CrossRef]
118. Ravikrishnan, R.; Rusia, S.; Ilamurugan, G.; Salunkhe, U.; Deshpande, J.; Shankaranarayanan, J.; Shankaranarayana, M.L.; Soni, M.G. Safety Assessment of Lutein and Zeaxanthin (Lutemax^{TM} 2020): Subchronic Toxicity and Mutagenicity Studies. *Food Chem. Toxicol.* **2011**, *49*, 2841–2848. [CrossRef] [PubMed]

119. Firdous, A.P.; Kuttan, G.; Kuttan, R. Anti-Inflammatory Potential of Carotenoid Meso-Zeaxanthin and Its Mode of Action. *Pharm. Biol.* **2015**, *53*, 961–967. [CrossRef] [PubMed]
120. Stahl, W.; Sies, H. Bioactivity and Protective Effects of Natural Carotenoids. *Biochim. Biophys. Acta - Mol. Basis Dis.* **2005**, *1740*, 101–107. [CrossRef]
121. Ma, L.; Lin, X.M. Effects of Lutein and Zeaxanthin on Aspects of Eye Health. *J. Sci. Food Agric.* **2010**, *90*, 2–12. [CrossRef]
122. Lourenço-Lopes, C.; Fraga-Corral, M.; Jimenez-Lopez, C.; Pereira, A.G.; Garcia-Oliveira, P.; Carpena, M.; Prieto, M.A.; Simal-Gandara, J. Metabolites from Macroalgae and Its Applications in the Cosmetic Industry: A Circular Economy Approach. *Resources* **2020**, *9*, 101. [CrossRef]
123. Murillo, A.G.; Hu, S.; Fernandez, M.L. Zeaxanthin: Metabolism, Properties, and Antioxidant Protection of Eyes, Heart, Liver, and Skin. *Antioxidants* **2019**, *8*, 390. [CrossRef]
124. Jin, E.; Feth, B.; Melis, A. A Mutant of the Green Alga *Dunaliella Salina* Constitutively Accumulates Zeaxanthin under All Growth Conditions. *Biotechnol. Bioeng.* **2003**, *81*, 115–124. [CrossRef]
125. Li, X.R.; Tian, G.Q.; Shen, H.J.; Liu, J.Z. Metabolic Engineering of *Escherichia Coli* to Produce Zeaxanthin. *J. Ind. Microbiol. Biotechnol.* **2015**, *42*, 627–636. [CrossRef]
126. Jiao, Y.; Reuss, L.; Wang, Y. β-Cryptoxanthin: Chemistry, Occurrence, and Potential Health Benefits. *Curr. Pharmacol. Rep.* **2019**, *5*, 20–34. [CrossRef]
127. Gammone, M.A.; Riccioni, G.; D'Orazio, N. Marine Carotenoids against Oxidative Stress: Effects on Human Health. *Mar. Drugs* **2015**, *13*, 6226–6246. [CrossRef]
128. Burri, B.J.; La Frano, M.R.; Zhu, C. Absorption, Metabolism, and Functions of β-Cryptoxanthin. *Nutr. Rev.* **2016**, *74*, 69–82. [CrossRef]
129. Ganesan, P.; Noda, K.; Manabe, Y.; Ohkubo, T.; Tanaka, Y.; Maoka, T.; Sugawara, T.; Hirata, T. Siphonaxanthin, a Marine Carotenoid from Green Algae, Effectively Induces Apoptosis in Human Leukemia (HL-60) Cells. *Biochim. Biophys. Acta - Gen. Subj.* **2011**, *1810*, 497–503. [CrossRef]
130. Manabe, Y.; Hirata, T.; Sugawara, T. Suppressive Effects of Carotenoids on the Antigeninduced Degranulation in RBL-2H3 Rat Basophilic Leukemia Cells. *J. Oleo Sci.* **2014**, *63*, 291–294. [CrossRef]
131. Novoveská, L.; Ross, M.E.; Stanley, M.S.; Pradelles, R.; Wasiolek, V.; Sassi, J.F. Microalgal Carotenoids: A Review of Production, Current Markets, Regulations, and Future Direction. *Mar. Drugs* **2019**, *17*, 640. [CrossRef] [PubMed]
132. Kallscheuer, N.; Moreira, C.; Airs, R.; Llewellyn, C.A.; Wiegand, S.; Jogler, C.; Lage, O.M. Pink- and Orange-Pigmented Planctomycetes Produce Saproxanthin-Type Carotenoids Including a Rare C45 Carotenoid. *Environ. Microbiol. Rep.* **2019**, *11*, 741–748. [CrossRef] [PubMed]
133. Shindo, K.; Misawa, N. New and Rare Carotenoids Isolated from Marine Bacteria and Their Antioxidant Activities. *Mar. Drugs* **2014**, *12*, 1690–1698. [CrossRef] [PubMed]
134. Shindo, K.; Kikuta, K.; Suzuki, A.; Katsuta, A.; Kasai, H.; Yasumoto-Hirose, M.; Matsuo, Y.; Misawa, N.; Takaichi, S. Rare Carotenoids, (3R)-Saproxanthin and (3R,2′S)-Myxol, Isolated from Novel Marine Bacteria (Flavobacteriaceae) and Their Antioxidative Activities. *Appl. Microbiol. Biotechnol.* **2007**, *74*, 1350–1357. [CrossRef] [PubMed]
135. Hertzberg, S.; Liaaen-Jensen, S.; Siegelman, H.W. The Carotenoids of Blue-Green Algae. *Phytochemistry* **1971**, *10*, 3121–3127. [CrossRef]
136. Marasco, E.K.; Vay, K.; Schmidt-Dannert, C. Identification of Carotenoid Cleavage Dioxygenases from Nostoc Sp. PCC 7120 with Different Cleavage Activities. *J. Biol. Chem.* **2006**, *281*, 31583–31593. [CrossRef]
137. Francis, G.W.; Hertzberg, S.; Andersen, K.; Liaaen-Jensen, S. New Carotenoid Glycosides from *Oscillatoria Limosa*. *Phytochemistry* **1970**, *9*, 629–635. [CrossRef]
138. Hamidi, M.; Safarzadeh Kozani, P.; Safarzadeh Kozani, P.; Pierre, G.; Michaud, P.; Delattre, C. Marine Bacteria versus Microalgae: Who Is the Best for Biotechnological Production of Bioactive Compounds with Antioxidant Properties and Other Biological Applications? *Mar. Drugs* **2020**, *18*, 28. [CrossRef] [PubMed]
139. Gastineau, R.; Davidovich, N.; Hansen, G.; Rines, J.; Wulff, A.; Kaczmarska, I.; Ehrman, J.; Hermann, D.; Maumus, F.; Hardivillier, Y.; et al. Haslea Ostrearia -like Diatoms. Biodiversity out of the Blue. *Adv. Bot. Res.* **2014**, *71*, 441–465. [CrossRef]
140. Kooistra, W.H.C.F.; Gersonde, R.; Medlin, L.K.; Mann, D.G. The Origin and Evolution of the Diatoms. Their Adaptation to a Planktonic Existence. *Evol. Prim. Prod. Sea* **2007**, 207–249. [CrossRef]
141. Tanno, Y.; Kato, S.; Takahashi, S.; Tamaki, S.; Takaichi, S.; Kodama, Y.; Sonoike, K.; Shinomura, T. Light Dependent Accumulation of β-Carotene Enhances Photo-Acclimation of *Euglena Gracilis*. *J. Photochem. Photobiol. B Biol.* **2020**, *209*, 111950. [CrossRef] [PubMed]
142. Faraloni, C.; Torzillo, G. Synthesis of Antioxidant Carotenoids in Microalgae in Response to Physiological Stress. *IntechOpen* **2017**, 143–157. [CrossRef]
143. Rao, A.V.; Rao, L.G. Carotenoids and Human Health. *Pharmacol. Res.* **2007**, *55*, 207–216. [CrossRef]
144. Kotake-Nara, E.; Nagao, A. Absorption and Metabolism of Xanthophylls. *Mar. Drugs* **2011**, *9*, 1024–1037. [CrossRef]
145. Sugawara, T.; Baskaran, V.; Tsuzuki, W.; Nagao, A. Brown Algae Fucoxanthin Is Hydrolyzed to Fucoxanthinol during Absorption by Caco-2 Human Intestinal Cells and Mice. *J. Nutr.* **2002**. [CrossRef]
146. Asai, A.; Sugawara, T.; Ono, H.; Nagao, A. Biotransformation of Fucoxanthinol into Amarouciaxanthin a in Mice and HepG2 Cells: Formation and Cytotoxicity of Fucoxanthin Metabolites. *Drug Metab. Dispos.* **2004**. [CrossRef]

147. Yim, M.J.; Hosokawa, M.; Mizushina, Y.; Yoshida, H.; Saito, Y.; Miyashita, K. Suppressive Effects of Amarouciaxanthin A on 3T3-L1 Adipocyte Differentiation through down-Regulation of PPARγ and C/EBPα MRNA Expression. *J. Agric. Food Chem.* **2011**, *59*, 1646–1652. [CrossRef] [PubMed]
148. Hashimoto, T.; Ozaki, Y.; Taminato, M.; Das, S.K.; Mizuno, M.; Yoshimura, K.; Maoka, T.; Kanazawa, K. The Distribution and Accumulation of Fucoxanthin and Its Metabolites after Oral Administration in Mice. *Br. J. Nutr.* **2009**, *102*, 242–248. [CrossRef]
149. Wang, X.; Li, H.; Wang, F.; Xia, G.; Liu, H.; Cheng, X.; Kong, M.; Liu, Y.; Feng, C.; Chen, X.; et al. Isolation of Fucoxanthin from *Sargassum Thunbergii* and Preparation of Microcapsules Based on Palm Stearin Solid Lipid Core. *Front. Mater. Sci.* **2017**, *11*, 66–74. [CrossRef]
150. Li, H.; Xu, Y.; Sun, X.; Wang, S.; Wang, J.; Zhu, J.; Wang, D.; Zhao, L. Stability, Bioactivity, and Bioaccessibility of Fucoxanthin in Zein-Caseinate Composite Nanoparticles Fabricated at Neutral PH by Antisolvent Precipitation. *Food Hydrocoll.* **2018**, *84*, 379–388. [CrossRef]
151. Dai, J.; Kim, S.M.; Shin, I.S.; Kim, J.D.; Lee, H.Y.; Shin, W.C.; Kim, J.C. Preparation and Stability of Fucoxanthin-Loaded Microemulsions. *J. Ind. Eng. Chem.* **2014**, *20*, 2103–2110. [CrossRef]
152. Salvia-Trujillo, L.; Sun, Q.; Um, B.H.; Park, Y.; McClements, D.J. In Vitro and in Vivo Study of Fucoxanthin Bioavailability from Nanoemulsion-Based Delivery Systems: Impact of Lipid Carrier Type. *J. Funct. Foods* **2015**. [CrossRef]
153. Ravi, H.; Baskaran, V. Chitosan-Glycolipid Nanocarriers Improve the Bioavailability of Fucoxanthin via up-Regulation of PPARγ and SRB1 and Antioxidant Activity in Rat Model. *J. Funct. Foods* **2017**, *28*, 215–226. [CrossRef]
154. Barros, M.P.; Marin, D.P.; Bolin, A.P.; De Cássia Santos Macedo, R.; Campoio, T.R.; Fineto, C.; Guerra, B.A.; Polotow, T.G.; Vardaris, C.; Mattei, R.; et al. Combined Astaxanthin and Fish Oil Supplementation Improves Glutathione-Based Redox Balance in Rat Plasma and Neutrophils. *Chem. Biol. Interact.* **2012**, *197*, 58–67. [CrossRef]
155. Burgos-Díaz, C.; Opazo-Navarrete, M.; Soto-Añual, M.; Leal-Calderón, F.; Bustamante, M. Food-Grade Pickering Emulsion as a Novel Astaxanthin Encapsulation System for Making Powder-Based Products: Evaluation of Astaxanthin Stability during Processing, Storage, and Its Bioaccessibility. *Food Res. Int.* **2020**, *134*, 109244. [CrossRef]
156. Liu, C.; Tan, Y.; Xu, Y.; McCleiments, D.J.; Wang, D. Formation, Characterization, and Application of Chitosan/Pectin-Stabilized Multilayer Emulsions as Astaxanthin Delivery Systems. *Int. J. Biol. Macromol.* **2019**, *140*, 985–997. [CrossRef]
157. Liu, G.; Hu, M.; Zhao, Z.; Lin, Q.; Wei, D.; Jiang, Y. Enhancing the Stability of Astaxanthin by Encapsulation in Poly (l-Lactic Acid) Microspheres Using a Supercritical Anti-Solvent Process. *Particuology* **2019**, *44*, 54–62. [CrossRef]
158. Fratter, A.; Biagi, D.; Cicero, A.F.G. Sublingual Delivery of Astaxanthin through a Novel Ascorbyl Palmitate-Based Nanoemulsion: Preliminary Data. *Mar. Drugs* **2019**, *17*, 508. [CrossRef] [PubMed]
159. Ligia Focsan, A.; Polyakov, N.E.; Kispert, L.D. Supramolecular Carotenoid Complexes of Enhanced Solubility and Stability — The Way of Bioavailability Improvement. *Molecules* **2019**, *24*, 3947. [CrossRef] [PubMed]
160. Tudor, C.; Bohn, T.; Iddir, M.; Dulf, F.V.; Focșan, M.; Rugină, D.O.; Pintea, A. Sea Buckthorn Oil as a Valuable Source of Bioaccessible Xanthophylls. *Nutrients* **2020**, *12*, 76. [CrossRef] [PubMed]
161. Bernaerts, T.M.M.; Verstreken, H.; Dejonghe, C.; Gheysen, L.; Foubert, I.; Grauwet, T.; Van Loey, A.M. Cell Disruption of *Nannochloropsis Sp.* Improves in Vitro Bioaccessibility of Carotenoids and Ω3-LC-PUFA. *J. Funct. Foods* **2020**, *65*, 103770. [CrossRef]
162. Choi, H.D.; Kang, H.E.; Yang, S.H.; Lee, M.G.; Shin, W.G. Pharmacokinetics and First-Pass Metabolism of Astaxanthin in Rats. *Br. J. Nutr.* **2011**, *105*, 220–227. [CrossRef] [PubMed]
163. Wolz, E.; Liechti, H.; Notter, B.; Oesterhelt, G.; Kistler, A. Characterization of Metabolites of Astaxanthin in Primary Cultures of Rat Hepatocytes. *Drug Metab. Dispos.* **1999**, *27*, 456–462.
164. Kistler, A.; Liechti, H.; Pichard, L.; Wolz, E.; Oesterhelt, G.; Hayes, A.; Maurel, P. Metabolism and CYP-Inducer Properties of Astaxanthin in Man and Primary Human Hepatocytes. *Arch. Toxicol.* **2002**, *75*, 665–675. [CrossRef]
165. Chen, G.; Wang, B.; Han, D.; Sommerfeld, M.; Lu, Y.; Chen, F.; Hu, Q. Molecular Mechanisms of the Coordination between Astaxanthin and Fatty Acid Biosynthesis in *Haematococcus Pluvialis* (Chlorophyceae). *Plant J.* **2015**, *81*, 95–107. [CrossRef]
166. Khachik, F.; Steck, A.; Pfander, H. Bioavailability, Metabolism, and Possible Mechanism of Chemoprevention by Lutein and Lycopene in Humans. *Food Factors Cancer Prev.* **1997**, 542–547. [CrossRef]
167. Arathi, B.P.; Sowmya, P.R.-R.; Vijay, K.; Baskaran, V.; Lakshminarayana, R. Biofunctionality of Carotenoid Metabolites: An Insight into Qualitative and Quantitative Analysis. In *Metabolomics - Fundamentals and Applications*; IntechOpen: London, UK, 2016; p. 19.
168. Khachik, F.; Englert, G.; Beecher, G.R.; Cecil Smith, J. Isolation, Structural Elucidation, and Partial Synthesis of Lutein Dehydration Products in Extracts from Human Plasma. *J. Chromatogr. B Biomed. Sci. Appl.* **1995**, *670*, 219–233. [CrossRef]
169. Giordano, E.; Quadro, L. Lutein, Zeaxanthin and Mammalian Development: Metabolism, Functions and Implications for Health. *Arch. Biochem. Biophys.* **2018**, *647*, 33–40. [CrossRef]
170. Berg, J.; Lin, D. Lutein and Zeaxanthin: An Overview of Metabolism and Eye Health. *J. Hum. Nutr. Food Sci.* **2014**, *2*, 1039.
171. Eggersdorfer, M.; Wyss, A. Carotenoids in Human Nutrition and Health. *Arch. Biochem. Biophys.* **2018**, *652*, 18–26. [CrossRef] [PubMed]
172. Maiani, G.; Castón, M.J.P.; Catasta, G.; Toti, E.; Cambrodón, I.G.; Bysted, A.; Granado-Lorencio, F.; Olmedilla-Alonso, B.; Knuthsen, P.; Valoti, M.; et al. Carotenoids: Actual Knowledge on Food Sources, Intakes, Stability and Bioavailability and Their Protective Role in Humans. *Mol. Nutr. Food Res.* **2009**, *53*, 194–218. [CrossRef] [PubMed]

173. Genç, Y.; Bardakci, H.; Yücel, Ç.; Karatoprak, G.Ş.; Akkol, E.K.; Barak, T.H.; Sobarzo-Sánchez, E. Oxidative Stress and Marine Carotenoids: Application by Using Nanoformulations. *Mar. Drugs* **2020**, *18*, 423. [CrossRef]
174. Fernández-García, E.; Carvajal-Lérida, I.; Pérez-Gálvez, A. In Vitro Bioaccessibility Assessment as a Prediction Tool of Nutritional Efficiency. *Nutr. Res.* **2009**, *29*, 751–760. [CrossRef] [PubMed]
175. Helena de Abreu-Martins, H.; Artiga-Artigas, M.; Hilsdorf Piccoli, R.; Martín-Belloso, O.; Salvia-Trujillo, L. The Lipid Type Affects the in Vitro Digestibility and β-Carotene Bioaccessibility of Liquid or Solid Lipid Nanoparticles. *Food Chem.* **2020**, *311*, 126024. [CrossRef]
176. Iddir, M.; Dingeo, G.; Porras Yaruro, J.F.; Hammaz, F.; Borel, P.; Schleeh, T.; Desmarchelier, C.; Larondelle, Y.; Bohn, T. Influence of Soy and Whey Protein, Gelatin and Sodium Caseinate on Carotenoid Bioaccessibility. *Food Funct.* **2020**, *11*, 5446–5459. [CrossRef] [PubMed]
177. Huo, T.; Ferruzzi, M.G.; Schwartz, S.J.; Failla, M.L. Impact of Fatty Acyl Composition and Quantity of Triglycerides on Bioaccessibility of Dietary Carotenoids. *J. Agric. Food Chem.* **2007**, *55*, 8950–8957. [CrossRef]
178. Bohn, T.; Mcdougall, G.J.; Alegría, A.; Alminger, M.; Arrigoni, E.; Aura, A.M.; Brito, C.; Cilla, A.; El, S.N.; Karakaya, S.; et al. Mind the Gap-Deficits in Our Knowledge of Aspects Impacting the Bioavailability of Phytochemicals and Their Metabolites-a Position Paper Focusing on Carotenoids and Polyphenols. *Mol. Nutr. Food Res.* **2015**, *59*, 1307–1323. [CrossRef]
179. Chitchumroonchokchai, C.; Failla, M.L. Bioaccessibility and Intestinal Cell Uptake of Astaxanthin from Salmon and Commercial Supplements. *Food Res. Int.* **2017**, *99*, 936–943. [CrossRef]
180. Tyssandier, V.; Lyan, B.; Borel, P. Main Factors Governing the Transfer of Carotenoids from Emulsion Lipid Droplets to Micelles. *Biochim. Biophys. Acta - Mol. Cell Biol. Lipids* **2001**, *1533*, 285–292. [CrossRef]
181. Borel, P.; Lietz, G.; Goncalves, A.; Szabo de Edelenyi, F.; Lecompte, S.; Curtis, P.; Goumidi, L.; Caslake, M.J.; Miles, E.A.; Packard, C.; et al. CD36 and Sr-Bi Are Involved in Cellular Uptake of Provitamin a Carotenoids by Caco-2 and Hek Cells, and Some of Their Genetic Variants Are Associated with Plasma Concentrations of These Micronutrients in Humans. *J. Nutr.* **2013**, *143*, 448–456. [CrossRef] [PubMed]
182. O'Connell, O.F.; Ryan, L.; O'Brien, N.M. Xanthophyll Carotenoids Are More Bioaccessible from Fruits than Dark Green Vegetables. *Nutr. Res.* **2007**, *27*, 258–264. [CrossRef]
183. Borel, P.; Grolier, P.; Armand, M.; Partier, A.; Lafont, H.; Lairon, D.; Azais-Braesco, V. Carotenoids in Biological Emulsions: Solubility, Surface-to-Core Distribution, and Release from Lipid Droplets. *J. Lipid Res.* **1996**, *37*, 250–261. [CrossRef]
184. Bohn, T.; Desmarchelier, C.; Dragsted, L.O.; Nielsen, C.S.; Stahl, W.; Rühl, R.; Keijer, J.; Borel, P. Host-Related Factors Explaining Interindividual Variability of Carotenoid Bioavailability and Tissue Concentrations in Humans. *Mol. Nutr. Food Res.* **2017**, *61*, 1–37. [CrossRef] [PubMed]
185. Sy, C.; Gleize, B.; Dangles, O.; Landrier, J.F.; Veyrat, C.C.; Borel, P. Effects of Physicochemical Properties of Carotenoids on Their Bioaccessibility, Intestinal Cell Uptake, and Blood and Tissue Concentrations. *Mol. Nutr. Food Res.* **2012**, *56*, 1385–1397. [CrossRef]
186. Reboul, E. Mechanisms of Carotenoid Intestinal Absorption: Where Do We Stand? *Nutrients* **2019**, *11*, 838. [CrossRef]
187. Guo, B.; Oliviero, T.; Fogliano, V.; Ma, Y.; Chen, F.; Capuano, E. Gastrointestinal Bioaccessibility and Colonic Fermentation of Fucoxanthin from the Extract of the Microalga *Nitzschia Laevis*. *J. Agric. Food Chem.* **2020**, *68*, 1844–1850. [CrossRef]
188. Sugawara, T.; Kushiro, M.; Zhang, H.; Nara, E.; Ono, H.; Nagao, A. Lysophosphatidylcholine Enhances Carotenoid Uptake from Mixed Micelles by Caco-2 Human Intestinal Cells. *J. Nutr.* **2001**, *131*, 2921–2927. [CrossRef]
189. Mikami, N.; Hosokawa, M.; Miyashita, K.; Sohma, H.; Ito, Y.M.; Kokai, Y. Reduction of HbA1c Levels by Fucoxanthin-Enriched Akamoku Oil Possibly Involves the Thrifty Allele of Uncoupling Protein 1 (UCP1): A Randomised Controlled Trial in Normal-Weight and Obese Japanese Adults. *Sapporo Med. J.* **2017**, *86*, 108–109. [CrossRef]
190. Asai, A.; Yonekura, L.; Nagao, A. Low Bioavailability of Dietary Epoxyxanthophylls in Humans. *Br. J. Nutr.* **2008**, *100*, 273–277. [CrossRef]
191. Mimoun-Benarroch, M.; Hogot, C.; Rhazi, L.; Niamba, C.N.; Depeint, F. The Bioavailability of Astaxanthin Is Dependent on Both the Source and the Isomeric Variants of the Molecule. *Bull. Univ. Agric. Sci. Vet. Med. Cluj-Napoca. Food Sci. Technol.* **2016**, *73*, 61. [CrossRef]
192. Yang, C.; Zhang, H.; Liu, R.; Zhu, H.; Zhang, L.; Tsao, R. Bioaccessibility, Cellular Uptake, and Transport of Astaxanthin Isomers and Their Antioxidative Effects in Human Intestinal Epithelial Caco-2 Cells. *J. Agric. Food Chem.* **2017**, *65*, 10223–10232. [CrossRef] [PubMed]
193. Park, J.S.; Chyun, J.H.; Kim, Y.K.; Line, L.L.; Chew, B.P. Astaxanthin Decreased Oxidative Stress and Inflammation and Enhanced Immune Response in Humans. *Nutr. Metab.* **2010**, *7*, 1–10. [CrossRef] [PubMed]
194. Vollmer, D.L.; West, V.A.; Lephart, E.D. Enhancing Skin Health: By Oral Administration of Natural Compounds and Minerals with Implications to the Dermal Microbiome. *Int. J. Mol. Sci.* **2018**, *19*, 3059. [CrossRef] [PubMed]
195. Odeberg, J.M.; Lignell, Å.; Pettersson, A.; Höglund, P. Oral Bioavailability of the Antioxidant Astaxanthin in Humans Is Enhanced by Incorporation of Lipid Based Formulations. *Eur. J. Pharm. Sci.* **2003**, *19*, 299–304. [CrossRef]
196. Liu, Y.; Huang, L.; Li, D.; Wang, Y.; Chen, Z.; Zou, C.; Liu, W.; Ma, Y.; Cao, M.J.; Liu, G.M. Re-Assembled Oleic Acid-Protein Complexes as Nano-Vehicles for Astaxanthin: Multispectral Analysis and Molecular Docking. *Food Hydrocoll.* **2020**, *103*, 105689. [CrossRef]
197. Olson, J.A. Absorption, Transport, and Metabolism of Carotenoids in Humans. *Pure Appl. Chem.* **1994**, *66*, 1011–1016. [CrossRef]

198. do Nascimento, T.C.; Pinheiro, P.N.; Fernandes, A.S.; Murador, D.C.; Neves, B.V.; de Menezes, C.R.; de Rosso, V.V.; Jacob-Lopes, E.; Zepka, L.Q. Bioaccessibility and Intestinal Uptake of Carotenoids from Microalgae Scenedesmus Obliquus. *LWT* **2021**, *140*, 110780. [CrossRef]
199. Dhuique-Mayer, C.; Borel, P.; Reboul, E.; Caporiccio, B.; Besancon, P.; Amiot, M.J. β-Cryptoxanthin from Citrus Juices: Assessment of Bioaccessibility Using an in Vitro Digestion/Caco-2 Cell Culture Model. *Br. J. Nutr.* **2007**, *97*, 883–890. [CrossRef]
200. Burri, B.J.; Chang, J.S.T.; Neidlinger, T.R. Bcryptoxanthin- and α-Carotene-Rich Foods Have Greater Apparent Bioavailability than Bcarotene-Rich Foods in Western Diets. *Br. J. Nutr.* **2011**, *105*, 212–219. [CrossRef] [PubMed]
201. Johnson, E.J. Role of Lutein and Zeaxanthin in Visual and Cognitive Function throughout the Lifespan. *Nutr. Rev.* **2014**, *72*, 605–612. [CrossRef]
202. Bernstein, P.S.; Li, B.; Vachali, P.P.; Gorusupudi, A.; Shyam, R.; Henriksen, B.S.; Nolan, J.M. Lutein, Zeaxanthin, and Meso-Zeaxanthin: The Basic and Clinical Science Underlying Carotenoid-Based Nutritional Interventions against Ocular Disease. *Prog. Retin. Eye Res.* **2016**, *50*, 34–66. [CrossRef] [PubMed]
203. Fernández-García, E.; Carvajal-Lérida, I.; Jarén-Galán, M.; Garrido-Fernández, J.; Pérez-Gálvez, A.; Hornero-Méndez, D. Carotenoids Bioavailability from Foods: From Plant Pigments to Efficient Biological Activities. *Food Res. Int.* **2012**, *46*, 438–450. [CrossRef]
204. Hempel, J.; Schädle, C.N.; Sprenger, J.; Heller, A.; Carle, R.; Schweiggert, R.M. Ultrastructural Deposition Forms and Bioaccessibility of Carotenoids and Carotenoid Esters from Goji Berries (*Lycium Barbarum* L.). *Food Chem.* **2017**, *218*, 525–533. [CrossRef]
205. Gille, A.; Neumann, U.; Louis, S.; Bischoff, S.C.; Briviba, K. Microalgae as a Potential Source of Carotenoids: Comparative Results of an in Vitro Digestion Method and a Feeding Experiment with C57BL/6J Mice. *J. Funct. Foods* **2018**, *49*, 285–294. [CrossRef]
206. Rodrigues, D.B.; Chitchumroonchokchai, C.; Mariutti, L.R.B.; Mercadante, A.Z.; Failla, M.L. Comparison of Two Static in Vitro Digestion Methods for Screening the Bioaccessibility of Carotenoids in Fruits, Vegetables, and Animal Products. *J. Agric. Food Chem.* **2017**, *65*, 11220–11228. [CrossRef] [PubMed]
207. Niranjana, R.; Gayathri, R.; Nimish Mol, S.; Sugawara, T.; Hirata, T.; Miyashita, K.; Ganesan, P. Carotenoids Modulate the Hallmarks of Cancer Cells. *J. Funct. Foods* **2015**, *18*, 968–985. [CrossRef]
208. Marco, G.J. A Rapid Method for Evaluation of Antioxidants. *J. Am. Oil Chem. Soc.* **1968**, *45*, 594–598. [CrossRef]
209. Kaulmann, A.; Bohn, T. Carotenoids, Inflammation, and Oxidative Stress-Implications of Cellular Signaling Pathways and Relation to Chronic Disease Prevention. *Nutr. Res.* **2014**, *34*, 907–929. [CrossRef]
210. Moloney, J.N.; Cotter, T.G. ROS Signalling in the Biology of Cancer. *Semin. Cell Dev. Biol.* **2018**, *80*, 50–64. [CrossRef]
211. Crusz, S.M.; Balkwill, F.R. Inflammation and Cancer: Advances and New Agents. *Nat. Rev. Clin. Oncol.* **2015**, *12*, 584–596. [CrossRef] [PubMed]
212. Heo, S.J.; Yoon, W.J.; Kim, K.N.; Oh, C.; Choi, Y.U.; Yoon, K.T.; Kang, D.H.; Qian, Z.J.; Choi, I.W.; Jung, W.K. Anti-Inflammatory Effect of Fucoxanthin Derivatives Isolated from *Sargassum Siliquastrum* in Lipopolysaccharide-Stimulated RAW 264.7 Macrophage. *Food Chem. Toxicol.* **2012**, *50*, 3336–3342. [CrossRef]
213. Kim, E.A.; Kim, S.Y.; Ye, B.R.; Kim, J.; Ko, S.C.; Lee, W.W.; Kim, K.N.; Choi, I.W.; Jung, W.K.; Heo, S.J. Anti-Inflammatory Effect of Apo-9′-Fucoxanthinone via Inhibition of MAPKs and NF-KB Signaling Pathway in LPS-Stimulated RAW 264.7 Macrophages and Zebrafish Model. *Int. Immunopharmacol.* **2018**, *59*, 339–346. [CrossRef] [PubMed]
214. Shiratori, K.; Ohgami, K.; Ilieva, I.; Jin, X.H.; Koyama, Y.; Miyashita, K.; Yoshida, K.; Kase, S.; Ohno, S. Effects of Fucoxanthin on Lipopolysaccharide-Induced Inflammation in Vitro and in Vivo. *Exp. Eye Res.* **2005**, *81*, 422–428. [CrossRef] [PubMed]
215. Kim, K.; Ahn, G.; Heo, S.; Kang, S.; Kang, M.; Yang, H.; Kim, D.; Woon, S.; Kim, S.; Jeon, B.; et al. Inhibition of Tumor Growth in Vitro and in Vivo by Fucoxanthin against Melanoma B16F10 Cells. *Environ. Toxicol. Pharmacol.* **2012**, *35*, 39–46. [CrossRef]
216. Hosokawa, M.; Wanezaki, S.; Miyauchi, K.; Kurihara, H.; Kohno, H.; Kawabata, J.; Odashima, S.; Takahashi, K. Apoptosis-Inducing Effect of Fucoxanthin on Human Leukemia Cell Line HL-60. *Food Sci. Technol. Res.* **1999**, *5*, 243–246. [CrossRef]
217. Farruggia, C.; Kim, M.B.; Bae, M.; Lee, Y.; Pham, T.X.; Yang, Y.; Han, M.J.; Park, Y.K.; Lee, J.Y. Astaxanthin Exerts Anti-Inflammatory and Antioxidant Effects in Macrophages in NRF2-Dependent and Independent Manners. *J. Nutr. Biochem.* **2018**, *62*, 202–209. [CrossRef]
218. Bi, J.; Cui, R.; Li, Z.; Liu, C.; Zhang, J. Astaxanthin Alleviated Acute Lung Injury by Inhibiting Oxidative/Nitrative Stress and the Inflammatory Response in Mice. *Biomed. Pharmacother.* **2017**, *95*, 974–982. [CrossRef]
219. Palozza, P.; Torelli, C.; Boninsegna, A.; Simone, R.; Catalano, A.; Mele, M.C.; Picci, N. Growth-Inhibitory Effects of the Astaxanthin-Rich Alga *Haematococcus Pluvialis* in Human Colon Cancer Cells. *Cancer Lett.* **2009**, *283*, 108–117. [CrossRef]
220. Yasui, Y.; Hosokawa, M.; Mikami, N.; Miyashita, K.; Tanaka, T. Dietary Astaxanthin Inhibits Colitis and Colitis-Associated Colon Carcinogenesis in Mice via Modulation of the Inflammatory Cytokines. *Chem. Biol. Interact.* **2011**, *193*, 79–87. [CrossRef] [PubMed]
221. Xu, X.R.; Zou, Z.Y.; Xiao, X.; Huang, Y.M.; Wang, X.; Lin, X.M. Effects of Lutein Supplement on Serum Inflammatory Cytokines, ApoE and Lipid Profiles in Early Atherosclerosis Population. *J. Atheroscler. Thromb.* **2013**, *20*, 170–177. [CrossRef] [PubMed]
222. Rubin, L.P.; Chan, G.M.; Barrett-Reis, B.M.; Fulton, A.B.; Hansen, R.M.; Ashmeade, T.L.; Oliver, J.S.; MacKey, A.D.; Dimmit, R.A.; Hartmann, E.E.; et al. Effect of Carotenoid Supplementation on Plasma Carotenoids, Inflammation and Visual Development in Preterm Infants. *J. Perinatol.* **2012**, *32*, 418–424. [CrossRef]

223. Narisawa, T.; Fukaura, Y.; Hasebe, M.; Ito, M.; Aizawa, R.; Murakoshi, M.; Uemura, S.; Khachik, F.; Nishino, H. Inhibitory Effects of Natural Carotenoids, α-Carotene, β-Carotene, Lycopene and Lutein, on Colonic Aberrant Crypt Foci Formation in Rats. *Cancer Lett.* **1996**, *107*, 137–142. [CrossRef]
224. Altieri, M.; Nicholls, C.; Molina, M.G.D.; Ugas, R.; Midas, P.; Méndez, V.E. Plan and Operation of the Third National Health and Nutrition Examination Survey, 1988-94. Series 1: Programs and Collection Procedures. *Vital Health Stat. 1.* **1994**, *7*, 1–407.
225. Min, K.B.; Min, J.Y. Serum Carotenoid Levels and Risk of Lung Cancer Death in US Adults. *Cancer Sci.* **2014**, *105*, 736–743. [CrossRef] [PubMed]
226. Gao, M.; Dang, F.; Deng, C. β-Cryptoxanthin Induced Anti-Proliferation and Apoptosis by G0/G1 Arrest and AMPK Signal Inactivation in Gastric Cancer. *Eur. J. Pharmacol.* **2019**, *859*, 172528. [CrossRef]
227. Iskandar, A.R.; Liu, C.; Smith, D.E.; Hu, K.Q.; Choi, S.W.; Ausman, L.M.; Wang, X.D. β-Cryptoxanthin Restores Nicotine-Reduced Lung SIRT1 to Normal Levels and Inhibits Nicotine-Promoted Lung Tumorigenesis and Emphysema in A/J Mice. *Cancer Prev. Res.* **2013**, *6*, 309–320. [CrossRef]
228. Liu, C.; Bronson, R.T.; Russell, R.M.; Wang, X.-D. β-Cryptoxanthin Supplementation Prevents Cigarette Smoke-Induced Lung Inflammation, Oxidative Damage, and Squamous Metaplasia in Ferrets. *Cancer Prev. Res.* **2011**, *4*, 1255–1266. [CrossRef]
229. Palozza, P.; Sestito, R.; Picci, N.; Lanza, P.; Monego, G.; Ranelletti, F.O. The Sensitivity to β-Carotene Growth-Inhibitory and Proapoptotic Effects Is Regulated by Caveolin-1 Expression in Human Colon and Prostate Cancer Cells. *Carcinogenesis* **2008**, *29*, 2153–2161. [CrossRef]
230. Rubin, L.P.; Ross, A.C.; Stephensen, C.B.; Bohn, T.; Tanumihardjo, S.A. Metabolic Effects of Inflammation on Vitamin A and Carotenoids in Humans and Animal Models. *Adv. Nutr. An Int. Rev. J.* **2017**, *8*, 197–212. [CrossRef] [PubMed]
231. Gallicchio, L.; Boyd, K.; Matanoski, G.; Tao, X.; Chen, L.; Lam, T.K.; Shiels, M.; Hammond, E.; Robinson, K.A.; Caulfield, L.E.; et al. Carotenoids and the Risk of Developing Lung Cancer: A Systematic Review. *Am. J. Clin. Nutr.* **2008**, *88*, 372–383. [CrossRef] [PubMed]
232. The ATBC Cancer Prevention Study Group. The Alpha-Tocopherol, Beta-Carotene Lung Cancer Prevention Study: Design, Methods, Participant Characteristics, and Compliance. *Ann. Epidemiol.* **1994**, *4*, 1–10. [CrossRef]
233. Lai, G.Y.; Weinstein, S.J.; Taylor, P.R.; McGlynn, K.A.; Virtamo, J.; Gail, M.H.; Albanes, D.; Freedman, N.D. Effects of α-Tocopherol and β-Carotene Supplementation on Liver Cancer Incidence and Chronic Liver Disease Mortality in the ATBC Study. *Br. J. Cancer* **2014**, *111*, 2220–2223. [CrossRef]
234. Huang, J.; Weinstein, S.J.; Yu, K.; Männistö, S.; Albanes, D. Serum Beta Carotene and Overall and Cause-Specific Mortality: A Prospective Cohort Study. *Circ. Res.* **2018**, *123*, 1339–1349. [CrossRef] [PubMed]
235. Erhardt, J.G.; Meisner, C.; Bode, J.C.; Bode, C. Lycopene, β-Carotene, and Colorectal Adenomas. *Am. J. Clin. Nutr.* **2003**, *78*, 1219–1224. [CrossRef] [PubMed]
236. Zhao, L.G.; Zhang, Q.L.; Zheng, J.L.; Li, H.L.; Zhang, W.; Tang, W.G.; Xiang, Y.B. Dietary, Circulating Beta-Carotene and Risk of All-Cause Mortality: A Meta-Analysis from Prospective Studies. *Sci. Rep.* **2016**, *6*, 1–10. [CrossRef]
237. Wang, Y.; Cui, R.; Xiao, Y.; Fang, J.; Xu, Q. Effect of Carotene and Lycopene on the Risk of Prostate Cancer: A Systematic Review and Dose-Response Meta-Analysis of Observational Studies. *PLoS One* **2015**, *10*, 1–20. [CrossRef]
238. Capelli, B.; Bagchi, D.; Cysewski, G.R. Synthetic Astaxanthin Is Significantly Inferior to Algal-Based Astaxanthin as an Antioxidant and May Not Be Suitable as a Human Nutraceutical Supplement. *Nutrafoods* **2013**, *12*, 145–152. [CrossRef]
239. Ambati, R.R.; Gogisetty, D.; Aswathanarayana, R.G.; Ravi, S.; Bikkina, P.N.; Bo, L.; Yuepeng, S. Industrial Potential of Carotenoid Pigments from Microalgae: Current Trends and Future Prospects. *Crit. Rev. Food Sci. Nutr.* **2019**, *59*, 1880–1902. [CrossRef]
240. Koller, M.; Muhr, A.; Braunegg, G. Microalgae as Versatile Cellular Factories for Valued Products. *Algal Res.* **2014**, *6*, 52–63. [CrossRef]
241. Li, J.; Zhu, D.; Niu, J.; Shen, S.; Wang, G. An Economic Assessment of Astaxanthin Production by Large Scale Cultivation of *Haematococcus Pluvialis*. *Biotechnol. Adv.* **2011**, *29*, 568–574. [CrossRef] [PubMed]
242. Barreiro, C.; Barredo, J.L. Carotenoids Production: A Healthy and Profitable Industry. *Methods Mol. Biol.* **2018**, *1852*, 45–55. [CrossRef] [PubMed]
243. Lourenço-Lopes, C.; Garcia-Oliveira, P.; Carpena, M.; Fraga-Corral, M.; Jimenez-Lopez, C.; Pereira, A.G.; Prieto, M.A.; Simal-Gandara, J. Scientific Approaches on Extraction, Purification and Stability for the Commercialization of Fucoxanthin Recovered from Brown Algae. *Foods* **2020**, *9*, 1113. [CrossRef] [PubMed]
244. Regulation (EU) 2015/2283 of the European Parliament and of the Council of 25 November 2015 on novel foods, amending Regulation (EU) No 1169/2011 of the European Parliament and of the Council and repealing Regulation (EC) No 258/97 of the European Parliam. In *Official Journal L*; Eur-lex: Luxembourg, 2015; Volume 327, pp. 1–22.
245. Regulation (EC) No 852/2004 of the European Parliament and of the Council of 29 April 2004 on the hygiene of foodstuffs. In *Official Journal L*.; Eur-lex: Luxembourg, 2004; Volume 139, pp. 1–54.
246. *Regulation (EC) No 1924/2006 of the European Parliament and of the Council of 20 December 2006 on Nutrition and Health Claims Made on Foods*; Eur-lex: Luxembourg, 2006; Volume 18, pp. 244–259.

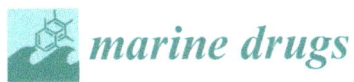

Review

On a Beam of Light: Photoprotective Activities of the Marine Carotenoids Astaxanthin and Fucoxanthin in Suppression of Inflammation and Cancer

Elena Catanzaro [1], Anupam Bishayee [2],* and Carmela Fimognari [1],*

1. Department for Life Quality Studies, Alma Mater Studiorum—Università di Bologna, corso d'Augusto 237, 47921 Rimini, Italy; elena.catanzaro2@unibo.it
2. Lake Erie College of Osteopathic Medicine, Bradenton, FL 34211, USA
* Correspondence: abishayee@lecom.edu or abishayee@gmail.com (A.B.); carmela.fimognari@unibo.it (C.F.)

Received: 29 September 2020; Accepted: 29 October 2020; Published: 30 October 2020

Abstract: Every day, we come into contact with ultraviolet radiation (UVR). If under medical supervision, small amounts of UVR could be beneficial, the detrimental and hazardous effects of UVR exposure dictate an unbalance towards the risks on the risk-benefit ratio. Acute and chronic effects of ultraviolet-A and ultraviolet-B involve mainly the skin, the immune system, and the eyes. Photodamage is an umbrella term that includes general phototoxicity, photoaging, and cancer caused by UVR. All these phenomena are mediated by direct or indirect oxidative stress and inflammation and are strictly connected one to the other. Astaxanthin (ASX) and fucoxanthin (FX) are peculiar marine carotenoids characterized by outstanding antioxidant properties. In particular, ASX showed exceptional efficacy in counteracting all categories of photodamages, in vitro and in vivo, thanks to both antioxidant potential and activation of alternative pathways. Less evidence has been produced about FX, but it still represents an interesting promise to prevent the detrimental effect of UVR. Altogether, these results highlight the importance of digging into the marine ecosystem to look for new compounds that could be beneficial for human health and confirm that the marine environment is as much as full of active compounds as the terrestrial one, it just needs to be more explored.

Keywords: photodamage; skin cancer; photoaging; marine carotenoids; astaxanthin; fucoxanthin

1. Introduction

Whether it is good weather or cloudy, every day we come into contact with ultraviolet radiation (UVR). UVR from the sun includes emissions with a wavelength range of 100–400 nm, which are divided into ultraviolet-A (UVA, 315–400 nm), ultraviolet-B (UVB, 280–315 nm), and ultraviolet-C (UVC, 100–280 nm). As sunlight travels through the atmosphere, all UVC and roughly 90% of UVB are trapped and blocked by the ozone. Thus, mostly UVA and, in a smaller amount UVB, reach the Earth's surface [1].

If under medical supervision, small amounts of UVR could be beneficial to help to treat certain diseases, such as psoriasis and eczema, and are fundamental in vitamin D production; the extremely dangerous effects dictate an unbalance towards the risks on the risk-benefit ratio [2]. Indeed, UVR acts as both tumor initiator and promoter and, for this reason, is defined as a "complete carcinogen." It is also the primary amendable risk factor for skin cancer [2]. Both UVA and UVB generate DNA lesions but in different sites and different ways. UVB radiations have shorter wavelengths than UVA. For this reason, they are more energetic, but they cannot penetrate the deepest layers of the skin and stop at the dermal stratum. They act directly on cells' DNA where they cause specific lesions, such as the formation of cyclobutane pyrimidine dimers (CPDs), which interfere with cell replication and promote melanogenesis and immunosuppression [3,4]. Besides, UVA reaches the most profound skin tissues. It does not trigger direct DNA damage, but it supports oxidative damage by interacting with intracellular components, such as the chromophore riboflavin or membrane-bound enzymes. This interaction alters both oxidative and nitrosative homeostasis. As a consequence, on the one hand, the reactive species that are created, such as the hydroxyl radical ($^{\bullet}OH$) or superoxide ($^{-}O_2$), can interact with DNA, generating single-strand breaks; on the other hand, singlet oxygen ($^1O_2$) is generated and, in turn, oxidizes DNA bases [5].

Besides cancer, UVR is the main character in perpetuating photodamage in terms of phototoxicity and photoaging. UVR exposure induces different types of harms, depending on whether the dose is acute or chronic. Both acute and chronic effects involve mainly the skin, the immune system, and the eyes [1,2]. The visible manifestation of acute damage comprises tanning, sunburn, and erythema. What is not tangible is that already after a single exposure to UVR, the genetic alterations occur together with the development of an inflammatory status, which comprises the basis for photoaging, immunodepression, and severe pathologies, including the above-mentioned skin cancer [1,2]. Chronic UVR exposure allows the accumulation of such alterations and leads to degenerative and irreversible changes in cells, tissues, and blood vessels that, if perpetuated, easily translate into non-reversible events [1,2].

Given the multifactorial nature of most types of neoplasms, and as not all neoplasms' causes are governable, prevention is not always an achievable therapeutic strategy. On the contrary, the best and most effective way to counteract skin cancer and, in general, photodamage is prevention. The best way to do so is the avoidance of UVR exposure [1]. The use of sunscreen lotions and clothes is the second most effective strategy. However, due to the rise of popularity of outdoor activities, the concept of a beautifying tan, the low compliance of sunscreen users, and the lack of correct and univocal information about UVR effects, it is challenging to achieve effective prevention [1].

The mid-ocean ridge covers 23% of the earth, of which only 3% has been explored. In other words, almost one-quarter of our planet is a single mountain range, and we did not enter it until after Neil Armstrong and Buzz Aldrin performed the "giant leap for mankind". Considering that 1600 years of ocean explorations costs can barely cover the expenses of a single year of the National Aeronautics and Space Administration [6], it is clear that research and technologies were advancing already in the 20th century, but people's interest and, therefore, research has always been directed towards outer space instead of the deep sea [6]. Still, despite only very few parts of aquatic ecosystems having been explored, that 3% of known oceans currently represents a terrific source for natural agents with active biological activity.

Animals, plants, and even bacteria have been studied and used as a library where to search for new compounds that can counteract different pathologies. The marine environment is full of organisms that produce molecules with antioxidant activity, such as carotenoids that perfectly fit a photoprotective profile [7]. Algae synthesize and exploit carotenoids to pursue photosynthesis and protective roles against oxidative stress. Carotenoids are a heterogeneous class of tetraterpenoids that consist of 3–13 conjugates double bonds and, at times, of six carbon hydroxylated rings at one or both ends of the molecule. They fall into two categories, namely xanthophylls and carotenes. The first group is characterized by the presence of oxygen atoms and includes the marine astaxanthin (ASX) and fucoxanthin (FX) (Figures 1 and 2). Carotenes, on the contrary, are a pure hydrocarbons chain. The terrestrial β-carotene (BC) and lycopene belong to this class [8–10].

Thanks to their antioxidant and anti-inflammatory properties, carotenoids showed to prevent UV-mediated skin phototoxicity, photoaging, and skin cancer [11]. Indeed, they can scavenge free radicals and inactivate $^1O_2$. In particular, the presence of oxygenated carbon rings at the end of xanthophylls increases the effectiveness of singlet oxygen quenching [8–10].

This review will explore the photoprotective activity of ASX and FX on skin photodamage and the prevention of UV-mediated carcinogenesis and will discuss the potential use of these compounds in clinical and cosmetic fields. Several previous reviews explored the beneficial effects of these carotenoids [12–18]; however, to our knowledge, no one focused specifically on the prevention of all kinds of skin photodamage in great detail.

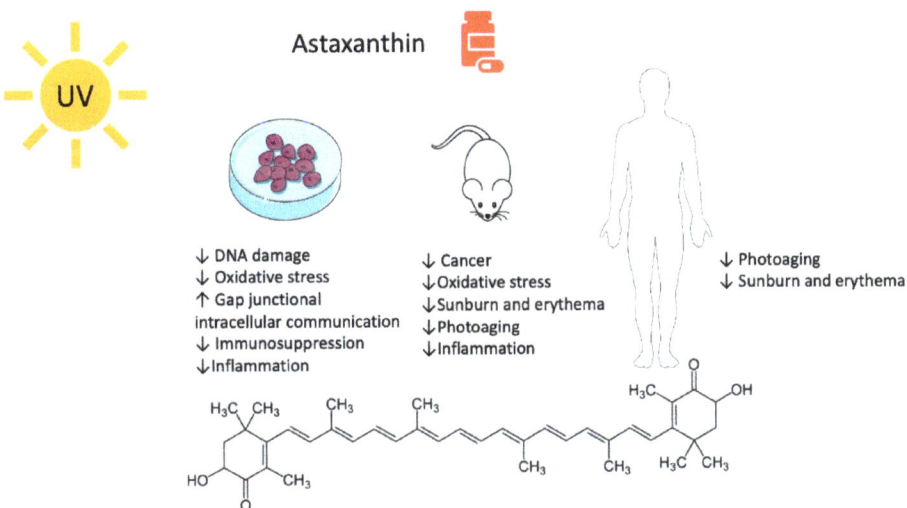

Figure 1. Molecular structure and biological activity of astaxanthin versus UV-mediated damage.

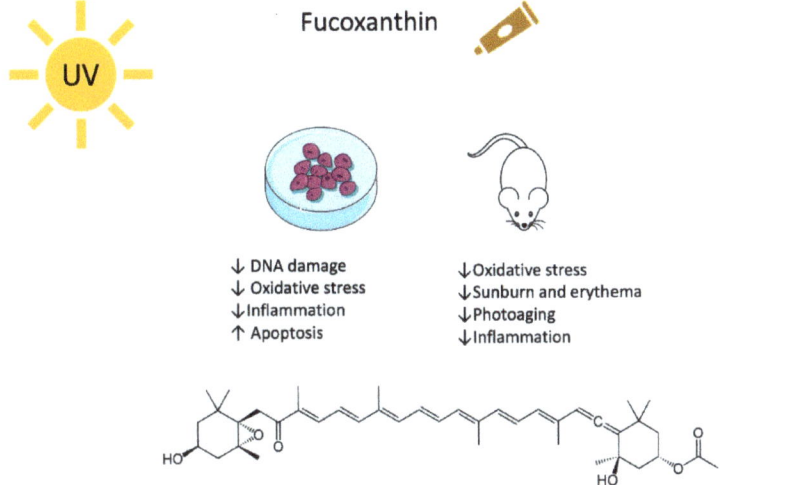

Figure 2. Molecular structure and biological activity of fucoxanthin versus UV-mediated damage.

2. Astaxanthin

Have you ever wondered why some crustaceans turn red when they are boiled? It is because of ASX. This carotenoid is stored in various crustaceans and other aquatic creatures fused into a protein complex known as crustacyanin. The intense and persistent heat of boiling water generates the liberation of free ASX, which confers the bright red color [19].

There are two primary natural sources of ASX: the microalgae that produce it and the numerous marine creatures that consume such algae, such as salmon, crustaceans, mollusks, and krill. Interestingly, the pink crustaceans, for which flamingos are greedy, confer the pink color to flamingos' feathers.

Usually, algal carotenoids have a photoprotective or light-harvesting role, or both of them [20]. ASX synthesis happens as a defense mechanism whenever the microalga *Haematococcus pluvialis* is stressed, for instance, when it is not fully covered by water. On that occasion, the UVRs, that are usually screened by water, can damage its tissues and vital parts, and *Haematococcus* activates one of the few strategies to protect itself, producing antioxidant substances [21,22].

ASX is one of the most efficient natural antioxidants in both marine and terrestrial environments. It is 65 times more potent than ascorbic acid, 100 times more than BC, and 10 times more than tocopherol [23–25]. Moreover, unlike BC, ASX does not have a rebound prooxidant effect [26,27]. It is much more efficient than BC in quenching radical and non-radical reactive species, such as singlet oxygen, which are responsible for damage caused by sunlight [25,28,29]. These outstanding properties derive from its particular molecular structure. ASX consists of two polar moieties (ionone rings) linked by a long conjugated double bonds carbon chain that represents the non-polar part of the molecule (Figure 1). If the polar moieties directly quench free radicals or other oxidants, the long unsaturated ramified carbon chain allows electron delocalization. In this way, the antioxidant effect is synergized [30–33]. More, this particular layout will enable ASX to slip and position itself within the cellular membrane, precisely fitting the polar–non-polar structure of the double phospholipidic layers and conferring protections through the interception of reactive molecular species before they can reach the inside of cells [30].

ASX exhibits a wide-ranging biological activity, including antioxidant, anticancer, and anti-inflammatory effects [28] (Figure 1). For these reasons, it has been identified as a perfect agent to counteract all photoinduced damage and to concur to regulate skin homeostasis.

2.1. Astaxanthin and UV-Mediated Skin Cancer

Given its high impact antioxidant properties, the role of ASX in cancer has been studied for a chemopreventive role more than as an antitumor agent. Different in vitro and in vivo models have been exploited to assess its potential in preventing tumorigenesis induced by both UVA and UVB radiations.

As mentioned above, the most common DNA lesion caused by UV, called "UV signature mutation," is the formation of CPDs. Upon exposure of DNA to UV, adjacent pyrimidines (CC, CT, or TT) create a saturated bond that, if not repaired, leads to those DNA mutations that initiate tumorigenesis [34]. UVB increases cutaneous ornithine decarboxylase (ODC) activity. ODC, the first enzyme in the polyamine-biosynthesis pathway, can cause sustained proliferation and clonal expansion of the initiated cells, leading to tumorigenesis [35]. For instance, high levels of ODC are crucial in promoting squamous cell carcinomas by driving the sustained proliferation and clonal expansion of v-Ha-ras–initiated cells [36]. In UV-exposed hairless mice, ASX negatively modulated the increased polyamine metabolism better than any other tested carotenoid, such as BC [37]. Furthermore, pretreatment with 5 µM ASX of human keratinocytes (HaCaT) 24 h before UVB exposure or a topical application of a 0.02% ASX gel after chronic UVB irradiation on male Wistar mice (3 irradiations per week per 4 weeks) impeded oxidative DNA damage [38,39].

Dermal fibroblasts are located within the dermis and hypodermis. For this reason, it is more probable that UVA more than UVB radiations reach these cells and create DNA lesions. ASX entirely prevented UVA-mediated DNA damage on a human skin fibroblast cell line (1BR-3) starting from 10 nM, 18 h prior 2 h of UVA irradiation. Predictably, this event was escorted by and probably due to ASX antioxidant activity [5].

To respond to UV-mediated insult due to the increased levels of reactive oxygen species (ROS), the skin itself deploys non-enzymatic and enzymatic antioxidants. Glutathione (GSH) is a tripeptide that shields cells from oxidative damage through self-oxidization. Thus, during oxidative stress, its reserves are depleted [40]. Differently, basal levels of superoxide dismutase (SOD) are increased in response to superoxide formation [41,42]. ASX was able to respond to oxidative stress sustaining the physiological redox homeostasis. In particular, preincubation (18 h) with ASX 10 µM counteracted both the GSH depletion and the SOD enhancement that were triggered by UVA [5].

The same antioxidant and DNA-protective effects were recorded replacing ASX with an algal extract enriched in ASX. However, the extract was able to match the impact of ASX only at the dose containing a 10^3 higher concentration than that of synthetic ASX (10 µM versus 10 nM, respectively) [5].

Firsthand, this result is surprising, since usually, extracts have a higher biological impact than single molecules due to the synergistic activity of all the compounds that compose it [43,44]. However, the authors of the study suggested that the differential activity is to ascribe to the low bioavailability of ASX in the extract [5]. Moreover, since it is not specified, we also wonder which form both commercial ASX and ASX in the extract are, whether they are in a free or an ester form. Many studies showed that ASX in the form of ester (ASXE) has a more powerful chemopreventive and anticancer activity, and this could be a further explanation for the effect of the extract [25]. For instance, ASX mono- and di-esters (ASXM and ASXD) showed better anticancer protection than ASX on healthy albino Wistar rats exposed to a combination of UV and 7,12-dimethylbenz(a)anthracene (DMBA) treatment. All ASX forms (free and esters) were able to significantly reduce the formation of malignant papillomas and slow down the onset of neoplastic lesions. Still, the esters almost completely reversed UVA effects (versus 44% of lessened tumor incidence and 65% reduction in tumor burden recorded for ASX). Both ASX and ASXE were able to counteract lipid peroxidation, SOD increment, and GSH depletion. The interesting fact is that the mere antioxidant potential did not mirror the chemopreventive activity, as ASXE have a higher impact in reducing UV-mediated lipid peroxidation. Thus, the anticancer potential of ASX and ASXE is probably not entirely caused by the direct antioxidant activity as ROS quenchers [25].

Different studies show the ability of ASX to act not only as antioxidants but also to directly target other tumorigenic pathways. For instance, ASX and ASXE counteracted the rise of tyrosinase activity caused by UV-DMBA treatment in rats [25]. Tyrosinase activity is physiologically upregulated as a consequence of GSH shortage and sustains the malignant transformation of normal melanocytes [45]. Of note, shrimp waste containing ASX had antioxidant potential and was able to lower tyrosinase activity on human dermal fibroblast cells [46]. In the context of promoting the recycling and re-use of waste materials to minimize the environmental impact, this finding is remarkable. Furthermore, both acute and chronic exposure of our body to UVR causes inflammation. As a result of UV-induced stress, inflammatory cytokines are released, and a protumorigenic environment is established [28]. On UV-DMBA treated mice, both ASX and ASXE 100 µg/kg body weight were able, at least in part, to avoid an inflammatory status thanks to the ability to restore physiological neutrophil to lymphocyte ratio and platelet to lymphocyte ratio [25], which represent clinical markers of inflammation and prognostic factors in different tumor types [47,48].

It is well acknowledged that an immunosuppressive environment supports tumor formation and progression and that UV exposure promotes the suppression of the immune system and favor skin cancer development [49,50]. If there is no evidence about the ability of ASX to prevent or counteract UV-mediated immunosuppression, ASX's general ability to boost the immune system has been highlighted in different studies. ASX boosted both humoral and cell-mediated immune response after polyvalent vaccination in beagle dogs and domestic shorthair cats [51,52]. Dogs were fed for 16 weeks with ASX 20 mg and at week 12, the polyvalent vaccine has been administered, while cats were fed for 12 weeks with ASX 10 mg and at week 8 the vaccine has been administered. In both animal models, ASX increased immune globulin (Ig) G production both pre- and post-vaccination but increased IgM production only after vaccination. A similar immunostimulant event occurs in murine spleen cells where ASX 20 nM increased IgG and IgM levels after 96 h treatment [53]. In dogs, but not in cats, ASX also mediated the cellular response increasing T-cell function, while in both cats and dogs it amplified natural killer (NK) cell cytotoxic activity both before and after vaccination [51,52].

The same effect on NK cytotoxic activity was recorded in humans' blood after a daily intake of 8 mg of ASX for 8 weeks [54]. Besides, the intake of ASX 100 mg/kg/day per os for 4 days counteracted the decrease in NK cell activity due to restraint stress in mice [55]. In another study, BALB/c mice were fed with ASX (0.02%, 40 µg/kg body weight/day in a beadlet form) mixed in a chemically defined diet three weeks before subcutaneous inoculation with transplantable methylcholanthrene-induced fibrosarcoma (Meth-A tumor) cells. These cancerous cells convey a tumor antigen that triggers T cell-mediated immune responses in syngeneic mice. The ASX antitumor activity was accompanied by higher cytotoxic T lymphocyte (CTL) activity and interferon-γ production by tumor-draining lymph node (TDLN) and spleen cells in the ASX-treated mice [56]. All these reports show that ASX boosts both humoral and cellular-mediated immune response in different models and represents the premises for the investigation of ASX's ability to counteract UV-mediated immunosuppression.

Furthermore, additional targets are hit by ASX that can concur with the mere antioxidant activity to confer the chemopreventive activity. The gap junctional intercellular communication (GJIC) is a system of aqueous channels that allow the communication between adjacent cells and the exchange of small metabolites to maintain tissue homeostasis. GIJC is involved in cell growth control and cancer progression [57,58]. A compromised GJIC characterizes many tumors, and its re-establishment supports the growth suppression of neoplastic foci [59]. Conflicting results have been recorded about the effect of ASX on GJIC. Concentrations of ASX higher than 0.1 μg/mL generated a detrimental reduction of GIJC on primary human fibroblasts, and this effect was reversed following ASX withdrawal [60]. However, two different ASX hydrosoluble derivatives, namely disodium disuccinate ASX and tetrasodium diphosphate ASX, upregulated GIJC on embryo fibroblasts from 0.001 to 0.1 μg/mL. At higher concentrations, such as 1 μg/mL, no modulation was recorded [61,62], excluding any detrimental effect. These controversial outcomes suggest that further studies are needed to sort this question out and highlight the necessity of assessing a risk/benefit analysis of this carotenoid.

To understand the ASX's potential therapeutic use, it is crucial to evaluate its toxicological profile. For the toxicological aspect of ASX, different outcomes have been generated in the past. A 22-year-old study [63] demonstrated that a diet containing 0.07% ASX exacerbated UV-induced tumorigenesis in female SKH-Hr-1 hairless mice, increasing the number of lesions and the rapid development of lethal complications. In the same study, a similar effect was recorded in animals fed with a diet containing 0.07% BC, but not in those fed with a diet containing 0.07% lycopene. However, as data about BC conflicted with many different studies, the authors of the study highlighted the importance of the diet in carotenoid bioavailability and hypothesized that dietary factors could interfere with ASX by fostering the protumorigenic effects [63]. Unfortunately, they did not measure the levels of ASX in serum or tissues to check the bioavailability nor perform the same experiment changing the diet of the experimental animals. For this reason, it is not possible to confirm this hypothesis. The latter study was the only one we found about ASX's protumorigenic potential, while its toxicological profile is typically very safe [24,64]. For instance, ASX and ASXE showed a favorable toxicological profile after oral administration at 100 and 200 μg/kg body weight to mice. No organ toxicity, changes in bodyweight, or behavior have been recorded together with unaffected biochemical serum parameters and skin homogenate profile [25].

ASX is commonly used as a food colorant and a supplement for its antioxidant activity and many other not scientifically confirmed uses. For this reason, very recently, the European Food Safety Authority (EFSA) carried out a scientific evaluation to assess the human health risks posed by ASX. Examining scientific literature, they concluded that the ingestion of 8 mg ASX per day is safe [65]. However, in the report, we could not find the protumorigenic effect that was depicted in the study mentioned above. Thus, it would be interesting to perform an epidemiological study to cross-correlate data about regular ASX consumers, type of diet, and skin tumors incidence.

Taken these results together, the outstanding direct antioxidant activity and the ability to modulate protumorigenic targets make ASX overpassing the antitumor potential of other carotenoids, such as BC and adonixanthin [25,29]. Nevertheless, clinical studies are certainly needed to confirm these impressive premises.

2.2. Astaxanthin, Photodamage, and Photoaging

2.2.1. Pre-Clinical Studies

As a consequence of UV irradiation, besides tumorigenesis, cells face an intense prooxidative and inflammatory reaction that gives rise to photodamage and photoaging. The most evident effect caused by acute toxic exposure to UVR is sunburn that manifests, for instance, as erythema [2]. As a result of sunburn, cells respond to the toxic insult by inducing apoptosis of damaged cells [66]. On HaCaT cells exposed to UVB, a 12 h-pretreatment with ASX (0.4–1 µM) was able to reduce oxidative stress via ROS quenching and counteract UVB-induced mitochondrial membrane depolarization and the consequential cell death [67]. Since the loss of mitochondrial potential is an early and irreversible event in the intrinsic apoptotic pathway [68], and as one of the most common triggers of the intrinsic apoptotic pathway is oxidative stress [69], ASX-mediated ROS quenching and apoptosis prevention were likely, at least in part, linked to each other.

Besides ROS, inflammatory stimuli can trigger UV-mediated apoptosis. When UVB reaches our body, keratinocytes which represent the first target act as sentinels, initiate the danger signal cascade. These events address the stress and promote apoptosis through the production of pro-apoptotic inflammatory factors, such as nitric oxide (NO) and the release of inflammatory cytokines, such as interleukins (ILs), migration inhibitory factor (MIF), and tumor necrosis factor α (TNF-α) [70–72]. Pretreatment or pre- and post-treatment of HaCaT cells with ASX at 5 µM reduced the upstream and downstream inflammatory response. It counteracted the increase in UVB-mediated inducible nitric oxide synthase (iNOS) and cyclooxygenase-2 (COX-2), and the production of prostaglandin E_2 (PGE_2). Furthermore, ASX restrained the UVB-induced release of IL-1α [73], IL-1β [38], IL-6, IL-8 [73], TNF-α [38,73], and MIF [38]. As a consequence, ASX was able to prevent apoptosis of UVB-exposed HaCaT cells [38].

The same inflammation cascade caused by UVA and UVB is one of the causes of photoaging. It can lead to an altered epithelial-mesenchymal paracrine communication between epidermal keratinocyte and dermal fibroblasts [74–76]. Metalloproteinases (MMPs) are zinc-containing endopeptidases that favor the deterioration of the extracellular matrix (ECM). UVR, oxidative stress, and cytokines trigger their release from keratinocytes and dermal fibroblasts. When UVR reaches the dermis, it directly triggers gene expression of metalloproteinase 1 (MMP-1), which degrades collagen I fibers and other elastic ones altering the healthy skin structure [76]. The impaired ECM structure results in skin sagging and wrinkling, and in the worst-case scenario, it can initiate tumor cell invasion in photocarcinogenesis [77].

In parallel, UVB- and UVA-exposed-keratinocytes secrete IL-1α that triggers the release of granulocyte macrophage-colony stimulatory factor (GM-CSF). Both IL-1α and GM-CSF reach the dermis and stimulate fibroblasts to secrete neutral endopeptidase (NEP), which in turn breaks the adjacent elastic fibers deteriorating the standard skin structure, reducing skin elasticity, and generating wrinkles [76]. Altogether, these events cause photoaging with various visible effects, such as wrinkles, dryness, and laxity [73,78,79].

ASX at 5 µM impeded MMP-1 secretion by dermal fibroblasts. In particular, epidermal keratinocyte pre-treated with ASX were exposed to UVB radiation. The medium was collected and then used to cultivate dermal fibroblasts, which, in turn, did not show any release of MMP-1, conversely to fibroblasts cultivated in UVB-exposed keratinocyte medium with no ASX treatment [73]. In a different study, it has been confirmed that ASX (1, 4 and 8 µM) blocks MMP-1 expression at gene and protein levels and blocked its enzymatic activity. This effect was accompanied by NEP inhibition. In a latter study, human fibroblasts were directly irradiated with UVA, and ASX was added after UV exposure [80]. This data is interesting because, as the authors of the study suggest, it excludes that only the antioxidant potential of ASX is responsible for its protective effect. Indeed, the most common and crucial reactive species have a life shorter than 4 µs [81], thus the effect of ASX post-treatment cannot be the result of its antioxidant activity. Besides, ASX post-treatment abrogated the release of GM-CSF and IL-1α in UVB-treated keratinocytes endorsing the alternative mechanism of action involving a cytokine release antagonism, instead of an antioxidant one [80].

On animals, the interesting photoprotective potential of ASX has been confirmed. Given that UVR causes skin damage through ROS formation, such as singlet oxygen, ASX would be expected to prevent UV-mediated skin damage. However, all ASX common preparations are high hydrophile in nature and not suitable for the common lipophile vehicle used for sunscreen. For this reason, a liposomal preparation was developed to include 6 mol% (% of the amount of ASX—expressed in moles - on the total amount of all constituents in the preparation) of ASX (Lipo-ASX). This preparation showed the same antioxidant properties of free ASX in terms of quenching singlet oxygen. Moreover, Lipo-ASX spread on Hos:HR-1 hairless mice dorsal skin before repeated UV irradiation overcame many morphological changes due to the UV-exposure, such as the thickness of the epidermal layer and cockle formation, as well as collagen destruction, preventing wrinkle formation. In parallel, transporting Lipo-ASX to the basal laminae through the creation of cationic liposomes containing ASX for iontophoretic transdermal delivery inhibited UV-melanin production, shielding melanocytes from UVR [82].

ASX's ability to prevent photodamage and photoaging has been confirmed in other models. UV-induced photoaging is a chronic process mostly driven by UVA. Komatsu and colleagues [83] tested chronic UVA exposure (20 J/cm^3, 5 times per week for 70 days) on hairless Hos:HR-1 mice while fed with or without ASXME (0.01% or 0.1% of the AIN-93G diet) purified from *Haematococcus pluvialis*. The first useful finding is that ASX reached and accumulated in both dermis and epidermis, thus letting presume an activity on both levels. The overall effect of ASXME was the avoidance of wrinkles, water loss, and visible aging signs. Confirming the in vitro studies, the ability to prevent wrinkles is ascribed to ASX's ability to keep MMP-13, the mice analogous of human MMP-1, at the same levels of unexposed mice as well as to suppress the decrease of transglutaminase 2 (TGM2). Indeed, a reduction in TGM2 would lead to the decline of epidermal-dermal integrity since it favors protein-cross linking within collagen VII [83]. Starting from day 56, both ASX groups showed lesser dryness with respect to control, in terms of transepidermal water loss (TWEL), probably due to the ability to suppress the UV-mediated increase in lymphoepithelial Kazal-type-related inhibitor (LEKTI), steroid sulfatase (STS), and aquaporin 3 (AOP3), restoring physiological levels [83].

LEKTI is a serine protease inhibitor that inhibits other serine proteases, such as different human kallikrein (KLK) isoforms. KLKs regulates skin desquamation and inflammation and is a marker of skin cancer [84]. ASX also increased the content of two natural moisturizing factors (NMFs), pyroglutamic acid (PCA), and urocanic acid (UCA), as if UVA-exposure did not happen [83]. Both STS and AOP3 play crucial roles in desquamation and water loss [85,86].

Topic application of a gel containing ASX on UVB-exposed Wistar mice significantly reduced photoaging effects. Mice received increasing energetic UVB irradiation for four weeks (50 mJ/cm^2 week 1; 70 mJ/cm^2 week 2; 80 mJ/cm^2 weeks 3 and 4), three times per week. A 0.02% ASX gel was applied on mice 20 min before and 4 h after irradiation. ASX, as usual, suppressed UVB-induced MMP-1 and counteracted the degradation of collagen fibers [39].

In another study, HR-1 hairless mice underwent UVA for 8 weeks. UVA intensity was increased to reach 100 mJ/cm^2 in 4 weeks. ASX was introduced in the diet at 100 mg/kg body weight. The supplementation decreased the visible sign of photoaging as wrinkling and skin thickening and maintained physiological ROS levels. Moreover, ASX increased collagen density overcoming non-irradiated group levels. It also prevented the reduction of capillaries diameter on UV-exposed skin through the upregulation of vascular endothelial growth factor (VEGF) and the downregulation of thrombospondin 1 (TSP-1) [87]. As the reduction of capillaries is correlated to ROS-mediated endothelial apoptosis [88], this data comes towards ASX's ability to prevent photocarcinogenesis, photodamage, and photoaging.

2.2.2. Clinical Studies

Since animal studies did not highlight any relevant toxic effect after acute or chronic UVA or UVB exposure, it was possible to proceed with studies on humans.

The American Food and Drug Administration (FDA) defines the minimal erythemal dose (MED) as "the smallest UV dose that produces perceptible redness of the skin (erythema) with clearly defined borders at 16 to 24 h after UV exposure". The ratio between MED of protected skin (MEDp), for instance with sunscreen, and MED of unprotected skin (MEDu) represents the famous sun protective factor (SPF) that is found on every sunscreen container [89].

To assess the effect of ASX on MED in humans, Ito et al. [90] performed a study in which 11 human subjects consumed 4 mg of ASX for 9 weeks. Then, small parts of their back were irradiated with UVB lamps, and their MED was compared to the one of the placebo group and to their MED measured irradiating their skin before the beginning of ASX supplementation. ASX administration significantly increased MED, which resulted 5 times higher than that observed in the placebo group. ASX supplementation also attenuated the UV-induced decrease in moisture in healthy subjects [90]. The only limitation of this promising study is the number of subjects recruited for the study. If these results were confirmed on a higher number of people, data would be more robust and pave the way for the use of ASX as a sunburn protector.

Different clinical studies have been performed to investigate ASX potential to prevent or cure photoaging signs. For these studies, no artificial UVR was applied to human subjects, but the effect of ASX supplementation in a standard skin deterioration scenario has been investigated. In a clinical trial involving 59 healthy female participants in a placebo-controlled, double-blind, randomized trial [73], two groups of 22 and 19 individuals received oral supplementation of 6 or 12 mg of ASX per day for 16 weeks, respectively. The remaining 18 people constituted the placebo group. Only at the end of 16 weeks some difference between the placebo group and the treated one was noticed. Wrinkle depths (measured through pictures of subjects and instrumental analysis), skin elasticity, and moisture were stable for both ASX groups, while deterioration was recorded for the placebo group. Furthermore, only the higher supplementation dose was able to maintain IL-1α levels steady from day 0 to week 16, while in both placebo and 6 mg ASX groups, those levels increased [73]. Of note, although the study did not show any toxic effect, an intake of 12 mg per day exceeded EFSA recommendations [65].

One study took place from August to December 2015 in Osaka [73], when the UV index (UVI) ranged from 6.6 and 2.0 [91]. UVI is an easy way to address the level of UV radiation. The World and Health Organization (WHO) states that until UVI 3, no protective measures are needed. Above 3, protection is necessary, and above 8 those protections should be reinforced [1]. In this study, 3 months of experimentation fall into the moderate category, and the other 2 in the low group [91]. This was the only study where the investigators specified both period of the year and city where the study took place. Still, this detail would be interesting to uniform and understand the applicability of the different studies outcomes. What emerges from this study and some similar ones is that ASX administration prevented general photoaging in terms of wrinkle, dryness, and elasticity at a dose ranging from 2 to 12 mg per day [73,92–95] and that ASX supplementation was safe during the whole duration of the study (16 weeks) at 12 mg/day. For instance, no alteration in blood or in the function of the liver, kidney, and serum cholesterol has been recorded [73]. An uncontrolled trial showed that a concomitant oral assumption of 6 mg ASX, together with topical use of a preparation containing the same carotenoid (78.9 μM) promoted a better effect on the same photoaging markers [93].

Whether the majority of these studies agree that ASX can prevent the formation of UV-related skin markers, research conducted by Chalyk et al. [94] claimed that ASX 4 mg orally taken for 4 weeks actively counteracted the pre-existing effect of photo- and physiological-aging. The residual skin analysis showed a decrease in corneocyte desquamation, and the blood test showed lower systemic malondialdehyde levels, which represent a marker of oxidative stress [94]. These promising results are not conclusive and, for sure, have to be confirmed. Indeed, usually, for all other reports we considered in this review, ASX's effect was visible following an extended period of supplementation (at least 16 weeks). Furthermore, we agree with Ng et al. [96] who, in their systematic review, point out that all these clinical studies are not without flaws. Whether because of the lack of placebo and/or control groups, or the low participant number, data are not conclusive. In addition, most of the research on humans has been funded by commercial entities, and a bias due to conflict of interests cannot be excluded [96].

Overall, more structured clinical studies are needed to understand the real photoprotective potential of ASX.

3. Fucoxanthin

FX represents more than 10% of the total carotenoids, counting within the terrestrial and marine environment [97]. It is a xanthophyll mainly produced by brown algae and stored in chloroplasts. It is present in edible algae commonly used in Japanese and Korean traditional food, such as Kombu (*Laminaria japonica*) and Wakame (*Undaria pinnatifida*) [98]. FX was isolated for the first time in 1914, and, 50 years later, its chemical structure was characterized [97]: the standard polyene chain links particular functional groups, such as an allenic bond, and hydroxyl, epoxy, carbonyl, and carboxyl moieties in the terminal rings (Figure 2). This complex structure explains the ability to quench singlet oxygen and to scavenge free radicals [99,100]. For instance, FX transforms the excess of energy that originates from singlet oxygen in heat. Mechanistically, a transition into the triplet state and consequent relaxation to the single state without changing the chemical structure happen. Besides, the high number of FX's conjugated bonds allows this carotenoid to donate electrons to free radicals forming adducts, with the result of quenching the reactive species [98,100]. In addition, conversely to most of all other carotenoids, FX quenches free radicals also in anoxic conditions, which is a very rare ability [98].

As for ASX, many studies show that FX has better antioxidant and photoprotective properties than the most common terrestrial origin antioxidants and carotenoids [101].

3.1. Fucoxanthin and UV-Mediated Skin Cancer

FX's preventive activity on UV-mediated carcinogenesis has been investigated only in vitro on keratinocytes and fibroblasts.

As previously reported, UVR in general and UVB, in particular, induce an inflammatory state that could promote detrimental effects, such as cutaneous inflammation, erythema, sunburn, photoaging, and, if the exposure is particularly vigorous or perpetuated, DNA damage and skin cancer [102]. In basal cell carcinoma and many other neoplastic lesions, tumorigenesis and cancer development can be perpetuated by forming the so-called inflammasome. Inflammasome, and specifically NLR family pyrin domain containing 3 (NLRP3), is a protein complex that mediates pyroptosis, an inflammatory regulated type of cell death. Diverse stimuli, such as oxidative stress and UVR, promote the activation of NLRP3 that results in caspase-1 activation, which in turn provokes the activation of immunostimulant and proinflammatory cytokines, such as IL-1ß, IL-1α, TNF-α, and COX-2. Those mediators are then responsible for the establishment of the protumorigenic environment [103,104]. A pretreatment with FX 5 μM could not break down inflammasome-related players on UV-exposed HaCaT human keratinocytes, such as NLRP3, caspase-1, and the inflammasome adaptor protein (ASC). Still, together with rosmarinic acid at a concentration of 5 μM, it gained this ability. Of note, neither rosmarinic acid alone counteracted pyroptosis. Besides, FX 5 μM alone slightly decreased UV-mediated cell death and cell-cycle alterations. These effects were again synergized by rosmarinic acid and accompanied by a strong antioxidant effect in terms of nuclear factor erythroid 2–related factor 2 (Nrf2) cascade activation [103]. Given that most of the studies that we are going to show in the next paragraphs exploit higher concentrations of FX, up to 50 μM, we wonder if the effects of rosmarinic acid could be produced by increasing the dose of FX alone.

In HaCaT cells, pretreatment with FX 10-50 μM lowered the release of IL-6 [101], which is prodrome for skin aging and carcinomas [105], and prevented the increase in ROS level due to UVA and UVB irradiation [101,106]. Moreover, compared to the UV-exposed group, FX at 10 μM lowered keratinocytes proliferation, which represents a marker of skin cancer [101]. Indeed, as a defense mechanism, skin counteracts the UV-mediated harm by arresting the cell cycle to repair the damaged cells or, if the damage is irreversible, by inducing apoptosis. When the toxic insult overcomes the organism's ability to respond, these mechanisms fail, and further UV exposure results in DNA damage and clonal cell expansion [107].

In human fibroblasts, FX showed an intense protective activity against UVB irradiations. In particular, it completely counteracted UVB-induced ROS formation and partially prevented UVB-mediated cell death. Starting from 50 µM, FX inhibited UVB-mediated DNA damage, probably thanks to its antioxidant activity, letting presume the ability to prevent the formation of neoplastic lesions [108].

Unfortunately, no in vivo nor clinical studies confirm the interesting in vitro results, lowering the impact of this compound as a chemopreventive agent.

3.2. Fucoxanthin, Photodamage and Photoaging

If ASX's potential to prevent photodamage is achieved mostly via oral integration, FX exerts a more effective photoprotection when incorporated in topical preparations. Unlike ASX, which accumulates well in the skin [83], FX hardly reaches an effective concentration in that organ after oral administration [109]. For this reason, a way to overcome this flaw and still exploit FX potential is to use this carotenoid in topic formulations, such as ointments, lotions, and emulsions.

An ointment containing 200 µg FX prevented UVB-induced erythema in female SHK-1 hairless mice. The pretreatment with FX after exposure to an acute proinflammatory dose of UVB (360 mJ/cm^2) improved skin conditions in terms of skin moisture and elasticity. At a molecular level, it counteracted the inflammation cascade through the decrease of COX-2 levels and the oxidative impairment through the upregulation of Nrf2 and its target gene heme oxygenase-1 (HO-1) [101]. The same FX-containing ointment prevented UVB-mediated skin edema and an increase in myeloperoxidase (MPO) [101].

A prevalent consequence of UVR exposure is the onset of hyperpigmentary disorders (HDs). To name one, the most common HD is solar lentigo. Solar lentigines are true and proper skin lesions and represent risk indicators for skin cancer (melanoma and non-melanoma). HDs are often the consequences of increased production of pro-melanogenic factors escorted by an altered expression or activity of receptors on melanocytes [110,111]. An interesting study showed that FX inhibited melanogenesis in vitro (B16 cells) and in vivo (guinea pigs). In vitro, FX slightly suppressed tyrosinase activity and theophylline-induced melanogenesis at 10 and 30 mg/mL by three-day treatment, but a more effective outcome was observed in the animal experiments. In vivo, the back of the skin of guinea pigs has been irradiated for 14 days with incremental UVB doses (7 days 160 mJ/cm^2 followed by 7 days 320 mJ/cm^2). FX, in the form of food (10 mg/kg) or ointment (50 µL of white petrolatum containing 0.01–1% of FX) applied after UVB irradiation, efficiently blocked cellular melanogenesis for six to ten days after the last irradiation session [11].

Many substances can trigger melanocyte receptors and start melanogenesis. Melanocyte stimulating hormones (MSH), prostaglandins, and common cytokines belong to this category and are specifically increased after UVB exposure. Both oral and topic application of FX decreased the mRNA levels of the PGE$_2$ precursor COX-2. Endothelin receptor A p75 neurotrophin receptor (NTR), that is a low-affinity receptor of NT-3, melanocortin 1 receptor (MC1R), that is MSH cognate receptor, and tyrosinase-related protein 1 (Tyrp1) are other melanogenesis stimulants increased by UV exposure and were all suppressed by FX, especially via the topical application at the same concentrations needed to block melanogenesis (0.01–1%) [11].

Interestingly, the antimelanogenic effect via both topic and oral administration was more efficient in vivo than in vitro (on B16 cells), where the entity of melanin reduction was similar to only a half of the effect of the gold-standard drug for many HDs, retinol. The reason behind this behavior is that FX is metabolized in several organs and tissues, and various metabolites reside in different organs. Since so far nobody characterized the FX metabolites that accumulate in the skin, the authors of the study suggested that they could be fucoxanthinol and amarouciaxanthin A, the most abundant and common metabolites of FX, and that those molecules should be investigated for antimelanogenic activity in vivo [11].

Matsui et al. [112] showed that application of a 0.5% FX vaseline-based cream at day 5 after 4 days of UVB chronic irradiation (1 h per day, 2.7 J/cm^2) on female ddY strain mice, efficiently cured the sunburn. The same protective effect was not recorded for the antioxidant N-acetylcysteine (NAC), the steroidal anti-inflammatory clobetasol, or BC nor its metabolite retinoic acid (RA). Thus, as for ASX, FX's photoprotective activity is probably not the result of the mere antioxidant potential, but the sum of the antioxidant activity and modulation of other pathways. To understand what made FX able to cure the photodamage, the authors of the study used a complementary approach. First, they excluded UVR absorption as FX showed an absorption peak mainly outside the UVA range (215–400 nm). Subsequently, they assessed whether and which substances were able to quench H_2O_2 and lessen oxidative stress through acellular bioassays and in vitro. They noticed that FX and NAC were able to do that; thus, as FX, but not NAC, cured the sunburn, they excluded that ROS quenching was the solely healing mechanism in mice.

The next step has been performing a microarray analysis of UV-exposed mice skin to identify which genes were mostly modulated by the irradiation. Filaggrin (Flg) is a protein fiber that acts as an essential mechanical support for the assembly of keratin filaments and regulates epidermal homeostasis [113]. The lipid envelope, which plays a crucial role in the skin barrier function, incorporates them within the stratum corneum. In the higher part of the stratum corneum, Flg is converted into its active form and takes part in the water retention process. A dysfunction of Flg and the barrier function of the epidermis generates various atopic disorders, such as atopic dermatitis. In the study of Matsui et al. [112], UVB exposure comported a dramatic downregulation of Flg gene levels with those of its promoters, the caudal type homeobox 1 (Cdx1) [112]. Indeed, in silico experiments showed that Cdx1 was downregulated by UV irradiation as well. FX, but not any other compound mentioned above, restored physiological levels of both Flg and Cdx1, suggesting a pivotal role of Flg in this fascinating carotenoid curative activity [112].

A less concentrated preparation of FX (80 μL of a solution containing 0.001% FX) prevented UVB-mediated photoaging on female Hos:HR-1 hairless mice. Applied 2 h before any session of incremental UVB irradiation doses (from 30 mJ/cm^2 to 65mj/cm^2) 5 times per week for 10 weeks, FX efficiently avoided wrinkle formation and epidermal hypertrophy. At a molecular level, in the epidermis, the same treatment lowered ROS levels and MMP-13 expression together with VEGF [114]. Angiogenesis in general and VEGF, in particular, are increased after UV irradiation [115,116] and actively sustain photoaging and wrinkle formation [117]. In this study too, the authors suggest that FX is not likely to exploit its photoprotective activity through the absorption of UVB [114] and other literature supports the fact that FX's absorption is relatively weak in UV wavelengths [98,114].

A very recent study showed that FX can be incorporated in sunscreen and efficiently synergize the effect of two common sunscreen compounds through UVR absorption. In a reconstructed skin model that mimics all different layers of human skin, 0.5% (weight/volume) FX enhanced the antioxidant properties of a standard sunscreen containing avobenzone and ethylhexyl methoxycinnamate [106]. In the same model, FX significantly exhibited the photoprotective activity of the same sunscreen. FX showed an acceptable degree of photodegradation that was accompanied by a 72% enhancement in UVA and UVB absorption compared to the only sunscreen. No phototoxic events have been reported on the skin model, conversely to the positive control ketoprofen, which promoted abundant cell death [106]. This latter information opens things up about the use of FX in sunscreen formulations and adds further elements to the discovery of FX's mechanism of action, especially from the perspective of increasing sunscreen efficacy. Indeed, although sunscreens rely on substances that filter UVB and UVA, recently, many studies show that antioxidants can improve the filter activity, probably by stabilizing them. Some of these combinations are indeed already on the market [118].

4. Current Challenges and Future Perspectives

Excluding the avoidance of UVR, the most effective way to protect from sun radiations is the use of sunscreen. However, sunscreen effectiveness is often inadequate due to low compliance. Thus, an alternative way to protect from the detrimental effect of sunlight, which includes all types of photodamage, such as sunburn, photoaging, immunosuppression, and the burden of skin cancer, should be taken into consideration [1]. So far, however, no supplement has been demonstrated to protect our skin from sunlight damage efficiently. Many natural antioxidant compounds, such as carotenoids, showed encouraging properties in terms of photoprotection [119]. Among them, the marine carotenoids ASX and FX stand out, overpassing the potential of the most efficient terrestrial carotenoids, such as BC.

As presented in this review, both ASX and FX protected from DNA damage and oxidative stress, exhibited an anti-inflammatory and immunostimulant activity, together with the activation of specific pathways involved in the prevention of UV-mediated phototoxicity, photoaging, and skin cancer (Figures 1 and 2). ASX is far more characterized than FX, which lacks entirely clinical studies. For ASX, a complete profile about its photoprotective potential in vitro and in vivo has been drawn, while for FX, some aspects have still to be investigated. For instance, the ability to protect from UV-induced carcinogenesis has been investigated in vivo only for ASX, while for FX the focus has been put on its ability to prevent phototoxicity in terms of sunburn and photoaging.

To be fair, it should not be underestimated that the cosmetic effects for both these carotenoids have been investigated. On the one hand, all UV damages are intertwined, and a simple sunburn or UV-induced lentigines can result in far more dangerous skin cancer. On the other hand, besides the physiopathologic correlation between UV-induced photoaging and cancer, we would like to highlight that the mere positive esthetic benefits of photoprotective supplements can indirectly help to counteract skin tumors. Usually, since wrinkle formation and brown spots are visible, while tumors are perceived as far events, the use of a photoprotective supplement that concurrently prevents photoaging, photodamage and tumorigenesis is a win-win condition. Indeed, people who are more aware of UV-mediated premature aging are also more prone to use sunscreen and protection from UVR [120,121]. Thus, since the low compliance often hampers the efficacy of measures concerning the protection from sunlight, a further incentive in the form of antiaging effect can only be beneficial.

Still, both FX and ASX showed a very high potential, but not conclusive results due to the lack of proper clinical studies. In the big picture, what is missing is the demonstration of the cause-effect relationship between the administration of ASX or FX and the protection and prevention of UV-mediated damage. Regarding ASX, this concept is reiterated by EFSA, which rejected the claim "protection of DNA, proteins, and lipids from oxidative damage" [122].

It is worth noting that in 2004 the World Intellectual Properties Organization approved a patent for the development of a method for reducing, preventing, ameliorating, or reversing oxidative DNA damage in animals and human subjects with ASX alone or in combination with other agents [123]. The study presented in the patent tried to demonstrate the antioxidant potential of ASX extracts, but no evidence has been produced about the overall effect deriving from these antioxidant properties, nor a straightforward cause-effect analysis between ASX intake and the antioxidant effect [123]. Moreover, we identified some pitfalls, such as lack of statistical analysis and experimental details (number of subjects), which limit the robustness of the study.

Given the even lower number of studies about FX and the complete lack of clinical ones, this issue is even more evident. However, this current situation does not change the high potential that these carotenoids have shown and that, according to the studies reported here, they have better activity than the most studied and promising carotenoids of terrestrial origin [25,28,29]. The properties that both carotenoids showed in vitro and on the animal in different photodamage models are outstanding. The antioxidant effect and the implication of different pathways make ASX and FX still good candidates for future therapeutic and cosmetic applications.

To better understand the potential benefits of high intakes of ASX and FX in food, or as a food supplement, bioavailability and pharmacokinetic analysis are necessary. As for all carotenoids, the bioavailability of ASX and FX is hampered by their lipophilic nature, and for this reason, they are better absorbed when ingested with other lipids that vehicle the substances in the organism [124]. After oral administration, ASX is absorbed by intestinal mucosal cells, assimilated with lipoproteins, and transported into the tissues where it is accumulated [125]. Its bioavailability is not high, but the use of lipophilic formulations expedites improvement. Indeed, in humans, after 4 h after the ingestion of

40 mg of ASX, its plasma concentration can range from 4% to 34% of the ingested dose depending on the formulation, where the high lipophilic preparation generates the better availability. At the maximum plasma peak (around 10 h after consumption), the same 40 mg of ASX generated a plasma concentration of 90.1 µg/L while the lipophilic formulation yielded a value of 191.5 µg/L [124]. This information is important when it comes to choosing the type of diet or formulation for ASX intake. While it is known that ASX accumulates in different tissues in mice, such as skin, liver, spleen, kidneys, and eyes [126], no evidence has been produced for humans, and this represents another missing piece for the evaluation of ASX's therapeutic potential. Of note, ASX's bioavailability studies did not include its metabolites because ASX's activity has been ascribed to its unchanged form [31,126].

On the contrary, FX is absorbed as fucoxanthinol, a hydrolyzed metabolite, in the small intestine that, in turn, is converted to amarouciaxanthin A [127]. For this reason, these two molecules have been used to monitor the pharmacokinetic properties of FX. In humans, the bioavailability of FX is even less efficient than that of ASX. After a single dose of an oral preparation of kombu extract containing 31 mg of FX, the plasma concentration of fucoxanthinol reached the highest concentration of 27.2 µg/L after 4 h after ingestion, while amarouciaxanthin A was not detected at all. In a different scenario, 0.31 mg FX daily for 28 days showed that FX did not lead to the accumulation of fucoxanthin metabolites in the body. As for ASX, the accumulation of FX nor its metabolites in the different tissues has not been analyzed in humans, but only in mice [127]. In particular, dietary FX preferentially accumulates as amarouciaxanthin A in the adipose tissue and as fucoxanthinol in the other tissues such as liver, kidney, spleen, heart, and lung, but not skin [109].

All the aforementioned information leads to the conclusion that with careful planning ASX is suitable to be used in oral preparation, while FX for its pharmacokinetic properties would be more efficient as a therapeutic drug if used as a topical preparation. It is interesting that the two carotenoids have different chemical-physical properties and can be exploited in different ways, in terms of oral integration, topical use, or even sunscreen preparation. Consequently, since personal habits play a crucial role in the compliance of photodamage protection, giving people the options of choosing between oral and topic administration could increase the number of individuals undergoing the prevention treatment.

Another aspect that has to be considered is that, besides the effectiveness of these carotenoids, it is necessary to assess their safety, whether they are used as a supplement or topical agent with curative or cosmetic effects. So far, both carotenoids showed a lack of toxicity. Oral administration of ASX proved to be safe on both animal and human tests, while for FX safety evidence arose only in vivo and on a model of reconstructed skin. A single and 13-week oral toxicity study on rats showed that up to 200 mg/kg body weight per day FX was safe, and no mortality nor abnormalities were observed [128]. Besides, following the organization for economic co-operation and development guideline number 439 "In Vitro Skin Irritation: Reconstructed Human Epidermis Test Method", the topical application of FX in the skin model proved to be a non-irritant [129]. Moreover, these data are promising, but not definitive. Bearing in mind the terrestrial xanthophyll canthaxanthin, used until 1990 as a tanning pill, but then withdraw from the market by FDA for canthaxanthin-induced retinopathy [130], attention should be paid to ASX and FX as well.

5. Conclusions

This review describes the photoprotective activity of ASX and FX on skin photodamage and the prevention of UV-mediated carcinogenesis and highlights the potential use of these compounds in the clinic and cosmetic fields. While a very favorable and nontoxic profile for both ASX and FX has been identified, further studies are needed to understand if this potential will translate into a concrete photoprotective effect in both oncology and cosmetology.

Author Contributions: Conceptualization, E.C. and C.F.; literature search and collection, E.C.; writing—original draft preparation, E.C.; writing—review and editing, E.C., C.F., and A.B.; supervision, C.F. All authors have read and agreed to the published version of the manuscript.

Funding: This research received no external funding.

Conflicts of Interest: The authors declare no conflict of interest.

References

1. Global Solar UV Index: A Practical Guide. Available online: https://www.who.int/uv/publications/en/UVIGuide.pdf (accessed on 7 May 2020).
2. D'Orazio, J.; Jarrett, S.; Amaro-Ortiz, A.; Scott, T. UV radiation and the skin. *Int. J. Mol. Sci.* **2013**, *14*, 12222–12248. [CrossRef]
3. Eller, M.S.; Ostrom, K.; Gilchrest, B.A. DNA damage enhances melanogenesis. *Proc. Natl. Acad. Sci. USA* **1996**, *93*, 1087–1092. [CrossRef]
4. Damian, D.L.; Barnetson, R.S.; Halliday, G.M. Effects of low-dose ultraviolet radiation on in vivo human cutaneous recall responses. *Aust. J. Dermatol.* **2001**, *42*, 161–167. [CrossRef]
5. Lyons, N.M.; O'Brien, N.M. Modulatory effects of an algal extract containing astaxanthin on UVA-irradiated cells in culture. *J. Dermatol. Sci.* **2002**, *30*, 73–84. [CrossRef]
6. Ballard, R. The Astonishing Hidden World of the Deep Ocean. Available online: https://www.ted.com/talks/robert_ballard_the_astonishing_hidden_world_of_the_deep_ocean (accessed on 28 April 2020).
7. Catanzaro, E.; Calcabrini, C.; Bishayee, A.; Fimognari, C. Antitumor Potential of Marine and Freshwater Lectins. *Mar. Drugs* **2019**, *18*, 11. [CrossRef] [PubMed]
8. Decker, E.A. Natural antioxidants in foods. In *Encyclopedia of Physical Science and Technology*, 3rd ed.; Meyers, R.A., Ed.; Academic Press: New York, NY, USA, 2003; pp. 335–342. ISBN 978-0-12-227410-7.
9. Hammond, B.R.; Renzi, L.M. Carotenoids. *Adv. Nutr. Bethesda Md* **2013**, *4*, 474–476. [CrossRef]
10. Merhan, O. The biochemistry and antioxidant properties of carotenoids. In *Carotenoids*; IntechOpen: Rijeka, Croatia, 2017; pp. 51–66.
11. Shimoda, H.; Tanaka, J.; Shan, S.-J.; Maoka, T. Anti-pigmentary activity of fucoxanthin and its influence on skin mRNA expression of melanogenic molecules. *J. Pharm. Pharmacol.* **2010**, *62*, 1137–1145. [CrossRef]
12. Mularczyk, M.; Michalak, I.; Marycz, K. Astaxanthin and other Nutrients from Haematococcus pluvialis-Multifunctional Applications. *Mar. Drugs* **2020**, *18*, 459. [CrossRef]
13. Wong, S.K.; Ima-Nirwana, S.; Chin, K.-Y. Effects of astaxanthin on the protection of muscle health (Review). *Exp. Ther. Med.* **2020**, *20*, 2941–2952. [CrossRef] [PubMed]
14. Genç, Y.; Bardakci, H.; Yücel, Ç.; Karatoprak, G.Ş.; Küpeli Akkol, E.; Hakan Barak, T.; Sobarzo-Sánchez, E. Oxidative Stress and Marine Carotenoids: Application by Using Nanoformulations. *Mar. Drugs* **2020**, *18*, 423. [CrossRef] [PubMed]
15. Xia, W.; Tang, N.; Kord-Varkaneh, H.; Low, T.Y.; Tan, S.C.; Wu, X.; Zhu, Y. The effects of astaxanthin supplementation on obesity, blood pressure, CRP, glycemic biomarkers, and lipid profile: A meta-analysis of randomized controlled trials. *Pharmacol. Res.* **2020**, *161*, 105113. [CrossRef] [PubMed]
16. Li, J.; Guo, C.; Wu, J. Astaxanthin in Liver Health and Disease: A Potential Therapeutic Agent. *Drug Des. Devel. Ther.* **2020**, *14*, 2275–2285. [CrossRef] [PubMed]
17. Hentati, F.; Tounsi, L.; Djomdi, D.; Pierre, G.; Delattre, C.; Ursu, A.V.; Fendri, I.; Abdelkafi, S.; Michaud, P. Bioactive Polysaccharides from Seaweeds. *Mol. Basel Switz.* **2020**, *25*, 3152. [CrossRef]
18. Bae, M.; Kim, M.-B.; Park, Y.-K.; Lee, J.-Y. Health benefits of fucoxanthin in the prevention of chronic diseases. *Biochim. Biophys. Acta Mol. Cell Biol. Lipids* **2020**, *1865*, 158618. [CrossRef]
19. Begum, S.; Cianci, M.; Durbeej, B.; Falklöf, O.; Hädener, A.; Helliwell, J.R.; Helliwell, M.; Regan, A.C.; Watt, C.I.F. On the origin and variation of colors in lobster carapace. *Phys. Chem. Chem. Phys.* **2015**, *17*, 16723–16732. [CrossRef]
20. Horton, P.; Ruban, A. Molecular design of the photosystem II light-harvesting antenna: Photosynthesis and photoprotection. *J. Exp. Bot.* **2005**, *56*, 365–373. [CrossRef]
21. Udayan, A.; Arumugam, M.; Pandey, A. Nutraceuticals from algae and cyanobacteria. In *Algal Green Chemistry*; Rastogi, R.P., Madamwar, D., Pandey, A., Eds.; Recent Process in Biotechnologies; Elsevier: Amsterdam, The Netherlands, 2017; pp. 65–89. ISBN 978-0-444-63784-0.
22. Schoefs, B.; Rmiki, N.-E.; Rachadi, J.; Lemoine, Y. Astaxanthin accumulation in Haematococcus requires a cytochrome P450 hydroxylase and an active synthesis of fatty acids. *FEBS Lett.* **2001**, *500*, 125–128. [CrossRef]

23. Yuan, J.-P.; Chen, F. Hydrolysis kinetics of astaxanthin esters and stability of astaxanthin of Haematococcus pluvialis during saponification. *J. Agric. Food Chem.* **1999**, *47*, 31–35. [CrossRef]
24. Stewart, J.S.; Lignell, A.; Pettersson, A.; Elfving, E.; Soni, M.G. Safety assessment of Astaxanthin-rich microalgae biomass: Acute and subchronic toxicity studies in rats. *Food Chem. Toxicol. Int. J. Publ. Br. Ind. Biol. Res. Assoc.* **2008**, *46*, 3030–3036. [CrossRef]
25. Rao, A.R.; Sindhuja, H.N.; Dharmesh, S.M.; Sankar, K.U.; Sarada, R.; Ravishankar, G.A. Effective inhibition of skin cancer, tyrosinase, and antioxidative properties by astaxanthin and astaxanthin esters from the green alga *Haematococcus pluvialis*. *J. Agric. Food Chem.* **2013**, *61*, 3842–3851. [CrossRef]
26. Palozza, P.; Serini, S.; Di Nicuolo, F.; Piccioni, E.; Calviello, G. Prooxidant effects of beta-carotene in cultured cells. *Mol. Aspects Med.* **2003**, *24*, 353–362. [CrossRef]
27. Martin, H.-D.; Jäger, C.; Ruck, C.; Schmidt, M.; Walsh, R.; Paust, J. Anti- and Prooxidant Properties of Carotenoids. *J. Für Prakt. Chem.* **1999**, *341*, 302–308. [CrossRef]
28. Davinelli, S.; Nielsen, M.E.; Scapagnini, G. Astaxanthin in skin health, repair, and disease: A comprehensive review. *Nutrients* **2018**, *10*, 522. [CrossRef]
29. Maoka, T.; Yasui, H.; Ohmori, A.; Tokuda, H.; Suzuki, N.; Osawa, A.; Shindo, K.; Ishibashi, T. Anti-oxidative, anti-tumor-promoting, and anti-carcinogenic activities of adonirubin and adonixanthin. *J. Oleo Sci.* **2013**, *62*, 181–186. [CrossRef]
30. Kidd, P. Astaxanthin, cell membrane nutrient with diverse clinical benefits and anti-aging potential. *Altern. Med. Rev. J. Clin. Ther.* **2011**, *16*, 355–364.
31. Goto, S.; Kogure, K.; Abe, K.; Kimata, Y.; Kitahama, K.; Yamashita, E.; Terada, H. Efficient radical trapping at the surface and inside the phospholipid membrane is responsible for highly potent antiperoxidative activity of the carotenoid astaxanthin. *Biochim. Biophys. Acta* **2001**, *1512*, 251–258. [CrossRef]
32. Britton, G. Structure and properties of carotenoids in relation to function. *FASEB J. Off. Publ. Fed. Am. Soc. Exp. Biol.* **1995**, *9*, 1551–1558. [CrossRef]
33. Pashkow, F.J.; Watumull, D.G.; Campbell, C.L. Astaxanthin: A novel potential treatment for oxidative stress and inflammation in cardiovascular disease. *Am. J. Cardiol.* **2008**, *101*, 58D–68D. [CrossRef] [PubMed]
34. Matsumura, Y.; Ananthaswamy, H.N. Short-term and long-term cellular and molecular events following UV irradiation of skin: Implications for molecular medicine. *Expert Rev. Mol. Med.* **2002**, *4*, 1–22. [CrossRef]
35. Tang, X.; Kim, A.L.; Feith, D.J.; Pegg, A.E.; Russo, J.; Zhang, H.; Aszterbaum, M.; Kopelovich, L.; Epstein, E.H.; Bickers, D.R.; et al. Ornithine decarboxylase is a target for chemoprevention of basal and squamous cell carcinomas in Ptch1+/- mice. *J. Clin. Investig.* **2004**, *113*, 867–875. [CrossRef]
36. Smith, M.K.; Trempus, C.S.; Gilmour, S.K. Co-operation between follicular ornithine decarboxylase and v-Ha-ras induces spontaneous papillomas and malignant conversion in transgenic skin. *Carcinogenesis* **1998**, *19*, 1409–1415. [CrossRef] [PubMed]
37. Savouré, N.; Briand, G.; Amory-Touz, M.C.; Combre, A.; Maudet, M.; Nicol, M. Vitamin A status and metabolism of cutaneous polyamines in the hairless mouse after UV irradiation: Action of beta-carotene and astaxanthin. *Int. J. Vitam. Nutr. Res. Int. Z. Vitam. Ernahrungsforschung J. Int. Vitaminol. Nutr.* **1995**, *65*, 79–86.
38. Yoshihisa, Y.; Rehman, M.U.; Shimizu, T. Astaxanthin, a xanthophyll carotenoid, inhibits ultraviolet-induced apoptosis in keratinocytes. *Exp. Dermatol.* **2014**, *23*, 178–183. [CrossRef] [PubMed]
39. Wiraguna, A.A.G.P.; Pangkahila, W.; Astawa, I.N.M. Antioxidant properties of topical Caulerpa sp. extract on UVB-induced photoaging in mice. *Dermatol. Rep.* **2018**, *10*, 7597. [CrossRef]
40. Chen, L.; Hu, J.Y.; Wang, S.Q. The role of antioxidants in photoprotection: A critical review. *J. Am. Acad. Dermatol.* **2012**, *67*, 1013–1024. [CrossRef]
41. Poswig, A.; Wenk, J.; Brenneisen, P.; Wlaschek, M.; Hommel, C.; Quel, G.; Faisst, K.; Dissemond, J.; Krieg, T.; Scharffetter-Kochanek, K.; et al. Adaptive antioxidant response of manganese-superoxide dismutase following repetitive UVA irradiation. *J. Investig. Dermatol.* **1999**, *112*, 13–18. [CrossRef] [PubMed]
42. Meewes, C.; Brenneisen, P.; Wenk, J.; Kuhr, L.; Ma, W.; Alikoski, J.; Poswig, A.; Krieg, T.; Scharffetter-Kochanek, K. Adaptive antioxidant response protects dermal fibroblasts from UVA-induced phototoxicity. *Free Radic. Biol. Med.* **2001**, *30*, 238–247. [CrossRef]
43. Fimognari, C.; Lenzi, M.; Ferruzzi, L.; Turrini, E.; Scartezzini, P.; Poli, F.; Gotti, R.; Guerrini, A.; Carulli, G.; Ottaviano, V.; et al. Mitochondrial pathway mediates the antileukemic effects of hemidesmus indicus, a promising botanical drug. *PLoS ONE* **2011**, *6*, e21544. [CrossRef]

44. Rasoanaivo, P.; Wright, C.W.; Willcox, M.L.; Gilbert, B. Whole plant extracts versus single compounds for the treatment of malaria: Synergy and positive interactions. *Malar. J.* **2011**, *10* (Suppl. 1), S4. [CrossRef]
45. Baum, A.; Cohen, L. Successful behavioral interventions to prevent cancer: The example of skin cancer. *Annu. Rev. Public Health* **1998**, *19*, 319–333. [CrossRef]
46. Chintong, S.; Phatvej, W.; Rerk-Am, U.; Waiprib, Y.; Klaypradit, W. In vitro antioxidant, antityrosinase, and cytotoxic activities of Astaxanthin from Shrimp Waste. *Antioxid. Basel Switz.* **2019**, *8*, 128. [CrossRef] [PubMed]
47. Cuello-López, J.; Fidalgo-Zapata, A.; López-Agudelo, L.; Vásquez-Trespalacios, E. Platelet-to-lymphocyte ratio as a predictive factor of complete pathologic response to neoadjuvant chemotherapy in breast cancer. *PLoS ONE* **2018**, *13*, e0207224. [CrossRef] [PubMed]
48. Faria, S.S.; Fernandes, P.C.; Silva, M.J.B.; Lima, V.C.; Fontes, W.; Freitas-Junior, R.; Eterovic, A.K.; Forget, P. The neutrophil-to-lymphocyte ratio: A narrative review. *Ecancermedicalscience* **2016**, *10*, 702. [CrossRef] [PubMed]
49. Rangwala, S.; Tsai, K.Y. Roles of the immune system in skin cancer. *Br. J. Dermatol.* **2011**, *165*, 953–965. [CrossRef]
50. Hart, P.H.; Norval, M. Ultraviolet radiation-induced immunosuppression and its relevance for skin carcinogenesis. *Photochem. Photobiol. Sci.* **2018**, *17*, 1872–1884. [CrossRef]
51. Chew, B.P.; Mathison, B.D.; Hayek, M.G.; Massimino, S.; Reinhart, G.A.; Park, J.S. Dietary astaxanthin enhances immune response in dogs. *Vet. Immunol. Immunopathol.* **2011**, *140*, 199–206. [CrossRef]
52. Park, J.S.; Mathison, B.D.; Hayek, M.G.; Massimino, S.; Reinhart, G.A.; Chew, B.P. Astaxanthin stimulates cell-mediated and humoral immune responses in cats. *Vet. Immunol. Immunopathol.* **2011**, *144*, 455–461. [CrossRef]
53. Okai, Y.; Higashi-Okai, K. Possible immunomodulating activities of carotenoids in in vitro cell culture experiments. *Int. J. Immunopharmacol.* **1996**, *18*, 753–758. [CrossRef]
54. Park, J.S.; Chyun, J.H.; Kim, Y.K.; Line, L.L.; Chew, B.P. Astaxanthin decreased oxidative stress and inflammation and enhanced immune response in humans. *Nutr. Metab.* **2010**, *7*, 18. [CrossRef]
55. Kurihara, H.; Koda, H.; Asami, S.; Kiso, Y.; Tanaka, T. Contribution of the antioxidative property of astaxanthin to its protective effect on the promotion of cancer metastasis in mice treated with restraint stress. *Life Sci.* **2002**, *70*, 2509–2520. [CrossRef]
56. Jyonouchi, H.; Sun, S.; Iijima, K.; Gross, M.D. Antitumor activity of astaxanthin and its mode of action. *Nutr. Cancer* **2000**, *36*, 59–65. [CrossRef] [PubMed]
57. Krutovskikh, V.A.; Piccoli, C.; Yamasaki, H.; Yamasaki, H. Gap junction intercellular communication propagates cell death in cancerous cells. *Oncogene* **2002**, *21*, 1989–1999. [CrossRef]
58. Mesnil, M.; Crespin, S.; Avanzo, J.-L.; Zaidan-Dagli, M.-L. Defective gap junctional intercellular communication in the carcinogenic process. *Biochim. Biophys. Acta* **2005**, *1719*, 125–145. [CrossRef] [PubMed]
59. Stahl, W.; Sies, H. The role of carotenoids and retinoids in gap junctional communication. *Int. J. Vitam. Nutr. Res. Int. Z. Vitam. Ernahrungsforschung J. Int. Vitaminol. Nutr.* **1998**, *68*, 354–359.
60. Daubrawa, F.; Sies, H.; Stahl, W. Astaxanthin diminishes gap junctional intercellular communication in primary human fibroblasts. *J. Nutr.* **2005**, *135*, 2507–2511. [CrossRef]
61. Hix, L.M.; Frey, D.A.; McLaws, M.D.; Østerlie, M.; Lockwood, S.F.; Bertram, J.S. Inhibition of chemically-induced neoplastic transformation by a novel tetrasodium diphosphate astaxanthin derivative. *Carcinogenesis* **2005**, *26*, 1634–1641. [CrossRef]
62. Zhang, L.X.; Acevedo, P.; Guo, H.; Bertram, J.S. Upregulation of gap junctional communication and connexin43 gene expression by carotenoids in human dermal fibroblasts but not in human keratinocytes. *Mol. Carcinog.* **1995**, *12*, 50–58. [CrossRef]
63. Black, H.S. Radical interception by carotenoids and effects on UV carcinogenesis. *Nutr. Cancer* **1998**, *31*, 212–217. [CrossRef]
64. Spiller, G.A.; Dewell, A. Safety of an Astaxanthin-rich Haematococcus pluvialis algal extract: A randomized clinical trial. *J. Med. Food* **2003**, *6*, 51–56. [CrossRef]
65. Turck, D.; Castenmiller, J.; de Henauw, S.; Hirsch-Ernst, K.I.; Kearney, J.; Maciuk, A.; Mangelsdorf, I.; McArdle, H.J.; Naska, A.; Pelaez, C.; et al. Safety of Astaxanthin for its use as a novel food in food supplements. *EFSA J.* **2020**, *18*, e05993. [CrossRef]

66. Khalil, C.; Shebaby, W. UVB damage onset and progression 24 h post exposure in human-derived skin cells. *Toxicol. Rep.* **2017**, *4*, 441–449. [CrossRef]
67. Hu, F.; Liu, W.; Yan, L.; Kong, F.; Wei, K. Optimization and characterization of poly(lactic-co-glycolic acid) nanoparticles loaded with astaxanthin and evaluation of anti-photodamage effect in vitro. *R. Soc. Open Sci.* **2019**, *6*, 191184. [CrossRef] [PubMed]
68. Tait, S.W.G.; Green, D.R. Mitochondria and cell death: Outer membrane permeabilization and beyond. *Nat. Rev. Mol. Cell Biol.* **2010**, *11*, 621–632. [CrossRef] [PubMed]
69. Redza-Dutordoir, M.; Averill-Bates, D.A. Activation of apoptosis signalling pathways by reactive oxygen species. *Biochim. Biophys. Acta BBA Mol. Cell Res.* **2016**, *1863*, 2977–2992. [CrossRef]
70. Grandjean-Laquerriere, A.; Gangloff, S.C.; Le Naour, R.; Trentesaux, C.; Hornebeck, W.; Guenounou, M. Relative contribution of NF-kappaB and AP-1 in the modulation by curcumin and pyrrolidine dithiocarbamate of the UVB-induced cytokine expression by keratinocytes. *Cytokine* **2002**, *18*, 168–177. [CrossRef] [PubMed]
71. Honda, A.; Abe, R.; Yoshihisa, Y.; Makino, T.; Matsunaga, K.; Nishihira, J.; Shimizu, H.; Shimizu, T. Deficient deletion of apoptotic cells by macrophage migration inhibitory factor (MIF) overexpression accelerates photocarcinogenesis. *Carcinogenesis* **2009**, *30*, 1597–1605. [CrossRef] [PubMed]
72. Zhang, H.; Joseph, J.; Feix, J.; Hogg, N.; Kalyanaraman, B. Nitration and oxidation of a hydrophobic tyrosine probe by peroxynitrite in membranes: comparison with nitration and oxidation of tyrosine by peroxynitrite in aqueous solution. *Biochemistry* **2001**, *40*, 7675–7686. [CrossRef] [PubMed]
73. Tominaga, K.; Hongo, N.; Fujishita, M.; Takahashi, Y.; Adachi, Y. Protective effects of Astaxanthin on skin deterioration. *J. Clin. Biochem. Nutr.* **2017**, *61*, 33–39. [CrossRef] [PubMed]
74. Fisher, G.J.; Datta, S.C.; Talwar, H.S.; Wang, Z.Q.; Varani, J.; Kang, S.; Voorhees, J.J. Molecular basis of sun-induced premature skin ageing and retinoid antagonism. *Nature* **1996**, *379*, 335–339. [CrossRef]
75. Rabe, J.H.; Mamelak, A.J.; McElgunn, P.J.S.; Morison, W.L.; Sauder, D.N. Photoaging: Mechanisms and repair. *J. Am. Acad. Dermatol.* **2006**, *55*, 1–19. [CrossRef]
76. Imokawa, G.; Nakajima, H.; Ishida, K. Biological mechanisms underlying the ultraviolet radiation-induced formation of skin wrinkling and sagging II: Over-expression of neprilysin plays an essential role. *Int. J. Mol. Sci.* **2015**, *16*, 7776–7795. [CrossRef]
77. Pittayapruek, P.; Meephansan, J.; Prapapan, O.; Komine, M.; Ohtsuki, M. Role of matrix metalloproteinases in photoaging and photocarcinogenesis. *Int. J. Mol. Sci.* **2016**, *17*, 868. [CrossRef] [PubMed]
78. Gilchrest, B.A.; Yaar, M. Ageing and photoageing of the skin: Observations at the cellular and molecular level. *Br. J. Dermatol.* **1992**, *127* (Suppl. 41), 25–30. [CrossRef] [PubMed]
79. Gilchrest, B.A. A review of skin ageing and its medical therapy. *Br. J. Dermatol.* **1996**, *135*, 867–875. [CrossRef] [PubMed]
80. Nakajima, H.; Terazawa, S.; Niwano, T.; Yamamoto, Y.; Imokawa, G. The inhibitory effects of anti-oxidants on ultraviolet-induced up-regulation of the wrinkling-inducing enzyme neutral endopeptidase in human fibroblasts. *PLoS ONE* **2016**, *11*, e0161580. [CrossRef]
81. Redmond, R.W.; Kochevar, I.E. Spatially resolved cellular responses to singlet oxygen. *Photochem. Photobiol.* **2006**, *82*, 1178–1186. [CrossRef]
82. Hama, S.; Takahashi, K.; Inai, Y.; Shiota, K.; Sakamoto, R.; Yamada, A.; Tsuchiya, H.; Kanamura, K.; Yamashita, E.; Kogure, K. Protective effects of topical application of a poorly soluble antioxidant astaxanthin liposomal formulation on ultraviolet-induced skin damage. *J. Pharm. Sci.* **2012**, *101*, 2909–2916. [CrossRef]
83. Komatsu, T.; Sasaki, S.; Manabe, Y.; Hirata, T.; Sugawara, T. Preventive effect of dietary astaxanthin on UVA-induced skin photoaging in hairless mice. *PLoS ONE* **2017**, *12*, e0171178. [CrossRef]
84. Nauroy, P.; Nyström, A. Kallikreins: Essential epidermal messengers for regulation of the skin microenvironment during homeostasis, repair and disease. *Matrix Biol. Plus* **2020**, *6–7*, 100019. [CrossRef]
85. Elias, P.M.; Williams, M.L.; Choi, E.-H.; Feingold, K.R. Role of cholesterol sulfate in epidermal structure and function: Lessons from X-linked ichthyosis. *Biochim. Biophys. Acta* **2014**, *1841*, 353–361. [CrossRef]
86. Nakahigashi, K.; Kabashima, K.; Ikoma, A.; Verkman, A.S.; Miyachi, Y.; Hara-Chikuma, M. Upregulation of aquaporin-3 is involved in keratinocyte proliferation and epidermal hyperplasia. *J. Investig. Dermatol.* **2011**, *131*, 865–873. [CrossRef] [PubMed]
87. Li, X.; Matsumoto, T.; Takuwa, M.; Saeed Ebrahim Shaiku Ali, M.; Hirabashi, T.; Kondo, H.; Fujino, H. Protective effects of astaxanthin supplementation against ultraviolet-induced photoaging in hairless mice. *Biomedicines* **2020**, *8*, 18. [CrossRef] [PubMed]

88. Deng, M.; Xu, Y.; Yu, Z.; Wang, X.; Cai, Y.; Zheng, H.; Li, W.; Zhang, W. Protective effect of fat extract on UVB-induced photoaging in vitro and in vivo. *Oxid. Med. Cell. Longev.* **2019**, *2019*, e6146942. [CrossRef]
89. CFR—Code of Federal Regulations Title 21. Available online: https://www.accessdata.fda.gov/scripts/cdrh/cfdocs/cfCFR/CFRSearch.cfm?fr=201.327 (accessed on 12 July 2020).
90. Ito, N.; Seki, S.; Ueda, F. The protective role of Astaxanthin for UV-induced skin deterioration in healthy people-a randomized, double-blind, placebo-controlled trial. *Nutrients* **2018**, *10*, 817. [CrossRef]
91. Japan Meteorological Agency. Grafico della variazione annuale dell'indice UV massimo annuale (valore di analisi). Available online: https://www.data.jma.go.jp/gmd/env/uvhp/link_uvindex_month54.html (accessed on 9 May 2020).
92. Yamashita, E.Y. The effects of a dietary supplement containing Astaxanthin on skin condition. *Carot. Sci.* **2006**, *10*, 6.
93. Tominaga, K.; Hongo, N.; Karato, M.; Yamashita, E. Cosmetic benefits of astaxanthin on humans subjects. *Acta Biochim. Pol.* **2012**, *59*, 43–47. [CrossRef]
94. Chalyk, N.E.; Klochkov, V.A.; Bandaletova, T.Y.; Kyle, N.H.; Petyaev, I.M. Continuous Astaxanthin intake reduces oxidative stress and reverses age-related morphological changes of residual skin surface components in middle-aged volunteers. *Nutr. Res.* **2017**, *48*, 40–48. [CrossRef]
95. Yoon, H.-S.; Cho, H.H.; Cho, S.; Lee, S.-R.; Shin, M.-H.; Chung, J.H. Supplementating with dietary astaxanthin combined with collagen hydrolysate improves facial elasticity and decreases matrix metalloproteinase-1 and -12 expression: A comparative study with placebo. *J. Med. Food* **2014**, *17*, 810–816. [CrossRef] [PubMed]
96. Ng, Q.X.; De Deyn, M.L.Z.Q.; Loke, W.; Foo, N.X.; Chan, H.W.; Yeo, W.S. Effects of Astaxanthin supplementation on skin health: A systematic review of clinical studies. *J. Diet. Suppl.* **2020**, 1–14. [CrossRef]
97. Dembitsky, V.M.; Maoka, T. Allenic and cumulenic lipids. *Prog. Lipid Res.* **2007**, *46*, 328–375. [CrossRef]
98. D'Orazio, N.; Gemello, E.; Gammone, M.A.; de Girolamo, M.; Ficoneri, C.; Riccioni, G. Fucoxantin: A treasure from the sea. *Mar. Drugs* **2012**, *10*, 604–616. [CrossRef] [PubMed]
99. Zhang, H.; Tang, Y.; Zhang, Y.; Zhang, S.; Qu, J.; Wang, X.; Kong, R.; Han, C.; Liu, Z. Fucoxanthin: A promising medicinal and nutritional ingredient. *Evid. Based Complement. Altern. Med. ECAM* **2015**, *2015*, 723515. [CrossRef] [PubMed]
100. Sachindra, N.M.; Sato, E.; Maeda, H.; Hosokawa, M.; Niwano, Y.; Kohno, M.; Miyashita, K. Radical scavenging and singlet oxygen quenching activity of marine carotenoid fucoxanthin and its metabolites. *J. Agric. Food Chem.* **2007**, *55*, 8516–8522. [CrossRef] [PubMed]
101. Rodríguez-Luna, A.; Ávila-Román, J.; González-Rodríguez, M.L.; Cózar, M.J.; Rabasco, A.M.; Motilva, V.; Talero, E. Fucoxanthin-containing cream prevents epidermal hyperplasia and UVB-induced skin erythema in mice. *Mar. Drugs* **2018**, *16*, 378. [CrossRef] [PubMed]
102. Hatakeyama, M.; Fukunaga, A.; Washio, K.; Taguchi, K.; Oda, Y.; Ogura, K.; Nishigori, C. Anti-Inflammatory role of langerhans cells and apoptotic keratinocytes in ultraviolet-B-Induced cutaneous inflammation. *J. Immunol. Baltim. Md 1950* **2017**, *199*, 2937–2947. [CrossRef]
103. Rodríguez-Luna, A.; Ávila-Román, J.; Oliveira, H.; Motilva, V.; Talero, E. Fucoxanthin and Rosmarinic acid combination has anti-Inflammatory effects through regulation of NLRP3 inflammasome in UVB-exposed HaCaT keratinocytes. *Mar. Drugs* **2019**, *17*, 451. [CrossRef] [PubMed]
104. Ghiringhelli, F.; Apetoh, L.; Tesniere, A.; Aymeric, L.; Ma, Y.; Ortiz, C.; Vermaelen, K.; Panaretakis, T.; Mignot, G.; Ullrich, E.; et al. Activation of the NLRP3 inflammasome in dendritic cells induces IL-1β–dependent adaptive immunity against tumors. *Nat. Med.* **2009**. [CrossRef]
105. Leerach, N.; Yakaew, S.; Phimnuan, P.; Soimee, W.; Nakyai, W.; Luangbudnark, W.; Viyoch, J. Effect of Thai banana (Musa AA group) in reducing accumulation of oxidation end products in UVB-irradiated mouse skin. *J. Photochem. Photobiol. B* **2017**, *168*, 50–58. [CrossRef]
106. Tavares, R.S.N.; Kawakami, C.M.; de Pereira, K.C.; do Amaral, G.T.; Benevenuto, C.G.; Maria-Engler, S.S.; Colepicolo, P.; Debonsi, H.M.; Gaspar, L.R. Fucoxanthin for topical administration, a phototoxic vs. photoprotective potential in a tiered strategy assessed by In vitro methods. *Antioxidants* **2020**, *9*, 328. [CrossRef]
107. El-Abaseri, T.B.; Putta, S.; Hansen, L.A. Ultraviolet irradiation induces keratinocyte proliferation and epidermal hyperplasia through the activation of the epidermal growth factor receptor. *Carcinogenesis* **2006**, *27*, 225–231. [CrossRef]

108. Heo, S.-J.; Jeon, Y.-J. Protective effect of Fucoxanthin isolated from Sargassum siliquastrum on UV-B induced cell damage. *J. Photochem. Photobiol. B* **2009**, *95*, 101–107. [CrossRef] [PubMed]
109. Hashimoto, T.; Ozaki, Y.; Taminato, M.; Das, S.K.; Mizuno, M.; Yoshimura, K.; Maoka, T.; Kanazawa, K. The distribution and accumulation of fucoxanthin and its metabolites after oral administration in mice. *Br. J. Nutr.* **2009**, *102*, 242–248. [CrossRef] [PubMed]
110. Bastiaens, M.; Hoefnagel, J.; Westendorp, R.; Vermeer, B.-J.; Bouwes Bavinck, J.N. Solar lentigines are strongly related to sun exposure in contrast to ephelides. *Pigment. Cell Res.* **2004**, *17*, 225–229. [CrossRef]
111. Bastonini, E.; Kovacs, D.; Picardo, M. Skin pigmentation and pigmentary disorders: Focus on epidermal/dermal cross-talk. *Ann. Dermatol.* **2016**, *28*, 279–289. [CrossRef]
112. Matsui, M.; Tanaka, K.; Higashiguchi, N.; Okawa, H.; Yamada, Y.; Tanaka, K.; Taira, S.; Aoyama, T.; Takanishi, M.; Natsume, C.; et al. Protective and therapeutic effects of fucoxanthin against sunburn caused by UV irradiation. *J. Pharmacol. Sci.* **2016**, *132*, 55–64. [CrossRef]
113. Sandilands, A.; Sutherland, C.; Irvine, A.D.; McLean, W.H.I. Filaggrin in the frontline: Role in skin barrier function and disease. *J. Cell Sci.* **2009**, *122*, 1285–1294. [CrossRef] [PubMed]
114. Urikura, I.; Sugawara, T.; Hirata, T. Protective effect of Fucoxanthin against UVB-induced skin photoaging in hairless mice. *Biosci. Biotechnol. Biochem.* **2011**, *75*, 757–760. [CrossRef] [PubMed]
115. Yano, K.; Kajiya, K.; Ishiwata, M.; Hong, Y.-K.; Miyakawa, T.; Detmar, M. Ultraviolet B-induced skin angiogenesis is associated with a switch in the balance of vascular endothelial growth factor and thrombospondin-1 expression. *J. Investig. Dermatol.* **2004**, *122*, 201–208. [CrossRef]
116. Kim, M.-S.; Kim, Y.K.; Eun, H.C.; Cho, K.H.; Chung, J.H. All-trans retinoic acid antagonizes UV-induced VEGF production and angiogenesis via the inhibition of ERK activation in human skin keratinocytes. *J. Investig. Dermatol.* **2006**, *126*, 2697–2706. [CrossRef]
117. Yano, K.; Oura, H.; Detmar, M. Targeted overexpression of the angiogenesis inhibitor thrombospondin-1 in the epidermis of transgenic mice prevents ultraviolet-B-induced angiogenesis and cutaneous photo-damage. *J. Investig. Dermatol.* **2002**, *118*, 800–805. [CrossRef]
118. Lorigo, M.; Cairrao, E. Antioxidants as stabilizers of UV filters: An example for the UV-B filter octylmethoxycinnamate. *Biomed. Dermatol.* **2019**, *3*, 11. [CrossRef]
119. Balić, A.; Mokos, M. Do we utilize our knowledge of the skin protective effects of carotenoids enough? *Antioxid. Basel Switz.* **2019**, *8*, 259. [CrossRef]
120. Tuong, W.; Armstrong, A.W. Effect of appearance-based education compared with health-based education on sunscreen use and knowledge: A randomized controlled trial. *J. Am. Acad. Dermatol.* **2014**, *70*, 665–669. [CrossRef] [PubMed]
121. Mahler, H.I.M.; Kulik, J.A.; Harrell, J.; Correa, A.; Gibbons, F.X.; Gerrard, M. Effects of UV photographs, photoaging information, and use of sunless tanning lotion on sun protection behaviors. *Arch. Dermatol.* **2005**, *141*, 373–380. [CrossRef] [PubMed]
122. European Food Safety Authority (EFSA). Scientific Opinion on the substantiation of health claims related to astaxanthin and maintenance of joints, tendons, and connective tissue (ID 1918, 1978, 3142), protection of DNA, proteins and lipids from oxidative damage (ID 1449, 3141), maintenance of visual acuity (ID 1448), maintenance of blood cholesterol concentrations and maintenance of low plasma concentrations of C-reactive protein (ID 1450) pursuant to Article 13(1) of Regulation (EC) No 1924/2006. *EFSA J.* **2009**, *7*, 1–17. [CrossRef]
123. Chew, B.P.; Park, J.S. Natural Astaxanthin Extract Reduces DNA Oxidation. Available online: https://patents.google.com/patent/WO2005011712A1/en2005 (accessed on 22 October 2020).
124. Mercke Odeberg, J.; Lignell, A.; Pettersson, A.; Höglund, P. Oral bioavailability of the antioxidant astaxanthin in humans is enhanced by incorporation of lipid based formulations. *Eur. J. Pharm. Sci.* **2003**, *19*, 299–304. [CrossRef]
125. Ambati, R.R.; Siew Moi, P.; Ravi, S.; Aswathanarayana, R.G. Astaxanthin: Sources, extraction, stability, biological activities and its commercial applications—A review. *Mar. Drugs* **2014**, *12*, 128–152. [CrossRef] [PubMed]
126. Choi, H.D.; Kang, H.E.; Yang, S.H.; Lee, M.G.; Shin, W.G. Pharmacokinetics and first-pass metabolism of astaxanthin in rats. *Br. J. Nutr.* **2011**, *105*, 220–227. [CrossRef] [PubMed]
127. Hashimoto, T.; Ozaki, Y.; Mizuno, M.; Yoshida, M.; Nishitani, Y.; Azuma, T.; Komoto, A.; Maoka, T.; Tanino, Y.; Kanazawa, K. Pharmacokinetics of fucoxanthinol in human plasma after the oral administration of kombu extract. *Br. J. Nutr.* **2012**, *107*, 1566–1569. [CrossRef] [PubMed]

128. Iio, K.; Okada, Y.; Ishikura, M. Single and 13-week oral toxicity study of fucoxanthin oil from microalgae in rats. *Shokuhin Eiseigaku zasshi J. Food Hyg. Soc. Jpn.* **2011**, *52*, 183–189. [CrossRef]
129. Spagolla Napoleão Tavares, R.; Maria-Engler, S.S.; Colepicolo, P.; Debonsi, H.M.; Schäfer-Korting, M.; Marx, U.; Gaspar, L.R.; Zoschke, C. Skin irritation testing beyond tissue viability: Fucoxanthin effects on inflammation, homeostasis, and metabolism. *Pharmaceutics* **2020**, *12*, 136. [CrossRef] [PubMed]
130. FDA. Overview of Safety and Regulatory Issues Related to So-Called Tanning Pills. Available online: https://www.fda.gov/cosmetics/cosmetic-products/tanning-pills (accessed on 10 June 2020).

Publisher's Note: MDPI stays neutral with regard to jurisdictional claims in published maps and institutional affiliations.

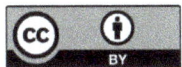

© 2020 by the authors. Licensee MDPI, Basel, Switzerland. This article is an open access article distributed under the terms and conditions of the Creative Commons Attribution (CC BY) license (http://creativecommons.org/licenses/by/4.0/).

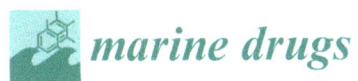

Review

Oxidative Stress and Marine Carotenoids: Application by Using Nanoformulations

Yasin Genç [1], Hilal Bardakci [2], Çiğdem Yücel [3], Gökçe Şeker Karatoprak [4], Esra Küpeli Akkol [5,*], Timur Hakan Barak [2] and Eduardo Sobarzo-Sánchez [6,7,*]

1. Department of Pharmacognosy, Faculty of Pharmacy, Hacettepe University, Sıhhiye, 06100 Ankara, Turkey; ygncyasin@gmail.com
2. Department of Pharmacognosy, Faculty of Pharmacy, Acibadem Mehmet Ali Aydınlar University, 34752 Istanbul, Turkey; hilal.bardakci@acibadem.edu.tr (H.B.); Timur.Barak@acibadem.edu.tr (T.H.B.)
3. Department of Pharmaceutical Technology, Faculty of Pharmacy, Erciyes University, 38039 Kayseri, Turkey; cyucel@erciyes.edu.tr
4. Department of Pharmacognosy, Faculty of Pharmacy, Erciyes University, 38039 Kayseri, Turkey; gskaratoprak@erciyes.edu.tr
5. Department of Pharmacognosy, Faculty of Pharmacy, Gazi University, Etiler, 06330 Ankara, Turkey
6. Instituto de Investigación e Innovación en Salud, Facultad de Ciencias de la Salud, Universidad Central de Chile, Santiago 8330507, Chile
7. Department of Organic Chemistry, Faculty of Pharmacy, University of Santiago de Compostela, 15782 Santiago de Compostela, Spain
* Correspondence: esrak@gazi.edu.tr (E.K.A.); eduardo.sobarzo@ucentral.cl (E.S.-S.); Tel.: +90-312-2023185 (E.K.A.); +90-569-53972783 (E.S.-S.); Fax: +90-312-2235018 (E.K.A.)

Received: 27 June 2020; Accepted: 11 August 2020; Published: 13 August 2020

Abstract: Carotenoids are natural fat-soluble pigments synthesized by plants, algae, fungi and microorganisms. They are responsible for the coloration of different photosynthetic organisms. Although they play a role in photosynthesis, they are also present in non-photosynthetic plant tissues, fungi, and bacteria. These metabolites have mainly been used in food, cosmetics, and the pharmaceutical industry. In addition to their utilization as pigmentation, they have significant therapeutically applications, such as improving immune system and preventing neurodegenerative diseases. Primarily, they have attracted attention due to their antioxidant activity. Several statistical investigations indicated an association between the use of carotenoids in diets and a decreased incidence of cancer types, suggesting the antioxidant properties of these compounds as an important factor in the scope of the studies against oxidative stress. Unusual marine environments are associated with a great chemical diversity, resulting in novel bioactive molecules. Thus, marine organisms may represent an important source of novel biologically active substances for the development of therapeutics. Marine carotenoids (astaxanthin, fucoxanthin, β-carotene, lutein but also the rare siphonaxanthin, sioxanthin, and myxol) have recently shown antioxidant properties in reducing oxidative stress markers. Numerous of bioactive compounds such as marine carotenoids have low stability, are poorly absorbed, and own very limited bioavailability. The new technique is nanoencapsulation, which can be used to preserve marine carotenoids and their original properties during processing, storage, improve their physiochemical properties and increase their health-promoting effects. This review aims to describe the role of marine carotenoids, their potential applications and different types of advanced nanoformulations preventing and treating oxidative stress related disorders.

Keywords: bioavailability; carotenoids; marine; nanoformulation; oxidative stress; reactive oxygen species

1. Introduction

The World Health Organization revealed that approximately 80% of the world's population count on medicinal plants, in order to maintain their health or for treatment purposes. Medicines and nature have been strictly linked through the utilization of traditional medicines as therapeutic agents for thousands of years. Plenty of studies were performed on traditional medicines, which were primarily plants, constituting the basis of most early medicines (such as aspirin, digitoxin, morphine, quinine, etc.) and providing a pivotal role in today's drug discovery [1]. Even today, natural metabolites play a crucial role as one of the major sources of novel medicines due to their incomparable structural diversity, relatively small dimensions (<2000 Da), and their drug-like properties (absorption and metabolism) as well [2].

Marine flora and fauna, such as algae, bacteria, sponges, fungi, seaweeds, corals, diatoms, etc. serve as a generous source of bioactive metabolites with a great difference and complexity. The variance of marine environments, sea, and oceans offer a limitless biodiversity in compounds obtained from marine species. In order to survive in extreme habitats, they have developed particular secondary metabolic pathways to produce molecules to accommodate their lifestyles. For example, despite the unusual environmental conditions (light and oxygen exposure) that might lead oxidative damage, marine organisms do not undergo any serious photodynamic damage. Hence, it is known that marine organisms are able to synthesize molecules with bioactivity, especially antioxidant molecules, to protect themselves from external factors, such as ultraviolet (UV) radiation, stress, and herbivores [3,4]. Marine organisms attracted the interest of scientists due to the substantial bioactivities of their extracts and isolates. In this purpose, a number of metabolites of a wide variety of chemical classes, including terpenes, shikimates, polyketides, acetogenins, peptides, alkaloids, and many unidentified and uncharacterized structures, were purified from marine bio resources and exhibited several utilizations as nutraceuticals and pharmaceuticals [2]. Those compounds have various pharmacological activities, such as antioxidant, antibacterial, antitumor, antiviral, anti-inflammatory, antidiabetic, antihypertensive, anticoagulant [4]. Amongst them carotenoids have become the topic of great interest for pharmaceutical industry; thus, they have significant antioxidant activities and anticancer activities [5–8].

Carotenoids are naturally occurring lipophilic pigments responsible for the red, orange and yellow color of some species of archaea and fungi, algae, plants, and photosynthetic bacteria as well. They are in the structure of tetraterpene and capable of absorbing light primarily between 400 nm and 500 nm. They are encountered in macroalgae, bacteria, and unicellular phytoplanktons and perform diverse and notable functions such as protecting chlorophyll via absorbing light energy and transferring it to chlorophyll and scavenging free radicals of oxygen [9]. Animals are not capable of synthesizing carotenoids de novo since they need to ingest carotenoids via supplementation or in food. Aquatic animals ingest carotenoids from foods, such as algae and other animals, and convert their structure via metabolic reactions leading structural diversity. To date, more than 850 carotenoids were detected in nature, including up to 100 that are present in the food chain and human nutrition, and more than 250 are of marine origin [10–12]. The importance of carotenoids is due to their functional properties, not only as natural antioxidants and color enhancing agents in the food industry, but also as pharmaceuticals and as chemotaxonomic markers [8]. Carotenoids play significant role in eye, bone, and cardiovascular health; they are used in cancer prevention, to boost immune function and cognitive performance, as infant nutrition, and antioxidant, antitumour, antiaging, and anti-inflammatory agents. Carotenoids exert their activities via different mechanisms. For example, α-carotene and β-carotene are converted to vitamin A in the human body, and show its activity, lutein, and zeaxanthin protect human eye by absorbing blue and near UV light [8,9,11]. However, technically, the reason behind the other activities of carotenoids is thought to be due to their significant antioxidant activity.

Oxidative stress leads the formation of reactive oxygen species (ROS) against the endogenous and exogenous stimuli. Under physiological conditions, ROS are repeatedly generated and eliminated through ROS scavenging systems in order to maintain redox homeostasis. Change in redox balance leads altered ROS production, resulting in cell damage, aberrant cell signaling; thus, disruption of cell homeostasis [13]. ROS are extremely hazardous for living organisms, causing detrimental diseases, such as cardiovascular diseases, cancer, and diabetes. ROS involve in carcinogenesis through inducing persistent DNA injuries and mutations in p53, the tumor suppressor gene, genomic instability, and aberrant pro-tumorigenic signaling; thus, they might be considered as oncogenic. Thus, prevention of ROS production and balancing antioxidant system is thought to inhibit cancer development. On the contrary, many chemotherapeutic agents in cancer therapy, as well as ionizing radiation, function by promoting ROS production and promoting apoptosis and necrosis of the cells. For instance, some molecules, such as paclitaxel, are able to attack cancer cells via inducing ROS generation or interfering ROS metabolism [14]. Since high levels of ROS are also toxic to cancer cells and potentially induce cell death [13,14]. There are plenty of clinical researches revealing the anticancer and activity of antioxidants; hence, counterbalancing the ROS mediated injury is extremely important in the prevention of plenty of diseases, including cancer [15].

Antioxidants often refer to compounds that are able to donate an electron and neutralize free radicals resulting in scavenging and preventing cell injuries. Carotenoids are not only essential antioxidants, they are also crucial anticancer agents. They exert their anticancer activity via promoting gap junctional communication. Carotenoids initiate cell proliferation and differentiation by binding and regulating the receptors (retinoid acid receptor (RAR) and retinoid X receptor (RXR)). Although they have significant pharmacological activities, there are several limitations of carotenoids, such as low solubility in water, easy degradation, low shelf life, and unfavorable pH in digestive tract leading to alleviated bioavailability. To overcome these undesirable properties, various encapsulation methods are preferred for carotenoids [9]. In this paper, chemical structures, sources, bioavailability, and activities of carotenoids from marine organisms are overviewed.

2. Chemical Structures of Carotenoids

Most carotenoids are tetraterpenoid compounds consisted of a sequence of eight isoprene units. Biosynthesis of carotenoids include condensation reactions begin with the basic C5 unit dimethyl allyl diphosphate (DMADP) and isopentenyl diphosphate (IDP) units. Prenyl transferases lead the formation of several intermediates that are the origin of the biosynthesis branches for the formation of mono-, di-, and triterpenes. Subsequent tail to tail condensation of two geranylgeranyl diphosphate units to the head to tail condensation of DMADP and IDP to geranyl diphosphate evoke the synthesis of phytoene [16]. Nevertheless, the core structure is a polyene backbone with a series of conjugated C=C double bonds and an end group at both ends of this chain [12]. Typical structures of carotenoids are shown in Figure 1.

Currently, carotenoids are classified according to the presence of oxygen; carotenes without oxygen (pure hydrocarbon), and xanthophylls with oxygen in their chemical structure. Parent carotenoid lycopene is produced after stepwise desaturation of phytoene. Lycopene cyclases might interfere the formation of rings at both ends and produce carotenes such as α-carotene, β-carotene, β,ψ-carotene (γ-carotene) (Figure 2). There are about 50 types of carotenes detected in nature [12].

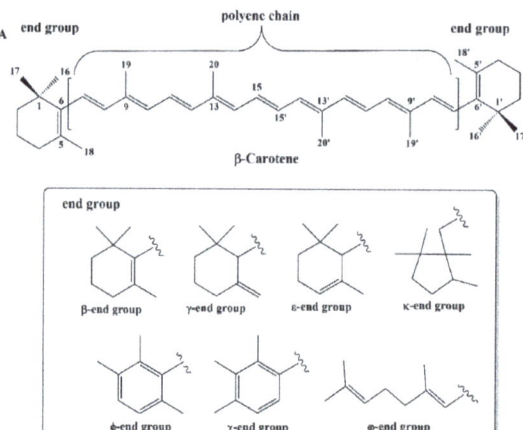

Figure 1. Typical structures of carotenoids.

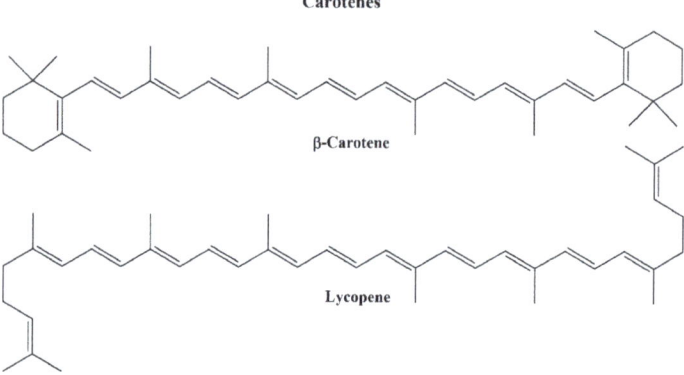

Figure 2. Structures of β-carotene and lycopene.

Xanthophylls are often characterized by the occurrence of carbonyl, carboxyl, hydroxyl, and epoxide groups in which pairs of hydrogen atoms are replaced with oxygen atoms. More than 800 kinds of xanthophylls have been reported in nature till today. β-cryptoxanthin, lutein, zeaxanthin, astaxanthin, fucoxanthin, and peridinin (Figure 3) are the examples of common xanthophylls. Although there are acyclic (e.g., lycopene) carotenoids are present, more common are with six membered (or rarely five-membered) ring at one end or both ends (bicyclic) of the molecule. [12,16,17]. Cis/trans isomerization is seen regarding to the stereochemistry of carotenoids. Biosynthetic pathways principally lead the *trans* configured carotenoids to be dominant in nature, although there are few examples of natural *cis* derivatives [16].

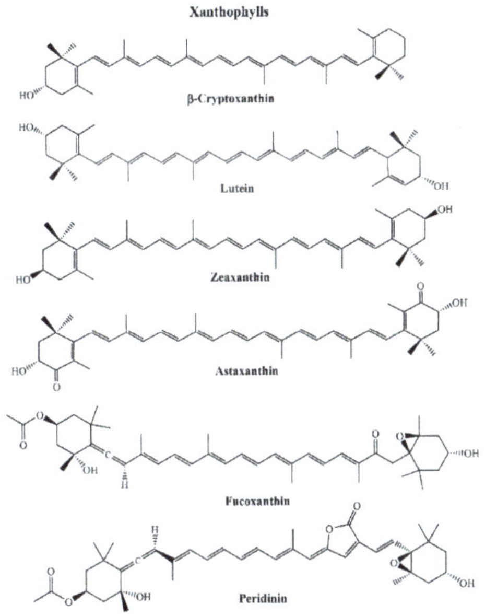

Figure 3. Structures of the examples of common xanthophylls.

Marine sponges are generally in brilliant colors due to the occurrence of carotenoids. They are often associated with symbionts such as bacteria or microalgae. Isorenieratene, renieratene, and renierapurpurin (Figure 4) are the frequently encountered aryl carotenoids in marine sponges.

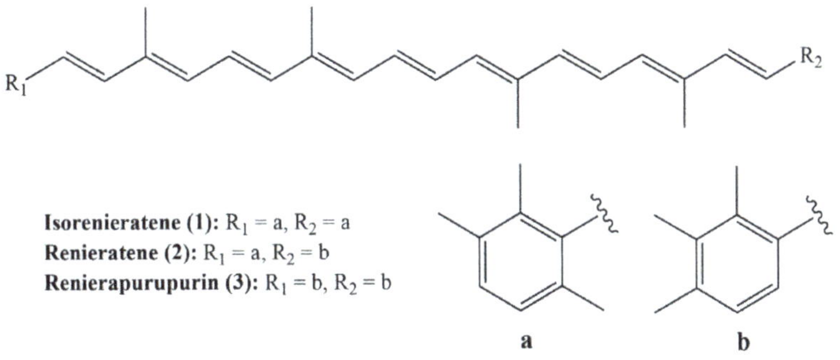

Isorenieratene (1): R_1 = a, R_2 = a
Renieratene (2): R_1 = a, R_2 = b
Renierapurupurin (3): R_1 = b, R_2 = b

Figure 4. Structures of isorenieratene, renieratene, and renierapurpurin.

To date, more than twenty aryl carotenoids have been detected in sponges. Since those compounds also reported in green sulfur bacteria, it was assumed that carotenoids in sponges originated from symbiosis with bacteria [10]. 2-nor-astaxanthin and actinioerythrin are the examples of characteristic carotenoids in sea anemones [10]. Lutein, zeaxanthin, fucoxanthin, and their metabolites are the mainly occurring carotenoids in chitons. β-carotene, α-carotene, zeaxanthin, lutein, and fucoxanthin are primarily encountered on the shells of abalone, and turban shell. Astaxanthin is the principle carotenoid synthesized from β-carotene by many crustaceans' algae. They ingest β-carotene from dietary algae astaxanthin—it is also widely encountered in both marine and fresh water fish [10].

3. Sources of Carotenoids from Marine Organisms

Carotenoids are very common in nature and can be found in highly diverse habitats. Terrestrial vegetables and fruits are important sources of carotenoids. Nonetheless, numerous marine organisms are likewise valuable sources for them. Both prokaryotic and eukaryotic divisions in marine environment may contain sufficient amount of various carotenoids. Prokaryotes are considered as primitive living organism in phylogenetic classification. However, there are several carotenoid containing members of this division. For example, Agrobacterium and Paracoccus genera in bacteria kingdom are favorable sources of astaxanthin [18]. In another study, two rare carotenoids with promising biological activities, saproxanthin and myxol were isolated from marine bacteria belonging to Flavobacteriaceae family. Members from Archaea division may also be valuable sources of carotenoids. Several studies demonstrated that, halophilic archaea from Haloferacaceae family can produce β-carotene, phytoene, lycopene, bacterioruberin, and salinixanthin [19]. *Cyanobacteria phylum*, photosynthetic microorganisms of prokaryotic division are widespread in various marine environments are also important carotenoid producers. Zeaxanthin, synechoxanthin, canthaxanthin, echinenone, nostoxanthin, caloxanthin, and myxoxanthophyll are some examples of carotenoids which were found in *Cyanobacteria phylum* [20].

Carotenoids are present in every kingdom of eukaryotes division: Protista, Fungi, Plantae and Animalia. Thraustochytrids family in Protista kingdom has carotenoid producers. Several strains from genera Thraustochytrium, Ulkenia, and Aurantiochytrium synthetize various carotenoids such as β-carotene, astaxanthin, zeaxanthin, canthaxanthin, phoenicoxanthin, and echinenone [21]. Furthermore, various yeast species were found from marine habitats that produce carotenoids especially Astaxanthin. Xanthophyllomyces, Rhodotorula, and Phaffi genera can be used for Astaxanthin production; however, amounts are lower when compared to algae [22].

Microalgae and macroalgae are considered main source of marine carotenoids. Their carotenoids accumulation can be due to their essential metabolism for survival (primary carotenoids) or precise ecological pressure (secondary carotenoids) [23]. The Chlorophyceae family contains most important genera for carotenoid production. *Dunaliella salina* from Chlorophyceae family is considered as a source of β-carotene production when it encounters with extreme conditions, such as high light density, nutrition deficiency, and salinity. It can also produce α-carotene, lutein, and zeaxanthin but is generally used for large scale β-carotene production [24]. Genus *Chlorella* and *Scenedesmus* genera are prominent sources of lutein therefore they are used in large scale of lutein production [25]. *Tetraselmis suecica* is marine green algae, which is generally used for aquaculture nutrition and rich for tocopherol [26]. *Haematococcus pluvialis* is widely used for astaxanthin production for a long period of time [27]. Chlamydomonas and Muriellopsis are some other examples of carotenoid producing microalgae and also lycopene, fucoxanthin, canthaxanthin, echinenone, and dinoxanthin are some examples of carotenoids from the Chlorophyceae family [28]. Macroalgae (seaweeds) are also noticeable sources of carotenoids, such as fucoxanthin, lutein, β-carotene and siphonaxanthin [29]. Especially brown algae species are important sources of fucoxanthin. *Hijikia fusiformis, Sargassum sp., Undaria pinnatifida, Fucus sp., Laminaria sp., Alaria crassifolia, Ishige okamurae, Cystoseira hakodatensis, Eisenia bicyclis, Myagropsis myagroides, Cladosiphon okamuranus, Petalonia binghamiae, Hijikia fusiformis, Kjellmaniella crassifolia,* and *Padina tetrastromatica* are important examples for their fucoxanthin content [30]. Seagrasses are also important carotenoid sources. Previous articles demonstrated that *Posidonia oceanica, Cymodocea nodosa, Zostera noltii, Halophila stipulacea, Cymodocea nodosa,* and *Zostera marina* are producers of several carotenoids such as β-carotene, lutein, lutein epoxide, zeaxanthin, violaxanthin, neoxanthin, siphonaxanthintype, and violaxanthin [31,32].

Even though marine animals do not synthetize carotenoids de novo, they can accumulate carotenoids via direct food intake or small metabolic transformations. Carotenoids are generally found in invertebrate marine animals in phylums Pomifera, Cnidaria, Mollusca, Crustacea, Echinodermata, and Tunicata. Sponges (Pomifera) contain more than 40 carotenoids, generally aryl carotenoids such as renierapurpurin, renieratene and isorenieratene which are assumed that occurs after biotransformation of fucoxanthin [33]. Phylum Cnidaria has small number of members contains carotenoids. *Actinia equine*, *Tealia feline*, and *Anemonia sulcata* are some examples that accumulate rare carotenoids such as 2-nor-astaxnthin, peridinin and actinioerythrin [34]. Mollusks contain numerous types of carotenoids. It has been shown that shellfishes contain β-carotene, lutein A, zeaxanthin, diatoxanthin, astaxanthin, etc. [34]. Bivalves and chitons also contain several carotenoids including fucoxanthin, zeaxanthin, lutein, diaxanthin, and peridinin [35]. In Crustacea phylum, crabs, shrimps, and lobsters generally accumulate astaxanthin, which is biotransformed from β-carotene after consumption of algae [35]. Sea urchins, holothurians, and starfishes from Echinodermata contain several carotenoids such as β-carotene, echinenone, canthaxanthin, astaxanthin and fucoxanthin [30]. Tunicates also biotransform carotenoid obtained from phytoplankton consumption, such as alloxanthin, fucoxanthin, mytiloxanthin, mytiloxanthinone, and halocynthiaxanthin [36]. Moreover, salmon fish accumulates astaxanthin in their muscles, which makes them valuable dietary carotenoid source [35].

4. Oxidative Stress and Cancer

Reactive oxygen species formed intracellular (mitochondria, the endoplasmic reticulum (ER), peroxisomes, microsomes, phagocytic cells, NAPDH oxidase (NOX) complexes, etc.), or extracellular sources. Specifically, mitochondria, produce significant amounts of reactive oxygen species (ROS), which can contribute to intracellular oxidative stress [37]. Another important source is NADPH oxidases found in various cells, especially phagocytes and endothelial cells, which are central to the formation of the inflammatory response [38]. Extracellular sources of ROS generation include ROS-inducing agents, are generally UV radiation, chemical compounds like drugs and toxins, pollutants, cigarette and alcohol [39]. The examples for the radicals include Superoxide ($O_2^{·-}$), Oxygen radical ($O_2^{··}$), Hydroxyl (OH$^·$), Alkoxy radical (RO$^·$), Peroxyl radical (ROO$^·$). The high reactivity of these radicals is due to the presence of an unpaired electron that tends to donate it or tends to obtain another electron to achieve stability. The non-radical species include hydrogen peroxide (H_2O_2), hypochlorous acid (HOCl), hypobromous acid (HOBr), ozone (O_3), singlet oxygen ($^1O_2$). Molecular oxygen (O_2) has two unpaired electrons with a parallel spin state and tends to form highly ROS. While molecular oxygen reacts slowly with non-radical substances, it reacts easily with other free radicals [40].

Molecular oxygen (O_2) has two unpaired electrons with a parallel spin state and tends to form highly ROS. While molecular oxygen reacts slowly with non-radical substances, it reacts easily with other free radicals. Reactive nitrogen types, like reactive oxygen species, occur in the biological environment when free radicals form more stable species with many effects [41].

These radicals damage DNA and proteins, causing cancer and oxidizing LDL, leading to cardiovascular diseases. Free radicals are not completely harmful in fact; our body also needs free radicals in the production and activation of some vital hormones [42]. Free radicals also come into play in the body in case of infection and removal of foreign substances, but they can also cause damage to the structure of healthy cells, such as DNA protein, and lipids and cause many diseases [43]. Bio membranes and intracellular organelles are sensitive to oxidative attacks due to the presence of unsaturated fatty acids in membrane phospholipids. When lipid peroxides formed by oxidation of lipids are destroyed, aldehydes, most of which are biologically active, are formed. These compounds are either metabolized at the cell level or diffuse from their original domains and spread damage to other parts of the cell. Malondialdehyde (MDA) occurs in the peroxidation of fatty acids containing three or more double bonds. MDA and 4-hydroxy-2-nonenal (4-HNE) formed as a result of lipid peroxidation are known to react with nucleotides and cause mutagenesis and carcinogenesis [44,45]. Amino acids that make up proteins tend to oxidize to a higher degree than lipids in general because they contain carboxyl and amino groups. These molecules contain reduced carbon atoms that will undergo oxidative transformation in their side chains. In many studies, diseases such as Parkinson's, diabetes, Alzheimer's, renal tumor formation and rheumatoid arthritis have been associated with increased protein carbonyl groups [46].

The main target of oxidative damage in the DNA chain is purine, pyrimidine bases and sugar structure [47]. Moreover, 8-hydroxy-2-deoxyguanosine is generated via reactive species and this product can produce mutations in DNA, which has carcinogenesis effect [48]. Disequilibrium between the production and elimination of ROS is defined as oxidative stress and numerous studies have shown the important roles of oxidative stress in propagation of cancer [49]. ROS can trigger many aspects of tumor development and progression, which can be divided into the cellular proliferation, evasion of apoptosis, tissue invasion and metastasis and angiogenesis. ROS can trigger number of signaling pathways like extracellular-regulated kinase 1/2 (ERK1/2), receptor tyrosine kinase (RTK), Wnt, Src, NF-κB, phosphatidylinositol-3 kinase (PI3K/Akt), matrix metalloproteinase (MMP), hypoxia inducible factor-1α (HIF-1α), and vascular endothelial growth factor (VEGF) [45,48]. Permanent oxidative stress due to high ROS level in antioxidant system weakness can activate Akt, ERK and c-MYC like oncogenes by inhibiting tumor suppressors such as p53 and Phosphatase and tensin homolog deleted on chromosome 10 (PTEN) [45]. ROS also play an important role in the spread of cancer and tumor formation in a secondary place. In the case of metastasis, ROS can interact with the cytoskeleton and extracellular matrix. In case of oxidative stress MMPs activated and they inhibit movement that suppresses metastasis (Scheme 1) [50].

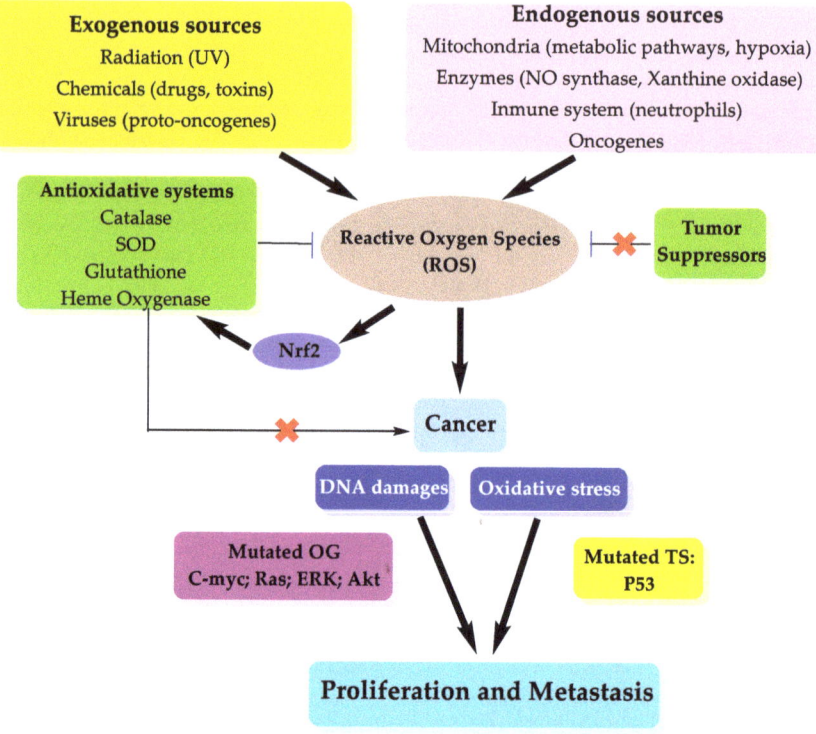

Scheme 1. Oxidative stress and cancer metastasis relation.

5. Carotenoids and Oxidative Stress

The capacity of carotenoids to quench O_2 and scavenge free radicals has been proposed as the main mechanism by which they afford their benign health effects [51]. Due to their triplet energy levels lying close to that of $^1O_2$ (1274 nm, 7849 cm^{-1} or 93.9 kJ/mole vs. 1380 nm, 7250 cm^{-1} or 86.7 kJ/mol for β-carotene, respectively, they are included in the group of the most effective physical quenchers of $^1O_2$ [52]. Carotenes with 11 conjugated double bonds have especially been shown to possess very strong extinguishing ability of $^1O_2$ quenching. In general terms, $^1O_2$ neutralization is based on transforming excess energy into heat through the lowest excited triple state ($^3Crt^*$) of carotenoids. The possible harmful effects of stimulated carotenoids can often be neglected due to their low energy and short life [53].

$$^1O_2 + \text{Carotenoid} \rightarrow {}^3O_2 + {}^3Crt^* (1)$$

$$^3Crt^* \rightarrow \text{Carotenoid} + \text{heat}$$

Radical scavenging mechanism of carotenoids are: (i) electron transfer, resulting with carotenoid radical cation (Carotenoid $^{\bullet+}$) or carotenoid radical anion (Carotenoid $^{\bullet-}$); (ii) radical addition/adduct formation, (R Carotenoid $^\bullet$); and (iii) allylic hydrogen removal with formation of neutral carotenoid radical (Carotenoid $^\bullet$) [52,54].

(i) $R^\bullet + \text{Carotenoid} \rightarrow R^- + \text{Carotenoid}^{\bullet+}$

$R^\bullet + \text{Carotenoid} \rightarrow R^+ + \text{Carotenoid}^{\bullet-}$

(ii) $R^\bullet + \text{Carotenoid} \rightarrow R \text{ Carotenoid}^\bullet$

(iii) $R^\bullet + \text{Carotenoid} \rightarrow RH + \text{Carotenoid}^\bullet$

However, some studies have shown that carotenes and xanthophylls have pro-oxidant properties under some conditions. When lipid peroxidation is in progression under high oxygen pressure [55], higher amount of carotene-peroxyl radical (Car-OO$^\bullet$) created, and as long as it is not eliminated by different antioxidant systems, Car-OO$\bullet$ will replicate lipid peroxidation with more attack on intact unsaturated fatty acid chains [54].

Because limited absorption and tissue specific accumulation of carotenes, it is wrong to assume that carotenoids will support health by scavenging ROS or RNS. Common belief that the removal of free radicals by antioxidants has a beneficial effect; however, the major contribution of carotenoids and their metabolites to cell protection is presumed to be stimulating endogenous antioxidant defenses like nuclear factor E_2-related factor 2 (Nrf2–Keap1) pathway [56–58]. Lycopene, phytoene, phytofluene, β-carotene and astaxanthin were evaluated for their effect on activation of antioxidant responsive elements (ARE) and their role in the induction of phase II enzymes. It was reported that the efficacy of carotenoids in ARE activation was not related to their effects on intracellular ROS and decreased glutathione level. The increase in Phase II enzymes like NAD(P)H:quinone oxidoreductase (NQO1) and γ-glutamylcysteine synthetase (GCS) has been removed by a dominant negative Nrf2, suggesting that carotenoid induction of these proteins is due to a functional Nrf2 and ARE transcription system [59].

Studies on the radical scavenging and antioxidant activities of various marine carotenoids have been summarized to understand the effects on oxidative stress. Astaxanthin, the xanthophyll carotenoid found in marine organisms, is one of the natural compounds with strong antioxidant activity. Astaxanthin, lycopene, β-carotene, and lutein carotenoids have been studied for their antioxidant activity with fluorometric assay. The 8-tetramethylchroman-2-carboxylic acid (Trolox) was employed as a calibrator in the assay. The results of the research highlighted that astaxanthin possess the highest antioxidant activity against peroxyl radicals [60].

Dose and colleagues studied the radical scavenging and antioxidant activity of synthetic astaxanthin with various methods. According to research, radical scavenging activities specified with 2,2-diphenyl-1-picrylhydrazyl (DPPH) radical scavenging, galvinoxyl radical scavenging, superoxide radical scavenging, and photon counting for singlet oxygen scavenging assays. In human hepatic cellular carcinoma (Huh7) cells, paraoxonase activity and Nrf2 transactivation and in HepG2 cells (hepatocellular carcinoma) glutathione assay and lipid peroxidation via BODIPY assay performed for cellular antioxidant activity. It has been reported that astaxanthin scavenge DPPH, galvinoxyl and singlet oxygen radicals in a concentration dependent manner but no effect on superoxide anion radicals. In cellular antioxidant activity astaxanthin increased the glutathione levels and also decreased lipid peroxidation in HepG2 cells [61].

A recent study also demonstrated the radical scavenging potential of astaxanthin with DPPH, 2,2′-azino-bis(3-ethylbenzothiazoline-6-sulfonic acid) (ABTS) radical scavenging activities and singlet oxygen quenching assays and also antioxidant potential with β-carotene bleaching activity. It was found that EC_{50} value in DPPH assay was 7.5 µg/mL and 7.7 µg/mL for ABTS assay. The research concluded that shrimp astaxanthin is a potent antioxidant agent and it has no cytotoxic effect on human dermal fibroblast cells [62].

Astaxanthin, zeaxanthin, lutein, ascorbic acid, and tocopherol acetate evaluated for their antioxidant activity with spectrophotometric, fluorimetric and chemiluminescence techniques. In dose dependent manner astaxanthin, lutein, and zeaxanthin showed near same activity against H_2O_2 and O_2^-. In this study, the strong antioxidant activity of xanthophylls was confirmed and it was also reported that they may be the first option to prevent the retinal oxidative stress due to their ability to pass the retina-blood barrier and their binding to the photoreceptor membranes [63]. In 2007, Santocono et al. conducted a new study to measure the protective effects of astaxanthin, lutein and zeaxanthin against K-N-SH human neuroblastoma cells against DNA damage caused by divergent reactive nitrogen species. Cells were treated with 20 and 40 µM of carotenoids. According to the comet assay, data revealed the ability of preventing DNA damage of carotenoids and it is also stated that this activity subjected to the type of RNOS donor and concentration [64].

Antioxidant activity of astaxanthin in the LS-180 cell line (human colorectal cancer). Cells were treated 50,100 and 150 µm astaxanthin. According to the results of the study, astaxanthin induced apoptosis, as well as decreased MDA levels and caused an increase in antioxidant activity with the effect of superoxide dismutase (SOD), catalase (CAT), and glutathione peroxidase (GPx). In the antioxidant activity tests, 150 µM astaxanthin showed significant effect among the other groups [65].

In UVA exposed human dermal fibroblasts, the effects of astaxanthin, canthaxanthin, and β-carotene on ROS and TBARS were evaluated. While radical scavenging activities of β-carotene and canthaxanthin are not observed, astaxanthin has been stated to have significant radical scavenging activity at both 5 and 10 µM doses. The increase in TBARS levels with UVA exposure decreased significantly (70%) compared to the control group with astaxanthin administration. In addition, the reduction of CAT and SOD enzymes in cells after UVA exposure was prevented by astaxanthin and β-carotene, while canthaxanthin had no effect [66].

Antioxidant effect of astaxanthin was evaluated against cyclophosphamide-induced oxidative stress and DNA damage. Rats were administered with 25 mg/kg (p.o) astaxanthin before or after administration of cyclophosphamide. In the control group, due to cyclophosphamide, an increase in MDA level and a decrease in Glutathione (GSH) amount were observed, whereas in pre- and post-treatment group, this situation resolved through astaxanthin [67].

DPPH radical scavenging capacity, microsomal lipid peroxidation inhibitory activity, and ROS scavenging activity in SH-SY5Y (human neuroblastoma) cells were performed in a study in which the antioxidant activities of 9-*cis* and 13-*cis* astaxanthin against all-*trans* isomer were measured (Figure 5). 9-*cis* astaxanthin and 13-*cis* astaxanthin scavenge the DPPH radical stronger than the *trans* isomer. In 2,2′-Azobis(2-amidinopropane) dihydrochloride (AAPH) and tert-butyl hydro peroxide (tBuOOH) induced lipid peroxidation, particularly 9-*cis* astaxanthin performed better antioxidant activity by inhibiting TBARS generation than all-*trans* isomer. In SH-SY5Y cells, 100 nM astaxanthin isomers were applied to the cells before 6-hydroxydopamine (6-OHDA) inducement. ROS generation was effectively suppressed by 9-*cis* astaxanthin [68].

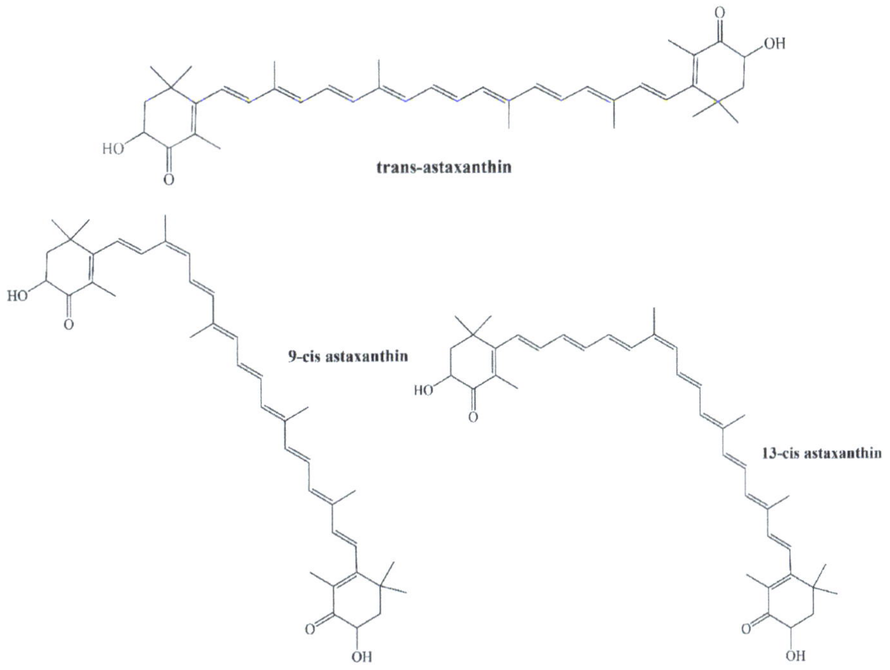

Figure 5. Structures of all-*trans* astaxanthin, 9-*cis* astaxanthin, and 13-*cis* astaxanthin.

Fucoxanthin is a carotenoid belonging to the class of xanthophylls, is common in brown seaweeds, and its effects on oxidative stress have been extensively studied. Iwasaki et al. (2012), conducted a study with purified fucoxanthin from seaweed *Undaria pinnatifida* to highlight the in vivo antioxidant activity. ICR mice and obese/diabetes KK-Ay mice were administered fucoxanthin (0.1%) with soybean oil. Lipid hydro peroxide levels in liver and abdominal white adipose tissue were measured. The 0.1% Fucoxanthin decreased the hydro peroxide amounts in KK-Ay mice. Little change in lipid hydro peroxide levels was observed in ICR mice with and without fucoxanthin administration. The activity of fucoxanthin on lowering lipid hydro peroxides in KK-Ay mice has been attributed to its decreasing effect on blood glucose level and hepatic lipid levels, not its radical scavenging feature [69].

Fucoxanthin purified from *Fucus vesiculosus*, *Fucus serratus* and *Laminaria digitata* brown algae and evaluated for its antioxidant activity. DPPH radical scavenging, iron (Fe^{2+})-chelating activity and reducing power activity were determined. Fucoxanthin had lower DPPH scavenging activity than BHT, while showed similar activity with EDTA in iron chelating activity. In reducing power assay fucoxanthin exhibited significantly lower ($p < 0.001$) activity than ascorbic acid at the same concentration. In the 5% fish oil-water emulsion containing iron as oxidation inducer, fucoxanthin showed better antioxidant activity compared with BHT with low levels of volatile oxidation products and reduction in tocopherol loss [70].

Antioxidant activity of fucoxanthin from *Phaeodactylum tricornutum* microalga examined by DPPH, hydrogen peroxide and superoxide anion radical scavenging activities and also reducing power was evaluated. IC_{50} value of DPPH scavenging activity was found to be 0.30 mM and it has been stated that fucoxanthin was more active than ascorbic acid, BHA, and α-tocopherol positive controls. When compared to positive controls fucoxanthin had lower effect in scavenging the hydrogen peroxide and superoxide anion radicals. In reducing power assay fucoxanthin showed higher activity than positive controls [71]. In a similar study, DPPH radical scavenging IC_{50} value of fucoxanthin was found 201.2 ± 21.4 µg/mL while β-carotene exhibited lower activity. In ferric reducing activity, fucoxanthin and astaxanthin were found to be more active than β-carotene. Results showed that fucoxanthin caused a 63% reduction in chemiluminescence in blood neutrophils and a 3.3-fold increase in reduced and oxidized glutathione in HeLa cells in a dose-dependent manner [72]. Xia et al. reported that fucoxanthin from *Odontella aurita* marine diatom showed potent antioxidant effects in DPPH and ABTS radical scavenging activities. EC_{50} values were found to be 140 and 30 μg/mL, respectively [73]. In a different study conducted by Sujatha et al. (2017), DPPH radical scavenging effect of fucoxanthin from brown seaweed *Sargassum wightii* with an EC_{50} value of 322.58 μg/mL was detected [74]. Fucoxanthin from *Sargassum filipendula* brown seaweed exhibited a strong DPPH radical scavenging activity with 1.4174 ± 0.0126 μg/L EC_{50} value [75].

In a study of Sudhakar et al. (2013), fucoxanthin purified from *Sargassum wightii*, *Sargassum ilicifolium*, *Sargassum longifolium*, *Padina gymnospora*, and *Turbinaria ornata* brown seaweeds. It was mentioned that fucoxanthin purified from *Padina gymnospora* exhibited better activity with 37% inhibition percentage than fucoxanthin isolated from *Sargassum ilicifolium* [76].

Antioxidant activity of fucoxanthin has been studied under anoxic and aerobic conditions via DPPH radical. In the same study also β-carotene, β- cryptoxanthin, zeaxanthin, lycopene and lutein evaluated for their antioxidant activity under anoxic conditions. It was concluded that other carotenoids except fucoxanthin reacted with DPPH at a low level. Under aerobic conditions to observe the stoichiometry of the reactions, 20–300 μM fucoxanthin was added to the 100 μM DPPH. Unlike anoxic reactions, fucoxanthin was found to react less with DPPH [77].

In high fat diet rats, antioxidant activity of fucoxanthin evaluated by Ha et al. (2013). Rats were administered 0.2% fucoxanthin with high fat during 4 weeks. Lipid peroxidation, plasma total antioxidant capacity (TAC), and activities of CAT, SOD, and GPx enzymes were identified. In plasma, total antioxidant capacity and GPx amounts were found to be significantly augmented in fucoxanthin treated group. In liver, CAT and GPx levels in fucoxanthin treated group were also found to be higher than control group. The effect of fucoxanthin on plasma lipid peroxidation did not differ statistically [78].

Fucoxanthin and, fucoxanthinol and halocynthiaxanthin metabolites were analyzed for their DPPH and ABTS radical scavenging activities and singlet oxygen quenching abilities (Figure 6). While fucoxanthin and fucoxanthinol scavenge the DPPH radical stronger than halocynthiaxanthin, fucoxanthinol had a stronger effect against the ABTS radical. In hydroxyl and superoxide radical scavenging activities fucoxanthin exhibited potent scavenging effect than both its metabolites. Moreover, β-carotene was found to be more effective in singlet oxygen quenching than fucoxanthin and its metabolites [79].

In mice with traumatic brain injury (TBI), the effects of fucoxanthin on oxidative stress were investigated by measuring MDA and GPx levels. Mice were administered intragastrically 50, 100, and 200 mg/kg fucoxanthin. Treatment of fucoxanthin, caused a decline in MDA levels and increase in GPx levels in the cerebral cortex tissue of TBI mice. Moreover, in the same study, fucoxanthin has been reported to increase in vitro neuron survival and decrease ROS level [80].

Maoka and colleagues synthesized mytiloxanthin, metabolite of fucoxanthin in shellfish and tunicates and evaluated its antioxidant activity by examining the quenching ability of scavenging singlet oxygen, hydroxyl radical and lipid peroxidation inhibition (Figure 7). In the same study, β-carotene, astaxanthin, and fucoxanthin were used as positive controls. Mytiloxanthin exhibited near same singlet oxygen quenching ability (61.6%) with astaxanthin (61.0%). Lower capacity of fucoxanthin in the same study was linked to the number of conjugated double bonds, polyene chain structures, and functional groups. Mytiloxanthin increased its activity by having an 11-conjugated double bond polyene system containing an acetylenic and a carbonyl group in its structure. In the lipid peroxidation experiment, mytiloxanthin exhibited slightly stronger activity than astaxanthin, while fucoxanthin and β-carotene showed higher activity [81].

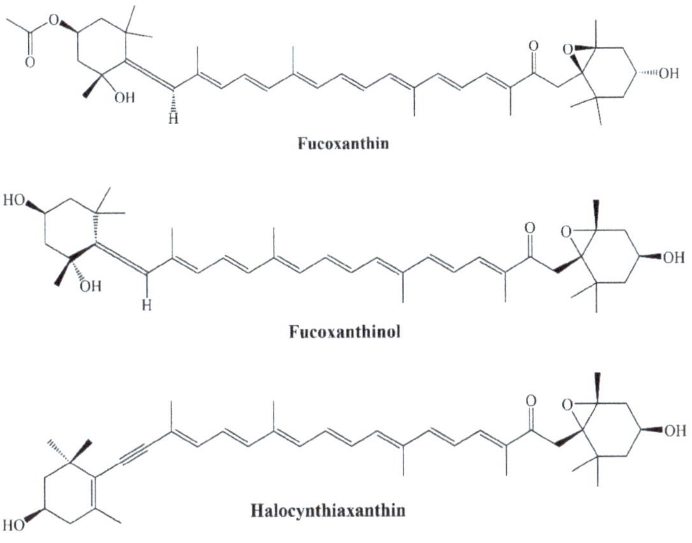

Figure 6. Structures of fucoxanthin and its metabolites.

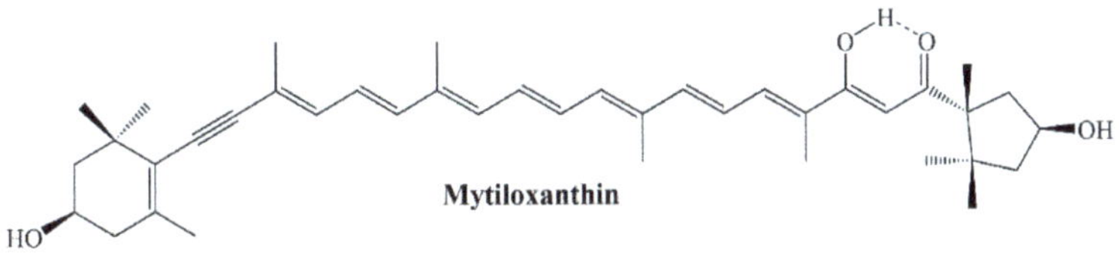

Figure 7. Structure of mytiloxanthin.

In the high fat diet rodent model, lutein and zeaxanthin isomers were investigated for their effects on lipid metabolism and anti-inflammatory activities on the retina. Lutein and zeaxanthin used in the experiment provided from Lutemax 2020™. Rats were administered lutein and zeaxanthin 100 mg/kg BW for 8 weeks. Lutein and zeaxanthin improved oxidative damage by decreasing the concentration of MDA and gaining the SOD, CAT, and GPx enzyme activities of the retina caused by high fat diet [82].

Zou et al., conducted a study for evaluating the regulation mechanism of zeaxanthin on phase II detoxification enzymes in human retinal pigment epithelium cells. It has been found that zeaxanthin is effective against mitochondrial dysfunction and apoptosis due to tert-butyl hydroperoxide, while it increases GSH by Nrf2 activation. In the same study, the effects of zeaxanthin were evaluated in the rat retina, liver and heart in vivo. Similar to in vitro results zeaxanthin was found to be effective in increasing GSH levels and decreasing markers of lipid and protein peroxidation, 4-hydroxynonenal and the carbonyl protein [83].

Bhosale et al., studied the antioxidant role of zeaxanthin and glutathione S-transferase (GSTP1) in egg yolk phosphatidylcholine liposomes. The two zeaxanthin diastereomers showed synergistic antioxidant effects against both azo lipid peroxyl radical producers [(2,2'-azobis(2-methyl-propionamidine) dihydrochloride and lipophilic 2,2'-azobis(2,4-dimethylvaleronitrile)] when bound to GSTP1. Non-dietary $(3R,3'S$-meso)-zeaxanthin was found to have strong activity than dietary $(3R,3'R)$-zeaxanthin in the presence of GSTP1 (Figure 8) [84].

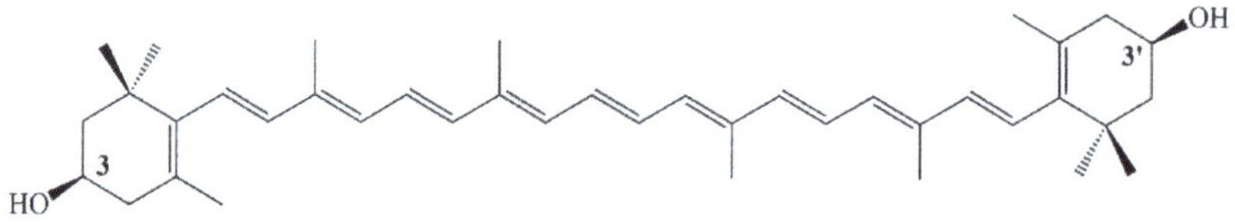

(3R, 3'R)-Zeaxanthin

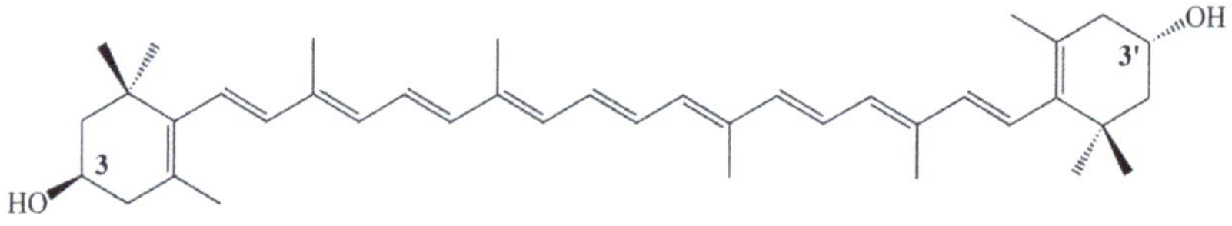

(3R, 3'S-meso)-Zeaxanthin

Figure 8. Structure of zeaxanthin.

Singlet oxygen quenching abilities of lycopene, β-carotene, zeaxanthin, astaxanthin, and canthaxanthin carotenoids evaluated by Cantrell et al. (2003). Lycopene showed the fastest quenching ability with 2.3×10^9 M^{-1} s^{-1} value, while the lowest activity is attributed to lutein 1.1×10^8 M^{-1} s^{-1} value. Interestingly, the ability of zeaxanthin to extinguish singlet oxygen decreases as concentration increases [85].

Several studies stated the beneficial effects of dietary supplementation of canthaxanthin the breeder's diet. Results clearly showed that increased antioxidative status in the egg yolk and newly hatched chicks and as a result hatching rate of chicken eggs was meaningfully increased. The common results of the studies focused on canthaxanthin providing great benefits for chicken eggs, embryos and chickens during postpartum development [86–90].

Canthaxanthin isomers which are purified from new soil *Dietzia* sp. evaluated for their antioxidant activity. DPPH and superoxide radical scavenging activities in addition ROS inhibitory activity in THP-1 (monocytic cell line) cells were performed. It was reported that the *cis* isomer of canthaxanthin showed 1.8-fold higher activity than *trans* isomer in DPPH radical scavenging activity. The *cis* isomer was found to be more active in superoxide radical scavenging activity and inhibiting the ROS formation in THP-1 cells as well [91].

In the study investigating the antioxidant activity of β-carotene used orally in patients with cystic fibrosis, groups were established with 24 patients and 14 healthy individuals. The total antioxidant capacity in the plasma of the 13 cystic fibrosis supplement group increased by 12% after 12 weeks of supplementation. Antioxidant activity has been demonstrated by a reduction in the amount of plasma MDA [92].

Allard et al. (1994) previously conducted a similar study on smoker and non-smoker volunteers. Lipid peroxidation was quantified by breath-pentane output and it was found that lipid peroxidation was significantly lower in smokers who received β-carotene compared to the control group [93]. However, it has been reported in several studies that high amounts of β-carotene supplementation cause adverse effects in people which exposed to high levels of oxidative stress [94].

Levin et al. (1997) studied with 9-*cis* β-carotene and all-*trans* β-carotene to compare their antioxidant activities. Isolated 9-*cis* β-carotene from *Dunaliella* and synthetic all-*trans* β-carotene administered to rats 1 g/kg. It has been reported that *cis* isomer has a greater affinity for free radicals in the liver. Levin et al. also reported the higher antioxidant activity of 9-*cis* β-carotene than all-trans β-carotene by avoiding methyl-linoleate peroxidation and algal carotene degradation in vitro. However, in some studies, it has been reported in contrasting results regarding the antioxidant activities of β-carotene and isomers (Figure 9) [95]. In the study of Mueller et al., it was explained that β-carotene isomers do not have ferric reducing activity. In addition, it has been reported that the ABTS and superoxide radical scavenging activities of all-E, 9Z and 13Z isomers did not differ statistically, while the 15Z isomer had lower activity [96].

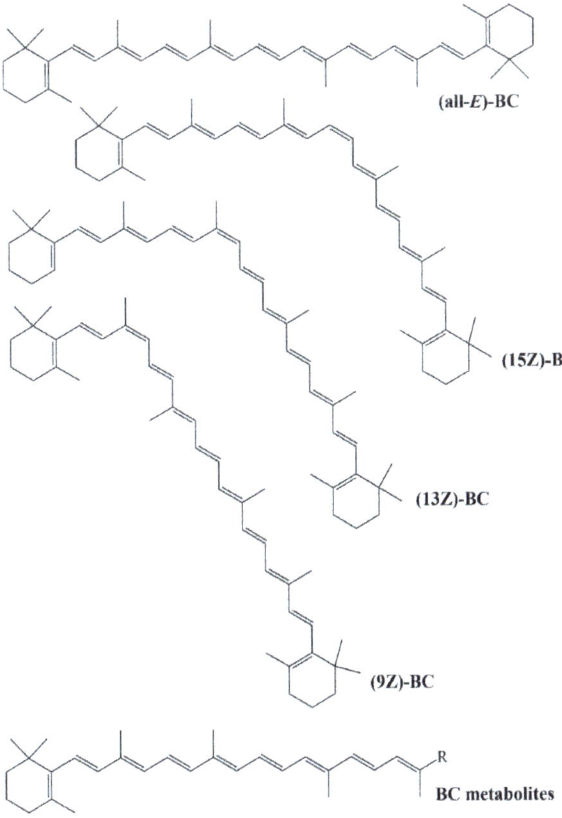

Figure 9. Structures of β-carotene isomers.

Similarly, in the study conducted by Rodrigues et al. (2012), it was reported that *cis*-β-carotene isomers have lower peroxyl radical scavenging activity than *trans*-isomers, and *trans* lycopene is the most active carotenoid among the studied carotenoids [97].

The rare marine carotenoids (3R)-saproxanthin and (3R,2'S)-myxol (Figure 10) have been isolated from 04OKA-13-27 (MBIC08261) and YM6-073 (MBIC06409) two marine bacteria strains and these strains have been classified in the Flavobacteriaceae family. Their inhibitory activity on lipid peroxidation in rat brain homogenate was evaluated and zeaxanthin was also studied in the same experiment. According to the results, IC_{50} values of saproxanthin, myxol, and zeaxanthin were found to be 2.1, 6.2, and 13.5 µM, respectively [98].

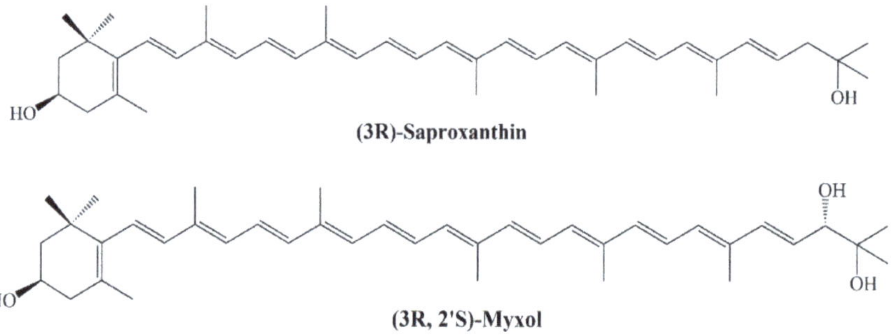

Figure 10. Structures of (3R)-saproxanthin and (3R,2′S)-myxol.

Conjugated double bond system forms most of the basic properties of carotenoids, also affects how these molecules are attached into biological membranes. Although the way these molecules interact with reactive oxygen species differs due to their chain length and end groups, their in vivo behavior may differ from that seen in solution. Some of them, especially β-carotene and lycopene may also lose their antioxidant effects at high concentrations or high partial oxygen pressures [44,99,100].

6. Marine Carotenoids and Bioavailability

There are more than 40 carotenoids that can be obtained from diet and there are various health benefits of carotenoids to human health [11]. However, it is essential for every metabolite to reach sufficient concentration in target tissues to exert its bioactivity. Thus, bioavailability is a key concept for evaluating health benefits of carotenoids. In this concept, effects of digestive system, absorption and biotransformation should be observed for clear understanding.

Fucoxanthin and astaxanthin are the most abundant carotenoids from marine organisms consequently these two are the most studied marine carotenoids for their bioavailability. Fucoxanthin is the most ample carotenoid in the nature and it is mostly found in marine environment [101]. Because of the health benefits of fucoxanthin, there are various in vitro, in vivo and clinical studies for its bioavailability. Sugawara et al. had investigated bioavailability of Fucoxanthin and ten other carotenoids in an in vitro study via using Caco-2 cellular line, which is originated from gastrointestinal system. Results demonstrated that Fucoxanthin has one of the lowest bioavailability among other studied carotenoids [102]. In a further study same cell line was used and results revealed that, even though cells successfully absorb fucoxanthin, it is rapidly deacetylated and converted to Fucoxanthinol [103]. Correspondingly, another further in vitro study had showed that fucoxanthinol had transformed to amarouciaxanthin A by human hepatoma HepG2 cells [104]. Pharmacokinetic parameters of Fucoxanthin were also studied in vivo model, 0.105 mg of Fucoxanthin was administered to 6 mice via intragastric route [105]. Results showed that Fucoxanthin was not accumulating in the studied parts of mice such as lung, kidney, heart, erythrocytes, liver and spleen. On the opposite, metabolites of fucoxanthin, fucoxanthinol and amarouciaxanthin A reached their maximum concentration in 4 h and decreased steadily for 24 h. In the adipose tissue metabolites were still detectable for after a week. These results were corresponding with previous in vitro studies. Moreover, in a subsequent study, fucoxanthinol and amarouciaxanthin A accumulation in adipose tissue were confirmed after feeding mice with Fucoxanthin for 14 days [106]. It was theorized that with application of higher doses of fucoxanthin, it is possible to accumulate Fucoxanthin in mammalian tissues without any transformation. In a study with rats, it was shown that after 65 mg/kg intake of fucoxanthin, it reaches its maximum plasma level after 7.7 h with concentration of 29.1 µg/L [107]. Few studies were conducted on bioavailability of fucoxanthin in humans. In a study, 18 volunteers were orally administered with Kambu extract which was containing 31 mg fucoxanthin and their blood samples were collected for 24 h. Results revealed that only fucoxanthinol was found in samples with maximum concentration of 44 nmol/L. Fucoxanthin and amarouciaxanthin A were not detected in plasma [108]. The outcome of the study declared by researchers was fucoxanthin in humans seems to have lower bioaccessibility in humans when compared to other carotenoids such as lutein and β-carotene. When considered the low bioavailability of fucoxanthin, different strategies were developed to increase it. In a study, rats were fed with brown seaweed, *Padina tetrastromatica* L., and chitosan-glycolipid hybrid nanogels were prepared for increasing the bioavailability. Results demonstrated that nanogels were improved the bioavailability more than 3-fold when compared to control group [109]. In addition, another study showed that fucoxanthin enriched *Phaeodactylum tricornutum* bioavailability can be increased with preparation of nanoparticles coated with casein and chitosan. C_{max} value was increased from 10.29 ± 0.1 to 33.66 ± 0.5 pmol/mL [110]. In a more recent study, it has been shown that digalactosylmonoacylglycerol and sulfoquinovosylmonoacylglycerol presence significantly increases both uptake and transport of fucoxanthin in Caco-2 cells [111].

There are numerous studies indicating that astaxanthin is highly valuable compound for human health [18]. This valuable potential of astaxanthin for human health leads to studies of its bioavailability. In a double blind randomized study, 28 health volunteers were ingested 250 g farmed or wild salmon which contain 5 μg Astaxanthin per gram for 2 weeks. The source of astaxanthin for wild salmon is krill while farmed ones were fed with synthetic type. Results showed that aqua cultured salmon leads to higher bioavailability; aquacultured salmon group reached 42 nmol/L while wild salmon group measured 27.3 nmol/L in day 3. It was reported that difference in bioavailability originated from isomerization [112]. In another study, pharmacokinetics of astaxanthin was examined in 3 middle-aged male volunteers with consumption of 100 mg racemic astaxanthin mixture in olive oil. Results demonstrated that astaxanthin concentration reached its maximum level after 7 h (1.3 mg/mL) and it was still observable in plasma for 72 h [113]. Results indicate that astaxanthin reaches significant levels in plasma without any biotransformation contrasting Fucoxanthin. Another clinical study was investigated the difference in bioavailability of astaxanthin between commercial food supplement and lipid-based formulation containing *Haematococcus pluvialis* green microalgae with 40 mg of astaxanthin [114]. Results revealed that lipid-based formulation achieved approximately 4-fold increment in bioavailability (1347 to 4960 μg h/L). In addition C_{max} value increased significantly from 55.2 to 191.5 μg/L. It is known that bioavailability may be affected various parameters such as sex, age, obesity, smoking, lifestyle, etc. In another study, effect of smoking on astaxanthin bioavailability and pharmacokinetic parameters was investigated on human volunteers. Results indicated that smoking significantly affected pharmacokinetic parameters for astaxanthin by reducing the half-life of elimination 30.5 h to 18.5 h. In addition, AUC value is lower in smoking group when compared to non-smoking volunteers, 6.52 and 7.53 μg h/L, respectively [115]. Even though, astaxanthin reaches sufficient plasma levels without biotransformation, still some metabolites of astaxanthin in human body were detected. 3-hydroxy-4-oxo-β-ionone, 3-hydroxy-4-oxo-β-ionone, 3-hydroxy-4-oxo-β-ionol, 3-hydroxy-4-oxo-7,8-dihydro-β-ionol was detected in two human volunteers via GC-MS analysis [116].

7. New Delivery Systems Used to Increase Marine Carotenoids Bioavailability

Encapsulation is one of the quality protection techniques of sensitive agents and is a method for production of them with new valuable properties. Recently, nanotechnology has contributed significantly to the development of drug carrier systems (biopolymeric and lipid-based carriers such as nanoliposomal formulations, surfactant-based nano-carriers, nanoemulsions, nano-structured lipid carriers) that can encapsulate compounds with poor stability, protect them from undesirable reactions, provide therapeutic effect at a low dose, improve targetability, and increase their activity [9,117]. In this regard, there are many studies on the application of encapsulated carotenoids in different nano-based drug delivery systems.

7.1. Application of Biopolymeric Nanocarriers for Encapsulation of Carotenoids

One of marine carotenoids, fucoxanthin has many effects, such as antioxidant, anti-obesity and anti-cancer effects [118] but it has high sensitivity when exposed to weather, thermal or light factors. Vo et al. evaluated to characterization and storage stability of encapsulated extracted fucoxanthin-rich oil (FO) from y using supercritical carbon dioxide with sunflower oil (SFO) and polyethylene glycol (PEG) as co-solvent and biodegradable coating at optimized conditions (mixing ratio of FO and PEG, temperature, and pressure). By using PEG as a biodegradable coating material, approximately 82% fucoxanthin encapsulation and a higher antioxidant activity of FO were found significantly than SFO and trolox [119].

Ravi et al. aimed to increase the stability and bioavailability of carotenoid such as fucoxanthin, encapsulated in chitosan, a biodegradable cationic polysaccharide, and glycolipid hybrid nanogels. Bioavailability studies were performed for investigate the effect of nanoencapsulation of fucoxanthin with glycolipid via micellization in vitro (simulated gastric and intestinal digestion). The bioavailability of fucoxanthin from chitosan-glycolipid hybrid nanogels was the highest compared to chitosan nanogels without glycolipid, mixture of fucoxanthin with glycolipid and control groups. The enhanced stability and bioavailability of fucoxanthin was observed by nanoencapsulation with chitosan and glycolipid [120].

As a continuation study, Ravi et al. prepared chitosan-glycolipid nanogels and investigated cellular uptake and anticancer efficacy of fucoxanthin on human colon cell line (Caco-2). They found that the low cell viability significantly at nanoencapsulated fucoxanthin with chitosan and glycolipid compared to without glycolipid for 48 h exposure. Chitosan-glycolipid hybrid nanogels successfully induced apoptosis in human colon cancer cells and suppressed ROS production by suppressing Bcl-2 protein associated increased levels of Bax through caspase-3 steps and suppressed cell viability [121].

Koo et al. developed casein nanoparticles (C-NP) and chitosan-coated nanoparticles (C-NP-CS) containing a valuable marine carotenoid, fucoxanthin which extracted from the microalga *Phaeodactylum tricornutum* for improvement of water solubility and its bioavailability. Nanoparticles characterized in terms of their size, morphology, structure, zeta potential, polydispersity index, encapsulation efficiency and adsorption to mucin. Increased retention and adsorption by mucin were observed with using cationic biopolymer chitosan coating and fucoxanthinol absorption to the blood circulation was found two-fold higher than with using C57BL/6 mice compared to C-NP [110].

Edelman et al. studied on new approach to improve the bioactivity of astaxanthin which is sensitive to oxidation and has very low bioavailability. Potato protein was approved by FDA and potato protein-based astaxanthin nanoparticles were designed because of be possible to reduce the dose of the required bioactive substance, to ensure the therapeutic effect and to increase solubility and oral bioavailability. Encapsulated astaxanthin was shown that ~80% simulated gastric and intestinal digestion and 11 times higher bioavailability was obtained compared to unencapsulated astaxanthin. Potato protein nanoparticles can be considered as a suitable drug delivery system to increase the bioavailability of hydrophobic compounds [122].

Application of biopolymeric nanocarriers for encapsulation of carotenoids is summarized in Table 1.

Table 1. Application of biopolymeric nanocarriers for encapsulation of carotenoids.

Nanocarriers	Carotenoids	Results and Benefits	References
Chitosan-glycolipid hybrid nanogels	Fucoxanthin	The bioavailability of fucoxanthin from chitosan-glycolipid hybrid nanogels was the highest compared to chitosan nanogels without glycolipid, mixture of fucoxanthin with glycolipid and control groups. Enhanced stability and bioavailability by nanoencapsulation.	[120]
		The low cell viability significantly at nanoencapsulated fucoxanthin compared to without using glycolipid and induced apoptosis in Caco-2 cells and suppressed ROS production.	[121]
PEG biodegradable coated nanoparticles		Approximately 82% fucoxanthin encapsulation and a higher antioxidant activity significantly than sunflower oil and trolox.	[122]
Casein nanoparticles and chitosan-coated nanoparticles		Increased retention and adsorption and two-fold higher absorption to the blood circulation than non-coated nanoparticles.	[110]
Potato protein-based polymeric nanoparticles	Astaxanthin	~80% simulated gastric and intestinal digestion and 11 times higher bioavailability compared to unencapsulated astaxanthin.	[122]

7.2. Application of Different Lipid-Based Nanocarriers for Encapsulation of Carotenoids

Many lipid based nanoformulations such as nanoliposomes, niosomes, solid lipid nanoparticles and nanostructured lipid carriers, were developed for improving biological activity, physicochemical stability, digestibility, antioxidant potential, resistibility and in vitro bioaccessibility.

Cordenonsi and co-workers aimed to develop nanostructured lipid carriers containing fucoxanthin for skin application to prevent skin hyperproliferative diseases. Hyperproliferation of the skin could be controlled and skin integrity could be restored with the presence of fucoxanthin. Nanostructured lipid carriers were coated with chitosan and biopharmaceutical properties (bio/mucoadhesion and wound healing) were improved by combining the advantages of chitosan. It stated that these nanostructured lipid carriers were promising approach with fucoxanthin to control skin hyperproliferation and maintain skin integrity in psoriatic skin [123].

Hama et al. evaluated the free radical scavenging effect of a useful antioxidant, astaxanthin loaded liposomes compared with the activity of the well-known antioxidants encapsulated β-carotene and α-tocopherol that stated that was the first report. The liposomal formulation provided encapsulation of high concentrations of astaxanthin and it was obtained that more potent hydroxyl radical scavenging activity significantly in aqueous solution was than either encapsulated β-carotene or α-tocopherol. Moreover, astaxanthin liposomes prevented cytotoxicity caused by hydroxyl radical in cultured NIH-3T3 cells [124].

Li et al. evaluated the protective effects of astaxanthin liposome (Asx-L) on photodamage by ultraviolet (UV)-B in mice skin. Topically treatment with 4 mL 0.2% astaxanthin or 4 mL 0.2% Asx-L were applied to groups (UVB light injury + astaxanthin and UVB light injury + Asx-L) 10 min before the irradiation for two weeks. The histological changes of skin, Ki-67, 8-hydroxy-2'-deoxyguanosine (8-OHdG), SOD activities and serum MMP-13 were measured. The pathological changes of skin tissues were significantly improved by topical Asx-L with decreased expressions of Ki-67, MMP-13 and 8-OHdG and increased SOD activity, due to strong antioxidation of Asx-L [125].

In the same study, Hama et al. designed Asx-L and evaluated prevention of UV-induced skin damage. Astaxanthin, which is accepted as a strong antioxidative carotenoid in biological membranes, is difficult to apply topically to the skin due to its poor water solubility. In this study, researchers tried to solve this problem by preparing Asx-L, which are suitable drug delivery systems for topical application to the skin. Asx-L has been shown to have strong cleaning ability against singlet oxygen production due to chemiluminescence in the water phase. When Asx-L was applied to the skin before UV exposure, skin thickening, and collagen reduction were prevented. The production of melanin was inhibited with topical application of Asx-L. As a result, application of a liposomal formulation containing Asx, it is possible to prevent skin damage caused by UV-induced [126].

Peng et al. prepared astaxanthin encapsulated in liposomes to eliminate such poor physicochemical properties of astaxanthin such as instability, low bioavailability and poor water solubility. Astaxanthin is a powerful oxygen radical scavenger and its efficacy on Hep3B and HepG2 cell lines was evaluated because of it was beneficial for carcinoma prognosis. Encapsulated astaxanthin showed apparently improved stability and permeability thus the total transport time is 7.55 h for encapsulates astaxanthin and 6.00 h for free astaxanthin. It was obtained that more antioxidant effect on intracellular antioxidant enzymes such as superoxide dismutase, catalase and glutathione S-transferase with astaxanthin liposomes compared to free astaxanthin and effectively facilitates apoptosis in the Hep3B cell line more than HepG2 cell line. The findings indicated that poor bioavailability of Asx can be improved and the prognosis of gamma radiation therapy with liposomal encapsulation [127].

In a previous study, Tamjidi et al. aimed to design nanolipid-based carriers (NLCs) containing astaxanthin which has instability, low bioavailability, and poor water solubility, to investigate the effect of contents of oil and surfactant on characteristics of astaxanthin-NLCs, and to optimize the characteristics and composition of formulation by response surface methodology. Tween 80 and lecithin and oleic acid, glyceryl behenate were selected as emulsifier and suitable lipids, respectively. The optimum formulation of Asx-NLCs with ideal properties was prepared with oleic acid Tween 80 and was different in terms of physical properties and storage stability. According to the data obtained in this study, NLCs could be used as a carrier system with potentially suitable physical stability for the administration of Asx and other lipophilic compounds into pharmaceutical products [128].

Barros et al. astaxanthin and peridinin, two typical carotenoids of marine microalgae included in phosphatidylcholine multilamellar liposomes and evaluated as inhibitor effects of lipid oxidation. Astaxanthin strongly decreased lipid damage when the lipoperoxidation promoters such as H_2O_2, tert-butyl hydroperoxide or ascorbate. Fe^{+2}:EDTA were added simultaneously to the liposomes which were prepared with egg yolk phosphatidylcholine which offers suitable oxidation targets for ROS. To check for antioxidant activity of carotenoids which was also associated with their effect about membrane permeability, peroxidation processes started by adding promoters to encapsulated Fe^{+2} in the inner aqueous solution in liposomes. Consequently, astaxanthin was a more effective antioxidant (26%) at H_2O_2 and ascorbate-induced lipoperoxidation at Fe^{+2} liposomes. Peridine showed a more moderate inhibition of the lipid oxidation process (17.7%) due to it could have limited the permeation of the peroxidation agents [129].

In another study, effect of astaxanthin on the structural properties of liposome membranes was evaluated by Pan et al. They stated that liposomal encapsulation could be greatly increased water dispersibility of astaxanthin and also an effective way to constantly supply astaxanthin in the body [130].

Rodriguez-Ruiz et al. developed nanostructured lipid carriers to improve antioxidant activity of Asx using a green process with SFO as liquid lipid. Antioxidant activity of encapsulated astaxanthin was measured using the physicochemical lipophilic α-tocopherol equivalent antioxidant capacity (TEAC). It was demonstrated that nanostructured lipid-based carriers have suitable potential to maintain or stabilize the antioxidant ability of astaxanthin and could be excellent candidates as antioxidant delivery systems for cosmetics and nutraceuticals [131].

Bhatt et al. conducted to intranasal delivery of astaxanthin-loaded solid lipid nanoparticles (Asx- solid lipid nanoparticles (SLNs)) to improve brain targeting for neurological disorders. Double emulsion solvent displacement method was used for preparing SLNs. SLN formulation (50 mg stearic acid, 6.11% bioactive, and poloxamer 188, lecithin ratio of 1:6) was optimized with a 213 nm particle size. On the pheochromocytoma-12 cell line, the antioxidant potential of Asx-SLNs was evaluated against H2O2 induced toxicity. Radiolabeled nanoparticles were found to be 96–98% stable even for 48 h and higher drug concentration in the brain was achieved by intranasal administration, which was compared to 99mTc labeled nanoparticles intravenous route and confirmed by gamma scintigraphy analysis. It was shown that this nasal system can provide the most neuroprotection in neurological disorders from oxidative stress under in vitro conditions [132]. Shanmugapriya and colleagues designed to emulsion-based delivery systems to increase the bioavailability of astaxanthin and α-tocopherol as active compounds for various biomedical applications. Anticancer potential of astaxanthin-α-tocopherol nanoemulsion prepared with spontaneous and ultrasonication emulsification methods was evaluated with optimizing production conditions for better resistance and toxicity testing against microbial infections. It could be said that this delivery system may be a starting point for prospective studies for cancer treatment applications [133].

Rostamabadi et al. summarized some nano-based drug delivery systems in review. One of them was nanoliposomal formulations, consisting of lutein, different lipids and cholesterol as a stabilizer were developed, characterized and evaluated in terms of microstructure analysis using TEM, particle size, polydispersity, zeta potential, in vitro release and stability and cytotoxicity studies. These formulations provided to increased physicochemical stability, water dispersibility, therapeutic effects (antioxidant and anticancer) of lutein. In other studies with nano-emulsion based delivery system, formulation components, process steps, emulsifier types and concentrations storage pH and temperature played a key role on stability and effectiveness of lutein. Emulsion formulation revealed proper stability thus coating oil droplets in emulsions was increased the physicochemical stability of lutein compared to uncoated. In vitro bioaccessibility and chemical stability of lutein emulsions were found higher than non-capsulated forms. Protection of bioactive lutein against UV irradiation was evaluated and in depression lutein was found that 14%, 6–8%, and only 0.06% from nanoemulsion, NLCs and SLNs. With these systems, highly antioxidant effect of lutein was found with 85% encapsulation efficiency and 98% suppressing free radicals [117].

It was stated that nutraceutical colorant of the carotenoid family, β-carotene has poor bioavailability and low physicochemical stability. To achieve sustained release, to target and to increase the application of β-carotene as a bioactive, numerous studies reported in some lipid-based and nano-scale carriers, such as nanoliposomes, SLNs, NLCs, nanoemulsions, and niosomes. In generally, β-carotene was encapsulated successfully into these nanocarriers and stability and biological activity of β-carotene were increased depending on the formulation components, interactions of β-carotene with them and methods [117].

Unlike other nanocarriers, in β-carotene loaded niosomal formulation, good resistibility to light, elevated temperatures and oxidative stress created by free radicals were obtained. In culture medium, β-carotene maintained resistant after 4 days and it was easily taken up through cells at 0.1–2 μM concentrations [134].

Similarly, lycopene which provides beneficial effect on human health, has low stability on different conditions such as light, high temperatures, oxygen, chemical reactions and environmental factors. Some nanocarriers (nanoliposomes, SLNs, NLCs, nanoemulsions and niosomes) were developed to eliminate the destructive effects and to enhance stability and bioactivity of lycopene. In one study, lycopene loaded niosomes were prepared successfully to protect the lycopene activity and increased its bioavailability. Antiproliferative activity was evaluated through MCF-7 and HeLa cell lines and niosomal formulation was shown perfect response in a dose-dependent manner. Therefore, anticancer activity of potential of lycopene was confirmed [135]. In another niosomal formulation containing lycopene, antidiabetic effect was assessed and effectiveness of formulation was stated [136].

Application of lipid-based nanocarriers for encapsulation of carotenoids is summarized in Table 2.

Table 2. Application of lipid-based nanocarriers for encapsulation of carotenoids.

Nanocarriers	Carotenoids	Results and Benefits	References
Nanostructured lipid carriers (NLCs)	Fucoxanthin	NLCs were promising approach with fucoxanthin to control skin hyperproliferation and maintain skin integrity in psoriatic skin.	[123]
Liposomes	Astaxanthin	More potent hydroxyl radical scavenging activity of astaxanthin significantly than either encapsulated β-carotene or α-tocopherol and prevented cytotoxicity on NIH-3T3 cells.	[124]
		The pathological changes of skin tissues were significantly improved and decreased expressions of Ki-67, MMP-13 and 8-OHdG and increased SOD activity were found.	[125]
		Singlet oxygen production could cleaned strongly. The production of melanin was inhibited.	[126]
		Improved stability and permeability, more antioxidant effect on intracellular antioxidant enzymes and effectively facilitated apoptosis.	[127]
		The suitable characteristics and composition of formulation, with ideal properties and storage stability were determined.	[128]
NLCs		Liposomal encapsulation could be greatly increased water dispersibility of astaxanthin.	[130]
		Improved antioxidant activity of astaxanthin was provided with NLCs that could be excellent candidates for cosmetics and nutraceuticals.	[131]
Liposomes	Astaxanthin and peridinin	Astaxanthin strongly decreased lipid damage with a more effective antioxidant at H_2O_2 and ascorbate-induced lipoperoxidation at Fe^{+2} liposomes.	[129]
Solid lipid nanoparticles (SLNs)	Astaxanthin	Radiolabeled nanoparticles were found to be 96–98% stable even for 48 h and higher drug concentration in the brain was achieved by intranasal administration, which was compared to 99mTc labeled nanoparticles intravenous route.	[133]
Liposomes	Lutein	Increased physicochemical stability, water dispersibility, therapeutic effects (antioxidant and anticancer) of lutein liposomal formulations.	[117]
Nanoemulsion NLCs SLNs		Highly antioxidant effect was found with 85% encapsulation efficiency and 98% suppressing free radicals.	
Liposomes NLCs SLNs	β-carotene	Successfully encapsulation of β-carotene and improved physicochemical stability during storage and increased biological activity of β-carotene.	
Niosomes		Good resistibility to light, elevated temperatures and oxidative stress with β-carotene loaded niosomal formulation. β-carotene maintained resistant after 4 days.	[134]

Table 2. *Cont.*

Nanocarriers	Carotenoids	Results and Benefits	References
Niosomes	Lycopene	Protecting the lycopene activity and increased bioavailability. Perfect response in a dose-dependent manner and confirmed anticancer activity with niosomal formulation.	[135]
		62% encapsulation efficiency as a reproducible and efficient technique could increase anti-diabetic property.	[136]

8. Application of Emulsion-Based Systems for Encapsulation of Different Carotenoids

Shu et al. prepared oil in water (O/W) thermo-stable nanoemulsions containing astaxanthin and stabilized with ginseng saponins as a natural surfactant via a high-pressure homogenization method to investigate the effects of pH, ionic strength, heat treatment and different temperatures (5, 25, and 40 °C) on the stability of droplets and/or astaxanthin nanoemulsions. A good long-term stability was shown against droplet growth during 15 days of storage at various temperatures (5, 25, and 40 °C) and the nanoemulsions were stable without droplet coalescence against thermal treatment (30–90 °C, 30 min), Their finding shown that nanoemulsion-based system could be suitable for delivering oil-soluble bioactive compounds such as astaxanthin and these studies need to be continued [137].

Khalid et al. evaluated the effect of modified lecithin (ML) and sodium caseinate (SC) on the formulation, stability and in vitro digestive behavior and bioavailability of astaxanthin-O/W nanoemulsions using high-pressure homogenization method. It was shown that successful formulation of astaxanthin-loaded nanoemulsions and emulsifiers effectively stabilized the O/W nanoemulsions but much higher bioaccessibility of astaxanthin was observed in ML-stabilized nanoemulsions mainly due to greater formation of mixed micelles compared to SC-stabilized nanoemulsions [138].

Liu et al. studied on effect of three long chain triglyceride (LCT) oils and evaluated bioactivity of using encapsulated astaxanthin in O/W nanoemulsions with simulated gastrointestinal tract (GIT) model. Astaxanthin-loaded nanoemulsions with greater bioaccessibility compared to free nanoemulsions, and this indicated that mixed micelles produced by LCT digestion resulted in greater solubility of this lipophilic bioactive substance [139].

In another nanoemulsion study, Affandi et al. investigated the effect of different surfactants on the physicochemical characteristics and stability of astaxanthin-loaded nanoemulsions over 90 days. Droplet size/size distribution of the nanoemulsions mentioned above depended on homogenization pressure/cycles and the type/concentration of surfactants (lecithin or Tween 80). For effective nanodelivery system of astaxanthin, it was found that 2% w/w astaxanthin and 4% w/w surfactant at 9000 rpm prehomogenization speed (~5 min) as optimized conditions [140].

Shanmugapriya and colleagues designed to emulsion-based delivery systems to increase the bioavailability of astaxanthin and α-tocopherol as active compounds for various biomedical applications. Anticancer potential of astaxanthin-α-tocopherol nanoemulsion prepared with spontaneous and ultrasonication emulsification methods was evaluated with optimizing production conditions for better resistance and toxicity testing against microbial infections. It could be said that this delivery system may be a starting point for prospective studies for cancer treatment applications [133].

Tan et al. designed a novel delivery system as named chitosan coated liposomes (chitosomes) containing lutein which included in the carotenoid family, for improving stability [141]. In another study, lutein loaded particle system was prepared with using polyvinylpyrrolidone and Tween 80 as a stabilizer and emulsifier respectively by Zhao et al. They found that this particle system had convenient water dispersibility and enhanced stability compared to free lutein [142].

In other studies with nano-emulsion based delivery system, formulation components, process steps, emulsifier types and concentrations storage pH and temperature played a key role on stability and effectiveness of lutein. Emulsion formulation revealed proper stability thus coating oil droplets in emulsions was increased the physicochemical stability of lutein compared to uncoated. In vitro bioaccessibility and chemical stability of lutein emulsions were found higher than non-capsulated forms. Protection of bioactive lutein against UV irradiation was evaluated and lutein depression was found that 14%, 6–8%, and only 0.06% from nanoemulsion, NLCs and SLNs. With these systems, highly antioxidant effect of lutein was found with 85% encapsulation efficiency and 98% suppressing free radicals [117].

Application of emulsion-based systems for encapsulation of different carotenoids is summarized in Table 3.

Table 3. Application of emulsion-based systems for encapsulation of different carotenoids.

Nanocarriers	Carotenoids	Results and Benefits	References
Nanoemulsion	Astaxanthin	A good long-term stability was shown against droplet growth during 15 days of storage at various temperatures and the nanoemulsions were stable without droplet coalescence against thermal treatment.	[137]
		Emulsifiers (modified lecithin (ML) and sodium caseinate (SC)) effectively stabilized the nanoemulsions and higher bioaccessibility was observed in ML-stabilized nanoemulsions.	[138]
		The greater bioaccessibility compared to free nanoemulsions and greater solubility.	[139]
		Optimum formulation components and conditions was selected that 2% w/w astaxanthin and 4% w/w surfactant at 9000 rpm prehomogenization speed (~5 min) for 90 days.	[140]
		Increased the bioavailability of astaxanthin.	[141]
Phospholipid-Chitosan vesicles (chitosomes)	Lutein	Increased the physicochemical stability of lutein with coating and higher in vitro bioaccessibility and chemical stability with nanoemulsions.	[117]
		Convenient water dispersibility and enhanced stability compared to free lutein.	[142]
	β-carotene Lutein Lycopene	Combination with chitosan with electrostatic attraction onto the membrane surface successfully Improved stability and controlled release of carotenoids by chitosomes.	[141]

9. Conclusions

There is a worldwide leaning on natural ingredients in food, nutraceutical, and cosmetics. It has been known that marine organisms serve as an extensive source for bioactive secondary metabolites due to their viability in extreme environments and conditions. In particular, carotenoids obtained from marine organisms displayed promising activity against various oxidative stress related disorders, and epidemiological studies revealed that the populations consuming carotenoid rich diets have lower oxidative stress related disorder risk. Although several activities of such compounds were shown by in vitro, in vivo, and several clinical studies, there is a need for advanced biological and molecular studies revealing the efficacy, activity mechanism, and metabolism. Bioavailability is an important factor to consider when developing suitable formulations with health benefits, since new delivery systems were produced for better bioavailability.

Author Contributions: Conceptualization, E.K.A.; drafting the manuscript, E.K.A., Y.G., G.Ş.K., H.B., Ç.Y., T.H.B.; review and editing the paper: E.K.A., and E.S.-S.; revising, E.K.A., Y.G., G.Ş.K., H.B., Ç.Y., T.H.B., E.S.-S. All authors have read and agreed to the published version of the manuscript.

Funding: This research received no external funding.

Conflicts of Interest: The authors declare no conflict of interest.

Abbreviations

$^1O_2$	Singlet oxygen
4-HNE	4-hydroxy-2-nonenal
5-Fu	5-Fluorouracil
6-OHDA	6-hydroxydopamine
8-OHdG	8-hydroxy-2′-deoxyguanosine
AAPH	2,2′-Azobis(2-amidinopropane) dihydrochloride
ABTS	2,2′-azino-bis(3-ethylbenzothiazoline-6-sulfonic acid
Akt	Protein kinase B
ARE	Antioxidant responsive elements
BHA	Butylated hydroxyanisole
Car-OO•	Carotene-peroxyl radical
CAT	Catalase
C-NP	Casein nanoparticles
C-NP-CS	Chitosan-coated nanoparticles
DMADP	Dimethyl allyl diphosphate
DPPH	2,2-diphenyl-1-picrylhydrazyl
EDTA	Ethylene diamine tetra acetic acid
ERK1/2	Extracellular-regulated kinase $\frac{1}{2}$
GCS	γ-glutamylcysteine synthetase
GPx	Glutathione peroxidase
GSH	Glutathione
GSTP1	Glutathione S-transferase
H_2O_2	Hydrogen peroxide
HIF-1α	Hypoxia inducible factor-1α
HOBr	Hypobromous acid
HOCl	Hypochlorous acid
Huh7	Human hepatic cellular carcinoma
IDP	Isopentenyl diphosphate
LDL	Low-density lipoprotein
LS-180	Human colorectal cancer cell line
MDA	Malondialdehyde
ML	Modified lecithin
MMP	Matrix metalloproteinase
MMPs	Matrix metallopeptidases
NADPH	Nicotinamide adenine dinucleotide phosphate
NF-κB	Nuclear Factor kappa B
NLCs	Nanolipid-based carriers
NOX	NAPDH oxidase
Nrf2–Keap1	Nuclear factor E_2-related factor 2
O2	Molecular oxygen
$O_2^{..}$	Oxygen radical
$O_2^{·-}$	Superoxide
O_3	Ozone
OH⁻	Hydroxyl
PI3K/Akt	Phosphatidylinositol-3 kinase
PTEN	Phosphatase and tensin homolog
RAR	Retinoid acid receptor

RNS	Reactive nitrogen species
RO·	Alkoxy radical
ROO·	Peroxyl radical
ROS	Reactive oxygen species
RTK	Receptor tyrosine kinase
RXR	Retinoid X receptor
SC	Sodium caseinate
SH-SY5Y	Human neuroblastoma cell line
SLNs	Solid lipid nanoparticles
SOD	Superoxide dismutase
TAC	Plasma total antioxidant capacity
TBARS	Thiobarbituric acid reactive substances
tBuOOH	Tert-butyl hydro peroxide
TEAC	α-tocopherol equivalent antioxidant capacity
Trolox	8-tetramethylchroman-2-carboxylic acid
UV	Ultraviolet
VEGF	Vascular endothelial growth factor

References

1. Butler, M.S. The role of natural product chemistry in drug discovery. *J. Nat. Prod.* **2004**, *67*, 2141–2153. [CrossRef]
2. Sarker, S.D.; Latif, Z.; Gray, A.I. *Natural Product Isolation*; Humana Press: Totowa, NJ, USA, 2006.
3. Kim, S.K. *Marine Pharmacognosy-Trends and Applications*; CRC Press-Taylor & Francis Group: Boca Raton, FL, USA, 2013.
4. Wali, A.F.; Majid, S.; Rasool, S.; Shehada, S.B.; Abdulkareem, S.K.; Firdous, A.; Beigh, S.; Shakeel, S.; Mushtaq, S.; Akbar, I.; et al. Natural products against cancer: Review on phytochemicals from marine sources in preventing cancer. *Saudi Pharm. J.* **2019**, *27*, 767–777. [CrossRef] [PubMed]
5. Kuppusamy, P.; Yusoff, M.M.; Maniam, G.P.; Ichwan, S.J.A.; Soundharrajan, I.; Govindan, N. Nutraceuticals as potential therapeutic agents for colon cancer: A review. *Acta Pharm. Sin. B* **2014**, *4*, 173–181. [CrossRef] [PubMed]
6. Shahidi, F.; Ambigaipalan, P. Novel functional food ingredients from marine sources. *Curr. Opin. Food Sci.* **2015**, *2*, 123–129. [CrossRef]
7. Correia-da-Silva, M.; Sousa, E.; Pinto, M.M.; Kijjoa, A. Anticancer and cancer preventive compounds from edible marine organisms. *Semin. Cancer Biol.* **2017**, *46*, 55–64. [CrossRef] [PubMed]
8. Huang, J.J.; Lin, S.; Xu, W.; Cheung, P.C.K. Occurrence and biosynthesis of carotenoids in phytoplankton. *Biotechnol. Adv.* **2017**, *35*, 597–618. [CrossRef] [PubMed]
9. Rehman, A.; Tong, Q.; Jafari, S.M.; Assadpour, E.; Shehzad, Q.; Aadil, R.M.; Iqbal, M.W.; Rashed, M.M.A.; Mushtaq, B.S.; Ashraf, W. Carotenoid-loaded nanocarriers: A comprehensive review. *Adv. Colloid Interface Sci.* **2020**, *275*, 102048. [CrossRef]
10. Maoka, T. Carotenoids in marine animals. *Mar. Drugs* **2011**, *9*, 278–293. [CrossRef]
11. Eggersdorfer, M.; Wyss, A. Carotenoids in human nutrition and health. *Arch. Biochem. Biophys.* **2018**, *652*, 18–26. [CrossRef]
12. Maoka, T. Carotenoids as natural functional pigments. *J. Nat. Med.* **2020**, *74*, 1–16. [CrossRef]
13. Glasauer, A.; Chandel, N.S. Targeting antioxidants for cancer therapy. *Biochem. Pharmacol.* **2014**, *92*, 90–101. [CrossRef] [PubMed]
14. Saeidnia, S.; Abdollahi, M. Antioxidants: Friends or foe in prevention or treatment of cancer: The debate of the century. *Toxicol. Appl. Pharmacol.* **2013**, *271*, 49–63. [CrossRef] [PubMed]
15. Nishino, H.; Tokuda, H.; Satomi, Y.; Masuda, M.; Osaka, Y.; Yogosawa, S.; Wada, S.; Mou, X.Y.; Takayasu, J.; Murakoshi, M.; et al. Cancer prevention by antioxidants. *Biofactors* **2004**, *22*, 57–61. [CrossRef] [PubMed]
16. Schieber, A.; Weber, F. *Carotenoids in Handbook on Natural Pigments in Food and Beverages Industrial Applications for Improving Food Color*; Carle, R., Schweiggert, R.M., Eds.; Woodhead Publishing: Duxford, UK, 2013.
17. Misawa, N. *1.20-Carotenoids in Comprehensive Natural Products II*; Liu, H.W., Mander, L., Eds.; Elsevier Science: London, UK, 2010.

18. Ambati, R.R.; Phang, S.M.; Ravi, S.; Aswathanarayana, R.G. Astaxanthin: Sources, extraction, stability, biological activities and its commercial applications—A review. *Mar Drugs* **2014**, *12*, 128–152. [CrossRef] [PubMed]
19. Rodrigo-Baños, M.; Garbayo, I.; Vílchez, C.; Bonete, M.J.; Martínez-Espinosa, R.M. Carotenoids from Haloarchaea and their potential in biotechnology. *Mar. Drugs* **2015**, *13*, 5508–5532. [CrossRef] [PubMed]
20. Zakar, T.; Laczko-Dobos, H.; Toth, T.N.; Gombos, Z. Carotenoids assist in cyanobacterial photosystem II assembly and function. *Front. Plant Sci.* **2016**, *7*, 295. [CrossRef]
21. Aasen, I.M.; Ertesvåg, H.; Heggeset, T.M.B.; Liu, B.; Brautaset, T.; Vadstein, O.; Ellingsen, T.E. Thraustochytrids as production organisms for docosahexaenoic acid (DHA), squalene, and carotenoids. *Appl. Microbiol. Biotechnol.* **2016**, *100*, 4309–4321. [CrossRef]
22. Mata-Gómez, L.C.; Montañez, J.C.; Méndez-Zavala, A.; Aguilar, C.N. Biotechnological production of carotenoids by yeasts: An overview. *Microb. Cell Fact.* **2014**, *13*, 12. [CrossRef]
23. Guedes, A.C.; Amaro, H.M.; Malcata, F.X. Microalgae as sources of carotenoids. *Mar. Drugs* **2011**, *9*, 625–644. [CrossRef]
24. Lamers, P.P.; Janssen, M.; De Vos, R.C.; Bino, R.J.; Wijffels, R.H. Exploring and exploiting carotenoid accumulation in Dunaliella salina for cell-factory applications. *Trends Biotechnol.* **2008**, *26*, 631–638. [CrossRef]
25. Sun, Z.; Li, T.; Zhou, Z.G.; Jiang, Y. Microalgae as a source of lutein: Chemistry, biosynthesis, and carotenogenesis. In *Microalgae Biotechnology*; Springer: Cham, Germany, 2015; pp. 37–58.
26. Sansone, C.; Galasso, C.; Orefice, I.; Nuzzo, G.; Luongo, E.; Cutignano, A.; Romano, G.; Brunet, C.; Fontana, A.; Esposito, F.; et al. The green microalga Tetraselmis suecica reduces oxidative stress and induces repairing mechanisms in human cells. *Sci. Rep.* **2017**, *7*, 41215. [CrossRef] [PubMed]
27. Khoo, K.S.; Lee, S.Y.; Ooi, C.W.; Fu, X.; Miao, X.; Ling, T.C.; Show, P.L. Recent advances in biorefinery of astaxanthin from *Haematococcus pluvialis*. *Biores. Technol.* **2019**, *288*, 121606. [CrossRef] [PubMed]
28. Raposo, M.F.D.J.; De Morais, A.M.M.B.; De Morais, R.M.S.C. Carotenoids from marine microalgae: A valuable natural source for the prevention of chronic diseases. *Mar. Drugs* **2015**, *13*, 5128–5155. [CrossRef] [PubMed]
29. Takaichi, S. Carotenoids in algae: Distributions, biosyntheses and functions. *Mar. Drugs* **2011**, *9*, 1101–1118. [CrossRef]
30. Galasso, C.; Corinaldesi, C.; Sansone, C. Carotenoids from marine organisms: Biological functions and industrial applications. *Antioxidants* **2017**, *6*, 96. [CrossRef]
31. Casazza, G.; Mazzella, L. Photosynthetic pigment composition of marine angiosperms: Preliminary characterization of Mediterranean seagrasses. *Bull. Mar. Sci.* **2002**, *71*, 1171–1181.
32. Silva, J.; Barrote, I.; Costa, M.M.; Albano, S.; Santos, R. Physiological responses of Zostera marina and Cymodocea nodosa to light-limitation stress. *PLoS ONE* **2013**, *8*, e81058. [CrossRef]
33. Abfa, I.K.; Radjasa, O.K.; Susanto, A.B.; Nuryadi, H.; Karwur, F.F. Exploration, isolation, and identification of Carotenoid from bacterial symbiont of sponge *Callyspongia vaginalis*. *Ind. J. Mar. Sci.* **2017**, *22*, 49–58.
34. Matsuno, T. Aquatic animal carotenoids. *Fish. Sci.* **2001**, *67*, 771–783. [CrossRef]
35. Maoka, T.; Mochida, K.; Kozuka, M.; Ito, Y.; Fujiwara, Y.; Hashimoto, K.; Nishino, H. Cancer chemopreventive activity of carotenoids in the fruits of red paprika *Capsicum annuum* L. *Cancer Lett.* **2001**, *172*, 103–109. [CrossRef]
36. Matsuno, T. The structural elucidation of two new marine carotenoids, amarouciaxanthin A and B. *J. Nat. Prod.* **1985**, *48*, 606–613. [CrossRef] [PubMed]
37. Starkov, A.A. The role of mitochondria in reactive oxygen species metabolism and signaling. *Ann. N.Y. Acad. Sci.* **2008**, *1147*, 37–52. [CrossRef] [PubMed]
38. Mittal, M.; Siddiqui, M.R.; Tran, K.; Reddy, S.P.; Malik, A.B. Reactive oxygen species in inflammation and tissue injury. *Antioxid. Redox. Sign.* **2014**, *20*, 1126–1167. [CrossRef] [PubMed]
39. Abdal Dayem, A.; Hossain, M.K.; Bin Lee, S.; Kim, K.; Saha, S.K.; Yang, G.M.; Choi, H.Y.; Cho, S.G. The role of reactive oxygen species (ROS) in the biological activities of metallic nanoparticles. *Int. J. Mol. Sci.* **2017**, *18*, 120. [CrossRef]
40. Phaniendra, A.; Jestadi, D.B.; Periyasamy, L. Free radicals: Properties, sources, targets, and their implication in various diseases. *Ind. J. Clin. Biochem.* **2015**, *30*, 11–26. [CrossRef]

41. Patel, R.P.; McAndrew, J.; Sellak, H.; White, C.R.; Jo, H.; Freeman, B.A.; Darley-Usmar, V.M. Biological aspects of reactive nitrogen species. *Biochim. Biophys. Acta* **1999**, *1411*, 385–400. [CrossRef]
42. Dröge, W. Free radicals in the physiological control of cell function. *Physiol. Rev.* **2002**, *82*, 47–95. [CrossRef]
43. Pham-Huy, L.A.; He, H.; Pham-Huy, C. Free radicals, antioxidants in disease and health. *Int. J. Biomed. Sci.* **2008**, *4*, 89–96.
44. Ayala, A.; Muñoz, M.F.; Argüelles, S. Lipid Peroxidation: Production, Metabolism, and Signaling Mechanisms of Malondialdehyde and 4-Hydroxy-2-Nonenal. *Oxid Med Cell Longev* **2014**, *2014*, 360438. [CrossRef]
45. Sajadimajd, S.; Khazaei, M. Oxidative stress and cancer: The role of Nrf2. *Curr. Cancer Drug Targets* **2018**, *18*, 538–557. [CrossRef]
46. Stadtman, E.R.; Levine, R.L. Protein Oxidation. *Ann. N.Y. Acad. Sci.* **2000**, *899*, 191–208. [CrossRef] [PubMed]
47. Cadet, J.; Wagner, J.R. DNA base damage by reactive oxygen species, oxidizing agents, and UV radiation. *Cold Spring Harb. Perspect. Biol.* **2013**, *5*, a012559. [CrossRef] [PubMed]
48. Sosa, V.; Moliné, T.; Somoza, R.; Paciucci, R.; Kondoh, H.; LLeonart, M.E. Oxidative stress and cancer: An overview. *Ageing Res. Rev.* **2013**, *12*, 376–390. [CrossRef] [PubMed]
49. Ahmed, O.M. Relationships between oxidative stress, cancer development and therapeutic interventions. *J. Can. Sci. Res.* **2016**, *12*, 376–390. [CrossRef]
50. Dasari, K.; O Madu, C.; Lu, Y. The role of oxidative stress in cancer. *Nov. Approach Can. Stud.* **2020**, *4*, 350–355.
51. Mordi, R.C.; Ademosun, O.T.; Ajanaku, C.O.; Olanrewaju, I.O.; Walton, J.C.; Kiokias, S.; Gordon, M.H. Free Radical Mediated Oxidative Degradation of Carotenes and Xanthophylls. *Molecules* **2020**, *25*, 1038. [CrossRef]
52. Fiedor, J.; Burda, K. Potential role of carotenoids as antioxidants in human health and disease. *Nutrients* **2014**, *6*, 466–488. [CrossRef]
53. Scheer, H. The Pigments. In *Light-Harvesting Antennas in Photosynthesis*; Green, B.R., Parson, W.W., Eds.; Kluwer Academic Publishers: Dordrecht, The Netherlands, 2003; pp. 29–81.
54. Young, A.J.; Lowe, G.M. Antioxidant and prooxidant properties of carotenoids. *Arch. Biochem. Biophys.* **2001**, *385*, 20–27. [CrossRef]
55. Barros, M.P.; Rodrigo, M.J.; Zacarias, L. Dietary carotenoid roles in redox homeostasis and human health. *J. Agric. Food Chem.* **2018**, *66*, 5733–5740. [CrossRef]
56. Ursini, F.; Maiorino, M.; Forman, H.J. Redox homeostasis: The golden mean of healthy living. *Redox Biol.* **2016**, *8*, 205–215. [CrossRef]
57. Pall, M.L.; Levine, S. Nrf2, a master regulator of detoxification and also antioxidant, anti-inflammatory and other cytoprotective mechanisms, is raised by health promoting factors. *Sheng Li Xue Bao* **2015**, *67*, 1–18. [PubMed]
58. Merhan, O. The biochemistry and antioxidant properties of carotenoids. In *Carotenoids*; Cvetkovic, D.J., Nikolic, G.S., Eds.; IntechOpen: London, UK, 2017; pp. 51–66.
59. Ben-Dor, A.; Steiner, M.; Gheber, L.; Danilenko, M.; Dubi, N.; Linnewiel, K.; Zick, A.; Sharoni, Y.; Levy, J. Carotenoids activate the antioxidant response element transcription system. *Mol. Cancer Ther.* **2005**, *4*, 177–186. [PubMed]
60. Naguib, Y.M. Antioxidant activities of astaxanthin and related carotenoids. *J. Agric. Food Chem.* **2000**, *48*, 1150–1154. [CrossRef] [PubMed]
61. Dose, J.; Matsugo, S.; Yokokawa, H.; Koshida, Y.; Okazaki, S.; Seidel, U.; Eggersdorfer, M.; Rimbach, G.; Esatbeyoglu, T. Free radical scavenging and cellular antioxidant properties of astaxanthin. *Int. J. Mol. Sci.* **2016**, *17*, 103. [CrossRef] [PubMed]
62. Chintong, S.; Phatvej, W.; Rerk-Am, U.; Waiprib, Y.; Klaypradit, W. In vitro antioxidant, antityrosinase, and cytotoxic activities of astaxanthin from shrimp waste. *Antioxidants* **2019**, *8*, 128. [CrossRef]
63. Santocono, M.; Zurria, M.; Paladino, G. Antioxidant activity of the xanthophylles astaxanthin, lutein and zeaxanthin: In vitro assays. *Investig. Ophthalmol. Vis. Sci.* **2003**, *44*, 1699.
64. Santocono, M.; Zurria, M.; Berrettini, M.; Fedeli, D.; Falcioni, G. Lutein, zeaxanthin and astaxanthin protect against DNA damage in SK-N-SH human neuroblastoma cells induced by reactive nitrogen species. *J. Photoch. Photobiol. B* **2007**, *88*, 1–10. [CrossRef]
65. Hormozi, M.; Ghoreishi, S.; Baharvand, P. Astaxanthin induces apoptosis and increases activity of antioxidant enzymes in LS-180 cells. *Artif. Cells Nanomed. Biotechnol.* **2019**, *47*, 891–895. [CrossRef]

66. Camera, E.; Mastrofrancesco, A.; Fabbri, C.; Daubrawa, F.; Picardo, M.; Sies, H.; Stahl, W. Astaxanthin, canthaxanthin and β-carotene differently affect UVA-induced oxidative damage and expression of oxidative stress-responsive enzymes. *Exp. Dermatol.* **2009**, *18*, 222–231. [CrossRef]
67. Tripathi, D.N.; Jena, G.B. Astaxanthin intervention ameliorates cyclophosphamide-induced oxidative stress, DNA damage and early hepatocarcinogenesis in rat: Role of Nrf2, p53, p38 and phase-II enzymes. *Mutat. Res. Genet. Toxicol. Environ. Mutagen.* **2010**, *696*, 69–80. [CrossRef]
68. Liu, X.; Osawa, T. Cis astaxhantin and especially 9-cis astaxhantin exhibits a higher antioxidant activity in vitro compared to the all-trans isomer. *Biochem. Biophys. Res. Commun.* **2007**, *357*, 187–193. [CrossRef] [PubMed]
69. Iwasaki, S.; Widjaja-Adhi, M.A.K.; Koide, A.; Kaga, T.; Nakano, S.; Beppu, F.; Hosokawa, M.; Miyashita, K. In vivo antioxidant activity of fucoxanthin on obese/diabetes KK-Ay Mice. *Food Nutr. Sci.* **2012**, *3*, 1491–1499.
70. Sathasivam, R.; Ki, J.S. A Review of the biological activities of microalgal carotenoids and their potential use in healthcare and cosmetic industries. *Mar. Drugs* **2018**, *16*, 26. [CrossRef] [PubMed]
71. Kawee-ai, A.; Kuntiya, A.; Kim, S.M. Anticholinesterase and antioxidant activities of fucoxanthin purified from the microalga Phaeodactylum tricornutum. *Nat. Prod. Commun.* **2013**, *8*, 1381–1386. [CrossRef]
72. Neumann, U.; Derwenskus, F.; Flaiz Flister, V.; Schmid-Staiger, U.; Hirth, T.; Bischoff, S.C. Fucoxanthin, a carotenoid derived from *Phaeodactylum tricornutum* exerts antiproliferative and antioxidant activities in vitro. *Antioxidants* **2019**, *8*, 183. [CrossRef]
73. Xia, S.; Wang, K.; Wan, L.; Li, A.; Hu, Q.; Zhang, C. Production, characterization, and antioxidant activity of fucoxanthin from the marine diatom Odontella aurita. *Mar. Drugs* **2013**, *11*, 2667–2681. [CrossRef]
74. Sujatha, M.; Suganya, P.; Pradeepa, V. Antioxidant and anticancerous activities of fucoxanthin isolated from brown seaweed *Sargassum wightii* against HepG2 Cell lines. *Int. J. Innov. Res. Sci. Eng. Technol.* **2017**, *6*, 16734–16742.
75. Zailanie, K.; Kartikaningsih, H.; Kalsum, U.; Sanjaya, Y.A. Fucoxanthin effects of pure *Sargassum filipendula* extract toward HeLa cell damage. *Int. J. Pharm. Technol. Res.* **2015**, *8*, 402–407.
76. Sudhakar, M.P.; Ananthalakshmi, J.S.; Nair, B.B. Extraction, purification and study on antioxidant properties of fucoxanthin from brown seaweeds. *J. Chem. Pharm. Res.* **2013**, *5*, 169–175.
77. Nomura, T.; Kikuchi, M.; Kubodera, A.; Kawakami, Y. Proton-donative antioxidant activity of fucoxanthin with 1,1-diphenyl-2-picrylhydrazyl (DPPH). *Biochem. Mol. Biol. Int.* **1997**, *42*, 361–370. [CrossRef]
78. Ha, A.W.; Na, S.J.; Kim, W.K. Antioxidant effects of fucoxanthin rich powder in rats fed with high fat diet. *Nutr. Res. Pract.* **2013**, *7*, 475–480. [CrossRef] [PubMed]
79. Sachindra, N.M.; Sato, E.; Maeda, H.; Hosokawa, M.; Niwano, Y.; Kohno, M.; Miyashita, K. Radical scavenging and singlet oxygen quenching activity of marine carotenoid fucoxanthin and its metabolites. *J. Agric. Food Chem.* **2007**, *55*, 8516–8522. [CrossRef]
80. Zhang, L.; Wang, H.; Fan, Y.; Gao, Y.; Li, X.; Hu, Z.; Ding, K.; Wang, Y.; Wang, X. Fucoxanthin provides neuroprotection in models of traumatic brain injury via the Nrf2-ARE and Nrf2-autophagy pathways. *Sci. Rep.* **2017**, *7*, 46763. [CrossRef] [PubMed]
81. Maoka, T.; Nishino, A.; Yasui, H.; Yamano, Y.; Wada, A. Anti-oxidative activity of mytiloxanthin, a metabolite of fucoxanthin in shellfish and tunicates. *Mar. Drugs* **2016**, *14*, 93. [CrossRef] [PubMed]
82. Tuzcu, M.; Orhan, C.; Muz, O.E.; Sahin, N.; Juturu, V.; Sahin, K. Lutein and zeaxanthin isomers modulates lipid metabolism and the inflammatory state of retina in obesity-induced high-fat diet rodent model. *BMC Ophthalmol.* **2017**, *17*, 129. [CrossRef]
83. Zou, X.; Gao, J.; Zheng, Y.; Wang, X.; Chen, C.; Cao, K.; Xu, J.; Li, Y.; Lu, W.; Liu, J.; et al. Zeaxanthin induces Nrf2-mediated phase II enzymes in protection of cell death. *Cell Death Dis.* **2014**, *5*, e1218. [CrossRef]
84. Bhosale, P.; Bernstein, P.S. Synergistic effects of zeaxanthin and its binding protein in the prevention of lipid membrane oxidation. *Biochim. Biophys. Acta Mol. Basis Dis.* **2005**, *1740*, 116–121. [CrossRef]
85. Cantrell, A.; McGarvey, D.J.; Truscott, T.G.; Rancan, F.; Böhm, F. Singlet oxygen quenching by dietary carotenoids in a model membrane environment. *Arch. Biochem. Biophys.* **2003**, *412*, 47–54. [CrossRef]
86. Surai, P. The antioxidant properties of canthaxanthin and its potential effects in the poultry eggs and on embryonic development of the chick, Part 1. *World Poult. Sci. J.* **2012**, *68*, 465–476. [CrossRef]
87. Zhang, W.; Zhang, K.Y.; Ding, X.M.; Bai, S.P.; Hernandez, J.M.; Yao, B.; Zhu, Q. Influence of canthaxanthin on broiler breeder reproduction, chick quality, and performance. *Poult. Sci.* **2011**, *90*, 1516–1522. [CrossRef]

88. Bonilla, C.E.V.; Rosa, A.P.; Londero, A.; Giacomini, C.B.S.; Orso, C.; Fernandes, M.O.; Paixão, S.J.; Bonamigo, D.V. Effect of broiler breeders fed with corn or sorghum diet and canthaxanthin supplementation on production and reproductive performance. *Poult. Sci.* **2017**, *96*, 1725–1734. [CrossRef]
89. Johnson-Dahl, M.L.; Zuidhof, M.J.; Korver, D.R. The effect of maternal canthaxanthin supplementation and hen age on breeder performance, early chick traits, and indices of innate immune function. *Poult. Sci.* **2017**, *96*, 634–646. [CrossRef] [PubMed]
90. Rosa, A.P.; Scher, A.; Sorbara, J.O.; Boemo, L.S.; Forgiarini, J.; Londero, A. Effects of canthaxanthin on the productive and reproductive performance of broiler breeders. *Poult. Sci.* **2012**, *91*, 660–666. [CrossRef] [PubMed]
91. Venugopalan, V.; Tripathi, S.K.; Nahar, P.; Saradhi, P.P.; Das, R.H.; Gautam, H.K. Characterization of canthaxanthin isomers isolated from a new soil Dietzia sp. and their antioxidant activities. *J. Microbiol. Biotechnol.* **2013**, *23*, 237–245. [CrossRef] [PubMed]
92. Rust, P.; Eichler, I.; Renner, S.; Elmadfa, I. Effects of long-term oral beta-carotene supplementation on lipid peroxidation in patients with cystic fibrosis. *Int. J. Vitam. Nutr. Res.* **1998**, *68*, 83–87.
93. Allard, J.P.; Royall, D.; Kurian, R.; Muggli, R.; Jeejeebhoy, K.N. Effects of β-carotene supplementation on lipid peroxidation in humans. *Am. J. Clin. Nutr.* **1994**, *59*, 884–890. [CrossRef]
94. Kiokias, S.; Gordon, M.H. Antioxidant properties of carotenoids in vitro and in vivo. *Food Rev. Int.* **2004**, *20*, 99–121. [CrossRef]
95. Levin, G.; Mokady, S. Antioxidant activity of 9-cis compared to all-trans β-carotene in vitro. *Free Rad. Biol. Med.* **1994**, *17*, 77–82. [CrossRef]
96. Mueller, L.; Boehm, V. Antioxidant activity of β-carotene compounds in different in vitro assay. *Molecules* **2011**, *16*, 1055–1069. [CrossRef]
97. Rodrigues, E.; Mariutti, L.R.; Chisté, R.C.; Mercadante, A.Z. Development of a novel micro-assay for evaluation of peroxyl radical scavenger capacity: Application to carotenoids and structure–activity relationship. *Food Chem.* **2012**, *135*, 2103–2111. [CrossRef]
98. Shindo, K.; Kikuta, K.; Suzuki, A.; Katsuta, A.; Kasai, H.; Yasumoto-Hirose, M.; Matsuo, Y.; Misawa, N.; Takaichi, S. Rare carotenoids, (3R)-saproxanthin and (3R,2′S)-myxol, isolated from novel marine bacteria (Flavobacteriaceae) and their antioxidative activities. *Appl. Microbiol. Biotechnol.* **2007**, *74*, 1350–1357. [CrossRef]
99. Martin, H.D.; Jäger, C.; Ruck, C.; Schmidt, M.; Walsh, R.; Paust, J. Anti-and Prooxidant Properties of Carotenoids. *J. Pract. Chem.* **1999**, *341*, 302–308. [CrossRef]
100. Yamashita, E. Astaxanthin as a medical food. *Funct. Food Health Dis.* **2013**, *3*, 254–258. [CrossRef]
101. Dembitsky, V.M.; Maoka, T. Allenic and cumulenic lipids. *Prog. Lipid Res.* **2007**, *46*, 328–375. [CrossRef]
102. Sugawara, T.; Kushiro, M.; Zhang, H.; Nara, E.; Ono, H.; Nagao, A. Lysophosphatidylcholine enhances carotenoid uptake from mixed micelles by Caco-2 human intestinal cells. *J. Nutr.* **2001**, *131*, 2921–2927. [CrossRef]
103. Sugawara, T.; Baskaran, V.; Tsuzuki, W.; Nagao, A. Brown algae fucoxanthin is hydrolyzed to fucoxanthinol during absorption by Caco-2 human intestinal cells and mice. *J. Nutr.* **2002**, *132*, 946–951. [CrossRef]
104. Asai, A.; Sugawara, T.; Ono, H.; Nagao, A. Biotransformation of fucoxanthinol into amarouciaxanthin A in mice and HepG2 cells: Formation and cytotoxicity of fucoxanthin metabolites. *Drug Metab. Dispos.* **2004**, *32*, 205–211. [CrossRef]
105. Hashimoto, T.; Ozaki, Y.; Taminato, M.; Das, S.K.; Mizuno, M.; Yoshimura, K.; Kanazawa, K. The distribution and accumulation of fucoxanthin and its metabolites after oral administration in mice. *Br. J. Nutr.* **2009**, *102*, 242–248. [CrossRef]
106. Yonekura, L.; Kobayashi, M.; Terasaki, M.; Nagao, A. Keto-carotenoids are the major metabolites of dietary lutein and fucoxanthin in mouse tissues. *J. Nutr.* **2010**, *140*, 1824–1831. [CrossRef]
107. Zhang, Y.; Wu, H.; Wen, H.; Fang, H.; Hong, Z.; Yi, R.; Liu, R. Simultaneous determination of fucoxanthin and its deacetylated metabolite fucoxanthinol in rat plasma by liquid chromatography-tandem mass spectrometry. *Mar. Drugs* **2015**, *13*, 6521–6536. [CrossRef]
108. Hashimoto, T.; Ozaki, Y.; Mizuno, M.; Yoshida, M.; Nishitani, Y.; Azuma, T.; Kanazawa, K. Pharmacokinetics of fucoxanthinol in human plasma after the oral administration of kombu extract. *Br. J. Nutr.* **2012**, *107*, 1566–1569. [CrossRef]

109. Ravi, H.; Baskaran, V. Chitosan-glycolipid nanocarriers improve the bioavailability of fucoxanthin via up-regulation of PPARγ and SRB1 and antioxidant activity in rat model. *J. Funct. Foods* **2017**, *28*, 215–226. [CrossRef]
110. Koo, S.Y.; Mok, I.K.; Pan, C.H.; Kim, S.M. Preparation of fucoxanthin-loaded nanoparticles composed of casein and chitosan with improved fucoxanthin bioavailability. *J. Agric. Food Chem.* **2016**, *64*, 9428–9435. [CrossRef]
111. Kotake-Nara, E.; Yonekura, L.; Nagao, A. Lysoglyceroglycolipids improve the intestinal absorption of micellar fucoxanthin by Caco-2 cells. *J. Oleo. Sci.* **2015**, *64*, 1207–1211. [CrossRef]
112. Rüfer, C.E.; Moeseneder, J.; Briviba, K.; Rechkemmer, G.; Bub, A. Bioavailability of astaxanthin stereoisomers from wild (Oncorhynchus spp.) and aquacultured (Salmo salar) salmon in healthy men: A randomised, double-blind study. *Br. J. Nutr.* **2008**, *99*, 1048–1054. [CrossRef]
113. Osterlie, M.; Bjerkeng, B.; Liaaen-Jensen, S. Plasma appearance and distribution of astaxanthin E/Z and R/S isomers in plasma lipoproteins of men after single dose administration of astaxanthin. *J. Nutr. Biochem.* **2000**, *11*, 482–490. [CrossRef]
114. Odeberg, J.M.; Lignell, Å.; Pettersson, A.; Höglund, P. Oral bioavailability of the antioxidant astaxanthin in humans is enhanced by incorporation of lipid based formulations. *Eur. J. Pharm. Sci.* **2003**, *19*, 299–304. [CrossRef]
115. Okada, Y.; Ishikura, M.; Maoka, T. Bioavailability of astaxanthin in Haematococcus algal extract: The effects of timing of diet and smoking habits. *Biosci. Biotechnol. Biochem.* **2009**, *73*, 1928–1932. [CrossRef]
116. Kistler, A.; Liechti, H.; Pichard, L.; Wolz, E.; Oesterhelt, G.; Hayes, A.; Maurel, P. Metabolism and CYP-inducer properties of astaxanthin in man and primary human hepatocytes. *Arch. Toxicol.* **2002**, *75*, 665–675. [CrossRef]
117. Rostamabadi, H.; Falsafi, S.R.; Jafari, S.M. Nanoencapsulation of carotenoids within lipid-based nanocarriers. *J. Controll. Rel.* **2019**, *298*, 38–67. [CrossRef]
118. Gammone, A.; Graziano Riccioni, G.; D'Orazio, N. Marine Carotenoids against oxidative stress: Effects on human health. *Mar. Drugs* **2015**, *13*, 6226–6246. [CrossRef]
119. Vo, D.T.; Saravana, P.S.; Woo, H.C.; Chun, B.S. Fucoxanthin-rich oil encapsulation using biodegradable polyethylene glycol and particles from gas-saturated solutions technique. *J. CO2 Util.* **2018**, *26*, 359–369. [CrossRef]
120. Ravi, H.; Baskaran, V. Biodegradable chitosan-glycolipid hybrid nanogels: A novel approach to encapsulate fucoxanthin for improved stability and bioavailability. *Food Hydrocoll.* **2015**, *43*, 717–725. [CrossRef]
121. Ravi, H.; Kurrey, N.; Manabe, Y.; Sugawara, T.; Baskaran, V. Polymeric chitosan-glycolipid nanocarriers for an effective delivery of marine carotenoid fucoxanthin for induction of apoptosis in human colon cancer cells (Caco-2 cells). *Mater. Sci. Eng. C* **2018**, *91*, 785–795. [CrossRef]
122. Edelman, R.; Engelberga, S.; Fahoumb, L.; Meyron-Holtzb, E.G.; Livneya, Y.D. Potato protein- based carriers for enhancing bioavailability of astaxanthin. *Food Hydrocoll.* **2019**, *96*, 72–80. [CrossRef]
123. Cordenonsi, L.M.; Faccendini, A.; Catanzaro, M.; Bonferoni, M.C.; Rossi, S.; Malavasi, L.; Raffin, R.P.; Schapoval, E.E.S.; Lanni, C.; Sandri, G.; et al. The role of chitosan as coating for nanostructured lipid carrier for skin delivery of fucoxanthin. *Int. J. Pharm.* **2019**, 118487. [CrossRef]
124. Hama, S.; Uenishi, S.; Yamada, A.; Ohgita, T.; Tsuchiya, H.; Yamashita, E.; Kogure, K. Scavenging of hydroxyl radicals in aqueous solution by astaxanthin encapsulated in liposomes. *Biol. Pharm. Bull.* **2012**, *35*, 2238–2242. [CrossRef]
125. Li, F.; Liu, Y.; Liao, J.; Duan, X. The preliminary study on anti-photodamaged effect of astaxanthin liposomes in mice skin. *Sichuan Da Xue Xue Bao Yi Xue Ban* **2018**, *49*, 712–715.
126. Hama, S.; Takahashi, K.; Inai, Y.; Shirota, K.; Sakamato, R.; Yamada, A.; Tsuchidya, H.; Kanamura, K.; Yamashita, E.; Kogure, K. Protective effects of topical application of a poorly soluble antioxidant astaxanthin liposomal formation on ultraviolet-induced skin damage. *J. Pharm. Sci.* **2012**, *101*, 2909–2916. [CrossRef]
127. Peng, C.H.; Chang, C.H.; Peng, R.Y.; Chyau, C.C. Improved membrane transport of astaxanthine by liposomal encapsulation. *Eur. J. Pharm. Biopharm.* **2010**, *75*, 154–161. [CrossRef]
128. Tamjidi, F.; Shahedi, M.; Varshosaz, J.; Nasirpour, A. Design and characterization of astaxanthin-loaded nanostructured lipid carriers. *Innov. Food Sci. Emerg.* **2014**, *26*, 366–374. [CrossRef]
129. Barros, M.P.; Pinto, E.; Colepicolo, P.; Pedersen, M. Astaxanthin and peridinin inhibit oxidative damage in Fe+2-loaded liposomes: Scavenging oxyradicals or changing membrane permeability? *Biochem. Biophys. Res. Commun.* **2001**, *288*, 225–232. [CrossRef] [PubMed]

130. Pan, L.; Wang, H.; Gu, K. Nanoliposomes as vehicles for astaxanthin: Characterization, in vitro release evaluation and structure. *Molecules* **2018**, *23*, 2822. [CrossRef] [PubMed]
131. Rodriguez-Ruiz, V.; Salatti-Dorado, J.; Barzegari, A.; Nicolas-Boluda, A.; Houaoui, A.; Caballo, C. Astaxanthin-loaded nanostructured lipid carriers for preservation of antioxidant activity. *Molecules* **2018**, *23*, 2601. [CrossRef] [PubMed]
132. Bhatt, P.C.; Srivastava, P.; Pandey, P.; Khan, W.; Panda, B.P. Nose to brain delivery of astaxanthin-loaded solid lipid nanoparticles: Fabrication, radio labeling, optimization and biological studies. *RSC Adv.* **2016**, *6*, 1000–10010.
133. Shanmugapriya, K.; Kim, H.; Saravana, P.S.; Chun, B.S.; Kang, H.W. Astaxanthin alpha tocopherol nanoemulsion formulation by emulsification methods: Investigation on anticancer, wound healing, and antibacterial effects. *Colloids Surf. B Biointerfaces* **2018**, *172*, 170–179. [CrossRef]
134. Palozza, P.; Muzzalupo, R.; Trombino, S.; Valdannini, A.; Picci, N. Solubilization and stabilization of β-carotene in niosomes: Delivery to cultured cells. *Chem. Phys. Lipids* **2006**, *139*, 32–42. [CrossRef]
135. Sharma, P.; Saxena, P.; Jaswanth, A.; Chalamaiah, M.; Tekade, K.R.; Balasubramaniam, A. Novel encapsulation of lycopene in niosomes and assessment of its anti-cancer activity. *J. Bioequiv. Bioavailab.* **2016**, *8*, 224–232.
136. Sharma, P.K.; Saxena, P.; Jaswanth, A.; Chalamaiah, M.; Balasubramaniam, A. Antidiabetic activity of lycopene niosomes: Experimental observation. *J. Pharm. Drug Dev.* **2017**, *4*, 103.
137. Shu, G.; Khalid, N.; Chen, Z.; Neves, M.A.; Barrow, C.J.; Nakajima, M. Formulation and characterization of astaxanthin-enriched nanoemulsions stabilized using ginseng saponins as natural emulsifiers. *Food Chem.* **2018**, *255*, 67–74. [CrossRef]
138. Khalid, N.; Shu, G.; Holland, B.J.; Kobayashi, I.; Nakajima, M.; Barrow, C.J. Formulation and characterization of O/W nanoemulsions encapsulating high concentration of astaxanthin. *Food Res. Int.* **2017**, *102*, 364–371. [CrossRef] [PubMed]
139. Liu, X.; Zhang, R.; McClements, D.J.; Li, F.; Liu, H.; Cao, Y.; Xiao, H. Nanoemulsionbased delivery systems for nutraceuticals: Influence of long-chain triglyceride (LCT) type on in vitro digestion and astaxanthin bioaccessibility. *Food Biophys.* **2018**, *13*, 412–421. [CrossRef]
140. Affandi, M.M.R.; Julianto, T.; Majeed, A. Development and stability evaluation of astaxanthin nanoemulsion. *Asian J. Pharm. Clin. Res.* **2011**, *41*, 142–148.
141. Tan, C.; Feng, B.; Zhang, X.; Xia, W.; Xia, S. Biopolymer-coated liposomes by electrostatic adsorption of chitosan (chitosomes) as novel delivery systems for carotenoids. *Food Hydrocoll.* **2016**, *52*, 774–784. [CrossRef]
142. Zhao, C.; Cheng, H.; Jiang, P.; Yao, Y.; Han, J. Preparation of lutein-loaded particles for improving solubility and stability by polyvinylpyrrolidone (PVP) as an emulsion-stabilizer. *Food Chem.* **2014**, *156*, 123–128. [CrossRef]

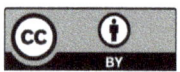

© 2020 by the authors. Licensee MDPI, Basel, Switzerland. This article is an open access article distributed under the terms and conditions of the Creative Commons Attribution (CC BY) license (http://creativecommons.org/licenses/by/4.0/).

MDPI
St. Alban-Anlage 66
4052 Basel
Switzerland
Tel. +41 61 683 77 34
Fax +41 61 302 89 18
www.mdpi.com

Marine Drugs Editorial Office
E-mail: marinedrugs@mdpi.com
www.mdpi.com/journal/marinedrugs